Contents

Section 3 Health Policy

Section 4 Protecting and Promoting Child Health

Child Health: A Reader

Edited by MARJORIE GOTT and BOB MOLONEY

With a Foreword by Yvonne Moores

RADCLIFFE MEDICAL PRESS
OXFORD and NEW YORK

15 Kings Meadow, Ferry Hinksey Road, Oxford OX2 0DP

141 Fifth Avenue, Suite N, New York, NY 10010, USA

British Library Cataloguing in Publication Data

A cataloguing record for this book is available from the British Library.

ISBN 1 85775 057 8

Typeset by Advance Typesetting Ltd
Printed and bound in Great Britain by
Biddles Ltd, Guildford and King's Lynn

Section 5 New Directions for Child Health

Section 6 A Partnership with Families

Section 7 Organizing for Change

Section 8 Changing Practice in Children's Nursing

List of Figures and Tables

Figures

Tables

Foreword

'Children have the right to be as healthy as possible.'
Article 24, United Nations Convention on the Rights of the Child

We have done much to promote health, and the Reader adds to our efforts. It looks purposefully to enhance the knowledge and skills of the nursing professions, who have a leading role in continuing to promote the health of children.

The nursing professions have contributed to an impressive decline in the incidence and severity of diseases associated with undernutrition, vitamin deficiences and infectious diseases.

One of our most encouraging successes in the UK's preventive health programmes is the increased uptake of childhood immunization. It has played an important part in reducing and sometimes eliminating a number of terrible diseases which many of us can still remember.

Looking for evidence of improved child health, the first and most basic indicator is the figure for infant mortality. For the fifth year running, infant mortality has fallen to a new low in England and Wales. We are well into single figures, a tremendous achievement and to the credit of modern medical science, and to the teams of doctors, nurses, midwives and health visitors. In addition, the 'Back to Sleep' campaign has dramatically reduced the rates of sudden, unexpected death rates in infants, a matter that has long concerned us.

What more can we do? 'A Vision for the Future – the Nursing, Midwifery and Health Visiting Contribution to Health and Health Care', launched by the Secretary of State, sets out an ambitious strategy for the nursing professions. It identifies five key areas and 12 targets for practice. The five key areas are: quality in practice; being accountable; clinical leadership of ourselves; focusing on purchasing; and underpinning with education and training. You, the reader, are in the forefront of nursing with a vision.

The 'Health of the Nation' provides a targeted focus, it is exciting because it is the first ever clear strategy in this country for securing real improvements in health, the foundations of which are laid in childhood. The key areas are coronary heart disease and stroke; cancers; mental health; accidents; and HIV/sexual health.

Clearly, there are big messages for improvement in the health of children and young people, for example, the importance of healthy lifestyles; healthy nutrition, physical exercise, rejection of smoking and substance abuse. Specifically, of course, there are targets for the reduction in childhood accidents and unwanted teenage pregnancies.

Child Health: A Reader sets health care in a broad setting recognizing the role that we in the nursing profession have to play, alongside others, to enable children to enjoy the best possible health and to develop their full potential. I commend this Reader to you.

Yvonne Moores, HON DSc, CIM
Chief Nursing Officer/Director of Nursing
Department of Health
February 1994

Acknowledgements

The authors and publishers wish to thank the following for permission to use copyright material:

Nursing Standard, Scutari Projects Ltd for material from Alison Kitson 'Getting started', *Nursing Standard*, February 12 1992, Vol. 6, No. 21;

Nursing Standard, Scutari Projects Ltd for material from E.S. Farmer 'Integrating research and practice', *Nursing Practice*, Vol. 5, No. 1, and E.S. Farmer, Reader in Nursing and Centre Director, Scottish Highlands Centre for Human Caring, Inverness;

Edward Arnold Publishers for material from Kim Manley 'Knowledge for nursing practice' and Jane Chapman 'Research – What it is and what it is not' (from Abigayl Perry and Moya Jolley: *Nursing: A knowledge base for practice*);

Royal College of Nursing, Scutari Projects Ltd for material from L. Ewles and I. Simnett: *Promoting Health*, 2nd Edition;

MCB University Press Ltd for material from Majorie Gott and Hester Packham The quality of community nursing services: Report of an exploratory study in a UK health authority', *International Journal of Health Care Quality Assurance*, Vol. 6, No. 1, 1993;

The Open University for Extracts from E206, Block 1, Unit 6;

Health Education Authority for material from P. Mares, A. Henley and C. Baxter, '*Health Care in Multiracial Britain*' 1985;

World Health Organization for material from '*Health for All, Targets 2000*';

'New World, New Opportunities' *Crown copyright. Reproduced with the permission of the Controller of Her Majesty's Stationery Office.*

The Open University Press for material from John Ashton and Howard Seymour 'The New Public Health' 1988;
Reproduced by permission from Children & Society, PO Box 872, London SE23 3HL. c. National Children's Bureau and Whiting & Birch Ltd;

'*The Health of the Nation*' Crown copyright. Reproduced with the permission of the Controller of Her Majesty's Stationery Office;

Radcliffe Medical Press for material from David Hall, Peter Hill and David Elliman '*The Child Surveillance Handbook*, 2nd edition' 1994;

Oxford University Press for material from R.S. Downie, C. Fyfe and A. Tannahill '*Health Promotion*' 1990;

Health Education Council for material from Geoffrey Pearson '*Young People and Heroin: An examination of heroin use in the north of England*' 1986;

King Edward's Hospital Fund for London for material from B. Jacobson, A. Smith and M. Whitehead '*The Nation's Health*' 1991;

Oxford University Press for material from Ilze Kalnins, David V. McQueen, Kathryn C. Backett, Lisa Curtice and Candace E. Currie 'Children, empowerment and health promotion: some new directions in research and practice', *Health Promotion International*, Vol. 7, No. 1, 1992;

E ZOOT: Health promotion by use of an electric bulletin board (Marjorie Gott) *Reproduced with kind permission of the copyright holder: the European Foundation for the Improvement of Living and Working Conditions (Shankill, Co. Dublin, Ireland)*;

Eastern Health Board, Dublin for article Community Mothers Programme;

The Macmillan Press Ltd for material from A.H. Bittles and D.F. Roberts '*Minority Populations*', ©The Galton Institute, 1992;

Blackwell Scientific Publications Ltd for material from Katri Vehviläinen-Julkunen 'Client-public health nurse relationships in child health care', *Journal of Advanced Nursing*, Vol. 17;

Blackwell Scientific Publications Ltd for material from Peter Callery and Lorraine Smith 'A study of role negotiation between nurses and the parents of hospitalized children', *Journal of Advanced Nursing*, Vol. 16;

Senior Nurse, Nursing Standard Publications, Scutari Projects Ltd, for material from Anne Casey 'A partnership with child and family', *Senior Nurse* 1988, 8, 4, 8–9;

Paediatric Nursing, Nursing Standard Publications, Scutari Projects Ltd for material from 'Towards a partnership in pain management', *Paediatric Nursing*, Vol. 5, No. 5, June 1993;

Blackwell Scientific Publications Ltd for material from Dorothy A. Whyte 'A family nursing approach to the care of a child with a chronic illness', *Journal of Advanced Nursing*, Vol. 17;

Churchill Livingstone for material from F.A. Carnevale, 'A description of stressors and coping strategies among parents of critically ill children – a preliminary study', *Journal of Intensive Care Nursing*, Vol. 6, 1990;

Senior Nurse, Nursing Standard Publications, Scutari Projects Ltd for material from Dawn Rafferty 'Team and primary nursing', *Senior Nurse*, Vol. 12, No. 1, 1992;

Paediatric Nursing, Nursing Standard Publications, Scutari Projects Ltd for material from Alan Glasper and Pauline Stradling 'Preparing children for admission', *Paediatric Nursing*, July 1989;

Paediaric Nursing, Nursing Standard Publications, Scutari Projects Ltd for material from Marion E. Broome 'Preparation of children for painful procedures', *Paediatric Nursing*, Vol. 16, No. 6, 1990;

Professional Nurse, Mosby-Year Book Europe Ltd for material from K. Martina Hannon 'Support can reduce the stress factor: Stress in neonatal nursing', *Professional Nurse*, May 1993;

World Health Organization for material from the booklet '*Changing nursing practice*', Health for All Nursing Series, No. 5;

Mrs Sue Williams, NHS Management Executive, for material from '*The future of paediatric nursing*';

Alan Glasper for material from '*Trends in child health nursing: A vision for the future*'. To be published in Child Health Nursing Journal.

General Introduction

Interest in child health has grown enormously in the last decade. Health policy makers nationally and internationally now recognize that children are a nation's future citizens, workers, taxpayers and parents, and, as such, are a highly valuable resource for the future. This recognition, and concomitant practice, training and policy shifts, are long overdue. The papers collected and newly commissioned for this Reader place child health firmly at the centre of health care practice and policy making.

The philosophy which underpins many of the papers selected for the Reader is the World Health Organization 'Health for All' (HFA) philosophy; we include extracts from recent HFA policy documents in two sections.

Each section is preceded by a short introductory guide to central themes, and to the papers selected and edited. Many of the papers selected for this Reader are difficult to categorize into a particular section, their impact is so overarching. Nonetheless an attempt has been made to group papers logically to ensure their readability. We hope that the reader appreciates this strategy, but does not feel constrained by it. Our main intention, in choosing and placing the papers as we have, is to stimulate thought, debate and change.

Over forty papers are presented. These include work previously published in journals, books or reports, extracts of policy documents, and newly commissioned papers. They have been drawn from an international body of work; their range represents a vast wealth of expertise.

In the editors' view the particular strengths of the Reader are:

- a strong theory base, with an emphasis on research and quality issues;
- a focus on teamwork and partnership in care, spanning the home, the hospital, the community and the workplace;
- a strong social policy focus, including national and international health and nursing policy issues;
- a focus on empowering children and families (as opposed to the traditional practice of requiring compliance with 'expert' opinion);
- an emphasis on health promotion, health protection and care in the community;
- identification of innovative 'new directions in child health';
- new approaches to the nursing of sick children, including the role of family centred care;
- changing practice in child health care.

The Reader supports a professional training course towards the award of a Diploma in Child Health Nursing. For those working towards this diploma, it is supplemented by an open learning teaching package and a supervised programme of clinical experience. The primary audience, therefore, is nurses working in child health settings, who are seeking professional updating. The focus of the Reader, however, is multi-disciplinary, as is the practice of child health. Papers included in the Reader are drawn from many disciplines and fields and it is believed that they will be of interest to other health care workers, social workers, teachers, youth leaders and health service policy makers.

SECTION 1

Nursing Practice

Introduction

The papers in this section have been chosen to represent themes and issues relevant to all those who practise nursing today, whatever the specialty.

The first issue addressed is that of quality. Quality of nursing care is a theme that recurs throughout this book. In an editorial (the first paper), Alison Kitson reflects on the fact that 'quality' is currently a fashionable 'buzz' word in nursing circles. She voices concern that, like many fashions, 'quality' might be adopted by nurses without the concept being fully understood. She also issues a challenge to educators to build understanding of quality issues into curricula.

The editors of this book (both educators) take up this challenge. In the selection and presentation of papers included there has been a deliberate attempt to challenge current attitudes and practices (in parenting, health promotion and service provision), to seek out 'quality' initiatives (in the 'New Directions' section), and to include users' views when measuring quality (both parents and children).

Papers by individual authors Farmer, Manley and Chapman outline the prerequisites of a sound knowledge base for nursing, and identify and locate research as fundamental to good nursing practice. Referring to Benner's work Farmer argues that nurturing and caring are the essence of nursing and call for a different type of scientific enquiry (research) than has been presented in the past (large scale, numerical, medical). Farmer also refers to the issue of quality, and makes a plea for a humanistic interpretation of quality based on nursing values, arrived at by analysis of nursing practice.

The nature of science is further explored in the paper by Manley, who traces key stages in the development of scientific (philosophical) thought. Manley concludes her paper by arguing for plurality in the research methods used to generate nursing knowledge.

The case for nursing research is argued convincingly by Chapman, who draws on a range of research studies to substantiate her views. A helpful discussion of the stages of the research process is provided for those who wish to understand published research more fully. In the final section, Chapman identifies strategies for implementation of research findings, a necessary stage for the development of high quality nursing care.

The quality of nursing care received is highly dependent on the relationship between nurses and patients. Central to this relationship is the quality of communication between nurses and patients. The Ewles and Simnett paper is reproduced in this book in the knowledge that it is widely recognised by nurse and health educators as the seminal work on this subject. In addition to providing guidelines for promoting effective verbal and non-verbal communication, Ewles and Simnett offer helpful advice for dealing with communication barriers. The general principles offered are appropriate for most communication situations, and are given here as an introduction to the topic. We focus again on communication in a later section, when we look at interactions between nurses and mothers of young children.

This final paper in this section is a report of a research project, designed to measure the quality of community nursing services. This piece of research explores user satisfaction with three different types of community nurse: district nurse, health visitor and school nurse. It is one of the few studies that have explored user satisfaction in a setting other than the hospital. It is included here because of this uniqueness, and also to reflect the move to the community that nursing and health care is currently witnessing. It concludes by advocating the use of a range of people (some voluntary) as resources for community nursing. This is an issue that we will explore in more detail in a later paper ('The Community Mothers Programme', 'New Directions' section).

1

Getting Started*

ALISON KITSON

Several people have said to me, in the course of learning about standards and quality assurance, that they don't want to make the same mistake as with the nursing process. Questioned further, they recall being told to go on a study day and learn 'how to do it'. Then they were expected to come back to the wards proficient forever in the ways of the process.

What seems to have stuck vividly in people's minds was the lack of sensitivity towards the needs of a huge body of professionals needing to acquire a new and complex skill in a short time. Looking back, we can be wise and philosophical about why things happened the way they did—for the majority of people.

However, I certainly cannot help feeling a little uneasy when I hear about nurses—and others—being told they have to set this and that standards by the end of the month. If they're lucky they might be 'sent' on a study day, after which they will be expected to have mastered the skills of standards, audit, quality and everything else to boot.

Haven't we gone through enough turmoil to realise that such quick learning fixes don't work? And if they did, then half the educational establishment would be out of a job. For a new idea, like the nursing process, or primary nursing, or quality, or audit to begin to infiltrate a mature mind, we are really talking about a slow, osmotic process where ideas and attitudes are challenged, new information is provided and then some practical experience is gained.

If we fall into that category of so-called 'adult learners', then we need the expert and sensitive guidance of professionals skilled in adult learning techniques; we certainly don't need anyone treating us like children or people with no sense and little experience. The demand for the right sort of partnership between practitioners and facilitators of learning is even more apparent with the arrival of the Post-registration Education and Practice (PREP) proposals.

I am more and more convinced that quality care is heavily reliant on how well staff have been kept up to date, and interested in and challenged by their work. There is a tremendous opportunity for staff of colleges of nursing, continuing education, and

---

*This is an abridged version of an article first published in *Nursing Standard*, Vol. 6, No. 21, p. 3, 1992.

practice development teams, to get together and provide the programmes practitioners really need.

And yet what I continue to find in a large number of nurse educators is a lack of real interest in or commitment to embracing such ideas. Quality still hasn't infiltrated the curriculum of even some of the Project 2000 courses, and if it does get a mention on RGN courses it is usually taught 'by the book' without any real passion or excitement.

Our job in the RCN Standards of Care Project and through the Quality Assurance Networks (QUAN) is to provide ideas and opportunities for practitioners and educators. But we can never hope to reach *all* the nurses who need some idea of the basics of quality. We can only go so far. So, you educators, will you take up the challenge?

2

Integrating Research and Practice*

E.S. FARMER

The opinion that research is not a legitimate activity for nurses has support in and outside the profession. It has been argued that nursing is a simple art that is not enhanced by science, and that research hinders rather than facilitates the provision of quality nursing services. This paper will examine these arguments and relate them to current controversies in nursing theory, education, research and practice.

The argument about whether nursing is an art or a science, or both, has a parallel in the history of medicine. Brody[1] suggests that rather than being a science, medicine is inherently a social activity and its values, aims and criteria for success are based on the wish to procure life improvements for individual people, whereas true science devotes itself to the discovery of truth regardless of whether that truth aids any human endeavour outside science.

Drawing on the work of Pellegrino and Thomasma, Brody contends that medicine has four features, making it:

> *A practical craft* that applies
> *scientific knowledge* to
> *individual cases* for purposes of a
> *right and good healing* action.[2]

If, indeed, medicine is not a science, the popular phrase 'the art of medicine' seems inappropriate as well as vague: medicine is not concerned with creating new works of beauty but with restoring. The idea of a practical craft captures this aim and assures a status somewhere between science and art.[1]

Parallels may be drawn between this view of the nature of medicine and the continuing debate on the essence of nursing. Brody argues that the practice of medicine is primarily a moral endeavour that should be open to whatever means are available to produce 'right and good healing actions'. This means recognising changing social perceptions on what is 'right and good', giving up cherished beliefs about what counts as knowledge and accepting that expert practice cannot be described or explained in the absolute sense.

---

*This is an abridged version of an article first published in *Nursing Practice*, Vol. 5, No. 1, pp. 2–7, 1991.

The shifting emphasis in society from disease to health has brought about something of a crisis in values, and the exposure and explosion of some of the myths surrounding the practice of medicine. The notion that medicine is somehow omniscient has dominated the activities of nurses and limited their presence for too long. It now needs to be firmly laid to rest so that we can move on and do what is required of us. As Benner notes: 'Contemporary medical practice no longer matches lay expectations. Modern physicians diagnose and treat diseases, whereas patients suffer illness and want more health promotion and illness prevention'.[3]

Benner defines health as 'the personal experience of relative well-being'. In contrast, illness is defined as 'the human experience of sickness, the experience of relative loss of well-being'. Illness includes the perception of pain, suffering, the fear of loss and the sense of interruption that comes when illness strikes. In further contrast to health and illness, disease is the manifestation of abnormalities in the function and structure(s) of cells, tissue, and organ system. 'Illness', says Benner, 'may occur in the absence of discernible disease, and the course of a disease can be quite distinct from the illness experience trajectory of the accompanying illness'.[3]

Descriptions of nursing

Travelbee[4] refers to nursing as an interpersonal process in which individuals, families and communities are assisted in preventing or coping with the experience of illness and suffering. She suggests that the realm of nursing includes helping individuals to find meaning in the experience of suffering and dying. Over the past 30 years, many other nurses have tried to describe the nature of nursing and delineate the boundaries of nursing practice, presenting their ideas in the form of models. Common to all these models of nursing are the concepts of person, environment, health and nursing, with caring the central concept.

Two major schools of thought which have influenced the philosophy of science are: natural science, which views reality as being reducible to separate variables and processes, any of which can be studied apart from the others; and human science, which views reality as a composite of multiple, inseparable realities that are irreducible and can only be studied holistically.

What we need is an acceptance of multiple modes of enquiry in our discipline. As Harman noted: 'It is not a question of which view is true in some ultimate sense. It is a matter of which picture is more useful in guiding human affairs.'[5]

Caring in nursing

What of these human affairs and the practice of nursing? According to Roach,[6] professions come into existence because societies have experienced a need for human services. These services, related to human development and welfare, are provided within unique human relationships. The nature of these relationships is a covenantal one, established and supported by faithfulness, justice, fairness and righteousness. The characteristics of the professional relationship are referred to by Roach as the 'Five Cs'. They are:

- **Compassion:** A way of living born out of an awareness of one's relationship to all living creatures; engendering a response of participation in the experience of another; a sensitivity to the pain and brokenness of the other; a quality of presence which allows one to share with and make room for the other.
- **Competence:** The state of having knowledge, judgement, skills, energy, experience and motivation required to respond adequately to the demands of one's professional responsibilities.

  Roach says competence without compassion can be brutal and inhumane, and compassion without competence may be no more than a meaningless, if not harmful, intrusion into the life of a person or persons needing help.
- **Confidence:** The quality which fosters trusting relationships. Roach argues that although much is being done in professional disciplines to foster trusting relationships, its absence in the everyday world creates the need to examine the quality of its presence in the field of services.
- **Conscience:** The state of moral awareness; a compass directing one's behaviour according to the moral fitness of things. Conscience is the caring person attuned to the moral nature of things. It is the morally conscious self in the actual state of moral awareness. Conscience grows out of experience, out of a process of valuing the self and others. Conscience is the call of care and manifests itself as care.
- **Commitment:** The willingness to enter into and sustain a caring relationship.

Benner[3] says the term 'caring' reflects interpersonal concern and liking, so that the other person's plight and fate matter to the carer. Caring is possible only from an involved stance: it sets up the condition of salience so that significant details are noticed. Caring, by its nature, does not seek to control or master but to facilitate and uncover the possibilities inherent in the situation and the person. Caring provides empowerment.

Education as the tool of caring

Roach[6] argues that if we care, in the professional sense, we need to develop professional education to provide the substance and environment required to nurture and encourage the capacity to care, and to foster the development of future professional leaders and practitioners who have the capacity to be there for others, and not exclusively for themselves. This development is at the heart of the current curriculum revolution in nursing in the United States, which is underpinned by the same kinds of concerns that prompted the reform of nurse education in the UK.

However, there is one significant difference. Although the Project 2000 proposals predominantly follow the behaviouristic training model of education, the American proposals are founded on humanism and caring.[7] Attention is focused on clarifying values, uncovering the assumptions and meanings that are part of daily nursing practice, and emphasis is placed on the freedom, openness and unpredictability of every learning experience.[8] Bevis and Murray noted that: 'In the conventional curriculum, the teacher relies heavily upon the lecture format and accepts the role of information provider, arbitrator of right and wrong, and benign dictator of content. These teaching roles subtly teach more than nursing. They teach an attitude toward self and authority that perhaps goes a long way toward sabotaging the very characteristics nurses must have to enhance nursing's ability to serve the public in ways that improve quality, [reduce] injustice, and promote uniform accessibility of health care.'[9]

Friere argues that 'knowledge emerges only through invention and reinvention, through the restless, impatient, continuing hopeful inquiry men pursue in the world, with the world, and with each other'.[10] In this regard, Bevis and Watson[11] propose that emancipatory education requires teachers to be problem posers, consultants and nurturers of curiosity, inquiry, caring and meaning. For these reasons they propose that the lecture be replaced by dialogue, argument, position papers, investigation, and other active strategies which have liberating and educating attributes.

This proposed emancipation of nurse education would require nurse educators to move from the surety of the formula-driven behaviourist curriculum to one of ambiguity,[11] and from the classroom to the places where nurses practise. Holmes[12] expressed doubts about the prospect of importing humanistic principles into British nurse education. He argues that it is difficult to reconcile the emancipatory education proposed by American nurse educators with the formal requirements of statutory training programmes which are characterised by unreflective 'banking' methods and traditional didacticism. Homes also criticises the highly prescriptive manner in which clinical experience is planned. There is, however, nothing in the statutory requirements for UK nurse education that prohibits innovative curriculum development. The greatest constraints are likely to be those of attitude and a failure to set up structures to facilitate the development of caring practices in both education and service.

There are two predictable responses to the curriculum revolution: the 'implement in haste and repent at leisure' phenomenon, a feature of British nursing, will recur, or it will be rejected because it is American. Either way, the Americans would be blamed for our lack of imagination and courage, and our failure to plan. Hopefully, neither of these will happen and we shall find a way to sensitively and actively support the humanistic principles underpinning the curriculum revolution.

Integrating research and practice

Moccia[7] contends that the failures of the US health care system are manifestations of the moral failure of a dominant world view within which caring values and nurses' work are positioned, at best, in the margins and shadows of the patriarchy's reality but which, more usually, are invisible.

If, as Benner[3] argues, health maintenance and illness require care and community, to achieve this we shall have to swim against the tide of prevailing political ideology that stresses the importance of self and autonomy. The fact that we live in a peopled world, and our connections with others are important to the way we exist in the world, is of little relevance in a society which has an economic view of people. Given this state of affairs, and all the consequences for nursing practice, how and why is research to be integrated into practice?

Central questions are raised by members of a profession when they have claimed a body of knowledge exemplified in common goals, language and approach.[13] It is clear from the literature that there are basically two types of knowledge needed and used by nurses. The first is what Benner calls 'know-how', which we cannot always theoretically account for, and the second (referred to by Benner as 'know-that') is what has been established through the systematic examination of a series of events. The 'know-how' knowledge is the perceptual awareness that begins with vague hunches and global assessments which initially bypass critical analysis: so conceptual clarity follows instead of precedes.[14] According to Benner, 'expert nurses often describe their perceptual abilities using phrases such as "gut feeling", "a sense of uneasiness" or a "feeling that things are not quite right". Expert nurses know that in all cases definitive evaluation of a patient's condition requires more than vague hunches, but through experience they have learned to allow their perceptions to lead to confirming evidence'. In this way there is an interaction between the 'know-how' and the 'know-that' types of knowledge.

The truths arrived at by intuition and introspection have not been valued. One of the main reasons for this is that nurses have not kept careful records of their own clinical learning. As Benner noted, 'although many single case studies have been published, few clinical comparisons of multiple case studies or clinical observations across patient populations exist'.[14] This failure to chart our practices and clinical observations has deprived nursing theory of the uniqueness and richness of the knowledge embedded in practice.

Uncovering this knowledge requires the use of qualitative, interpretive methods of inquiry as opposed to the linear, analytical and systems language which underpins the systematic method of nursing within nursing models. This is not, however, an invitation to abandon the nursing process. Problem solving and goal attainment are important functions, but understanding the experience of living with illness encompasses important issues that need to be addressed, and this needs a different approach and language that will be at odds with the reductionist techniques of standard setting and Diagnosis Related Groups (DRGs).

Implications for nurses

While Benner's work is relevant and appealing in its promise of excellence in clinical practice and in generating relevant theory, it needs careful consideration in the context of our political and social climate. We are witnessing the destruction of the nursing infrastructure, and while it may be welcomed by some it is not yet clear what, if anything, will replace it.

What is clear is that the kind of support needed to pursue a curriculum revolution and the development of practice theory is not widely available. The potential does exist, and the challenge we face is to create structures to support innovative practice. This has to be a collective effort by practising nurses, educators, managers and researchers.

Travelling the road to excellence requires daring but trail blazing, though exciting, is a lonely business and leadership will be needed if individual efforts are to be maximised. It is unlikely, and even undesirable, that one person will emerge as the guru of nursing. If caring is the core of nursing, then the connectedness that is implicit in caring must extend to those who deliver caring services.

The challenge is, therefore, one of collaboration and collective leadership, and it is a considerable one, requiring at least a mechanism to overcome the competitiveness foisted upon us by government dictat in the guise of cost-effectiveness and income generation. Add to that the implementation of Project 2000 programmes and planning to meet the needs identified in the UKCC Post-Registration and Practice Project, and it is not difficult to see that the responsibilities of leadership will be considerable. Our first responsibility is to our patients and clients, and this will increasingly involve sharing our ideas and talents, and embarking on collaborative research in the cause of 'right and good action'.

Producing curricula that are innovative and emancipatory needs collaboration, not only among staff in academic departments but also with those in colleges of nursing already facing enormous changes in the light of Project 2000 and government decisions on their future management. We need to create a climate of trust that will form the basis of our relationships with students, whose own life experiences must become the starting point of education in nursing. We have focused for too long on the content of education without due regard for the process. Bevis and Murray remind us that teaching is a political activity. 'Embedded in teaching are the hidden messages about what is valued, what learning is about and who is in power, in control.'[9]

Nurses have become accustomed to hearing words such as empathy, compassion, sympathy and holistic care without having internalised the values implicit in the terms. Consequently, we do not see the suffering patient or colleague, or perceive their needs.[3]

Recasting our educational programmes and practice on a philosophical foundation of humanism requires that we make the clarification of values a priority. We are conditioned to believe that the problems in health care are concerned with supply and demand, when they are more likely to be moral than practical, more about chosen ends in a particular political ideology than about managerial means. In a climate where autonomy and self-reliance are stressed, caring in both the personal and public domain is devalued and the need for care is seen as a sign of weakness, an embarrassment.[3]

The combination of a reductionist view of science and the advancement of self-interest lead very easily to a commercial view of health and disease. Patients soon become objects, disease categories to be manipulated, controlled or managed.[15] A technological understanding of the person renders health and wholeness inaccessible. This is dangerous. It encourages us to believe that there is a cake that has to be rationed, and to do this we have to place a value on life: to create persons and non-persons. There is a place for economics in health care, but it is dangerous when it becomes the tool of a particular political ideology.

One of the most contentious issues in health economics is that which concerns the use of Quality Adjusted Life Years (QALYs) for policy making. The underlying assumption of QALYs is that the expected benefit of an intervention can be related to the cost and yield of alternative interventions. The QALY is calculated by multiplying the gain in life years with a figure, between 0 and 1, that best reflects the quality of life over the same period. The obvious difficulties are those concerning what is included as cost and benefit, whose valuations are used and the notion that a tool used for policy making can also be used to make decisions about individual patient situations.

Rawles and Rawles,[16] among others, raise objections to the QALY. Their main objection is to the underlying argument about scarcity and the mismatch between supply and demand. They point out that, although resources are finite in an absolute sense, the demand for health care in the United Kingdom is far from infinite and the country's resources are adequate to meet those demands. The use of QALYs to make decisions about who lives and who dies is a reality, and nurses will be increasingly involved in ethical dilemmas forced upon them by political policies which have very suspect philosophical foundations. The self-interest of the health economist is easily dismissed. What is more difficult to deal with are the careless attitudes of nurses to the moral problems and dilemmas which their colleagues face daily. If we cannot care for each other, who will care for patients and clients?

A concentration on providing statistical evidence to support arguments for improved resources, rather than making assumptions based on experience and professional judgement, may work against nursing. If researchers have convinced practising nurses that they must no longer trust the evidence of their own eyes or value expert judgement, and if we as a discipline have devalued the caring in nursing, then our position is very serious indeed.

What is needed is intensive work to make explicit the values which underpin our practice so that we can avoid the painful, destructive divisions exemplified in far too many situations where self-interest, false premises and unworthy ambition are often the prime motivators. We need to articulate and communicate the rich theory which underlies clinical practice, and recognise that our students can make a major contribution to this work. To make this possible, educators and researchers will have to be where nursing is practised to facilitate this.

We need to consider the possibility that nursing models and the systematic method implicit in these models may perpetuate reductionism and hinder the uncovering of the knowledge embedded in practice. There is no suggestion that we should abandon the concepts set out in the models, but rather that we should find ways to test these in the various places where nursing is practised.

Given the accent on accountability and the sudden pressure for standard setting, it is important for us to promise only that which we can deliver. As Benner[3] noted, the perceptual recognitional abilities that daily make the difference in patient recovery do not translate into the language of standards. In the present climate of health care, therefore, the multidisciplinary clinical audit may be the safest holding position while we decide on the way forward within our discipline.

We must find methods to build research into the work of every practising nurse. This development will be of critical importance in a climate of multidisciplinary research geared towards policy making and cost containment rather than the building of knowledge in various disciplines.

If we cannot secure research funding from government, then we need to look elsewhere and to ask whether the money that our professional organisation ploughs into a host of entities for uncertain purposes is being well used. The establishment of an elitist RCN Nursing Research Advisory Group, whose membership is restricted to those who have higher degrees, is questionable and somewhat arrogant. The possession of a higher degree in nursing usually means that person has carried out one piece of research under supervision, and that makes nobody an expert.

In the words of Virginia Henderson, we have to nurse with our heads, our hands and our hearts. This requires the integration of research and practice, education and management. Finally, and most particularly, we need to trust each other if we are to build what is right and good in our discipline.

Notes

1. Brody, H. *Stories Of Sickness*, New Haven, Yale University Press, 1987.

2. Pellegrino, E.D., Thomasma, D.C. *A Philosophical Basis of Medical Practice*, New York, Oxford University Press, 1981.

3. Benner, P. 'Preserving caring in an era of cost-containment, marketing and high technology', *Yale Nurse*, 1985, August, 12–20.

4. Travelbee, J. *Interpersonal Aspects of Nursing*, Philadelphia, F.A. Davis, 1966.

5. Harman, W. *Symposium on Consciousness*, New York, Penguin, 1977.

6. Roach, S. *The Human Act of Caring: A Blueprint for the Health Professions*, Ottawa, Ontario, Canadian Hospital Association, 1987.

7. Moccia, P. 'No sire, it's a revolution', *Jnl Nurs Educ*, 1990, **29**(7), 307–311.

8. Tanner, C. 'Reflections on the curriculum revolution', *Jnl Nurs Educ*, 1990, **29**(7), 295–299.

9. Bevis, E.O., Murray, J.P. 'The essence of the curriculum revolution: Emancipatory teaching', *Jnl Nurs Educ*, 1990, **29**(7), 326–331.

10. Freire, N. *Pedagogy of the Oppressed*, New York, Herder and Herder, 1970.

11. Bevis, E.O., Watson, J. *Toward the Caring Curriculum: A New Pedagogy for Nursing*, New York, National League for Nursing, 1989.

12. Holmes, C.A. 'Alternative to natural science foundations for nursing', *Int J Nurs Stud*, 1990, **27**(3), 187–198.

13. Meleis, A.I., Price, M.J. 'Strategies and conditions for teaching theoretical nursing: An international perspective', *Journal of Advanced Nursing*, 1988, **13**, 592–604.

14. Benner, P. *From Novice to Expert. Excellence and Power in Clinical Nursing Practice*, California, Addison-Wesley, 1984.

15. Watson, J. 'The moral failure of the patriarchy', *Nursing Outlook*, **38**(2), 62–66.

16. Rawles, J., Rawles, K. 'The QALY argument: A physician's and a philosopher's view', *Journal of Medical Ethics*, 1990, **16**, 93–94.

3

Knowledge for Nursing Practice*

K. MANLEY

Knowledge and philosophy

> 'Philosophy provides a point of view: it is a belief construct, a speculation about the nature and value of things'
>
> (Bevis, 1982)

Philosophy is the 'seeking after wisdom or knowledge, especially that which deals with ultimate reality, or with the most general causes and principles of things and ideas and human perception and knowledge of them, physical phenomena and ethics' (Concise Oxford Dictionary, 1976).

A major concern of philosophy is the study of the nature of knowledge—this is called epistemology. Examples of epistemological questions could be, How one comes to know? or What is knowledge? In most other disciplines and in nursing to date the most valued approaches to developing knowledge have been the 'Scientific-Empirical' approach (Chinn and Jacobs, 1987). Chalmers (1982) however considers that this 'ideology of science' as it functions in society contains 'the dubious concept of science and the equally dubious concept of truth'. He further supports this belief with examples from behavioural psychology 'which encourages the treatment of people as machines' and 'the extensive use of the results of IQ studies in our educational system'. Chalmers states that 'bodies of knowledge such as these are defended by claiming or implying that they have been acquired by means of the "scientific method" and therefore must have merit'.

Philosophers do not have criteria which differentiate between knowledge that is scientific and that which is not. Each area of knowledge should be analysed for what it is, and for its purpose by considering the following questions:

- What is the aim of knowledge? (Chalmers states that this is different from what the aim is commonly thought to be or presented as)

*This is an abridged version of a chapter in A. Perry and M. Jolley (1991) *Nursing: a knowledge base for practice*, Edward Arnold, Sevenoaks, pp. 15–20.

PHILOSOPHY	EMPIRICAL SCIENCE
After Bevis (1982)	
Explores values	Describes facts
Looks at wholes and relationships with other wholes	Reduces phenomena to component parts to study, describe and explain how they operate
Answers questions why and queries the worth of experience	Answers how, when and where
Provides a value system for ordering priorities and selecting from various data	
After Sarter (1988)	
Unlimited totality 'the entire universe'	Domain delineated and definite

Figure 3.1 Differing characteristics of philosophy and empirical science

- What methods are used to accomplish the aims?
- To what degree have the aims been successfully accomplished?

(Chalmers, 1982)

This line of thought therefore focuses on knowledge itself, not whether knowledge can be claimed to be scientific or not. There have been many criticisms initially from outside nursing (Chalmers, 1982) and latterly from inside nursing (Suppe and Jacox, 1985) about the traditional approach to science and views about the nature of scientific knowledge (i.e. philosophy of science). Before these changes can be examined in more detail it is important to differentiate between philosophy and science. Figure 3.1 indicates more clearly how philosophy differs from empirical science.

Bergendal (1983) considers 'Such words as "knowledge" and "science" as not well defined' and goes on to state that 'one prevailing opinion is that knowledge and science are basically much the same'. Bergendal also states that another common opinion is that science is 'true' knowledge, the supreme form of knowledge. Science can be thought of in two ways: firstly as a body of knowledge, i.e. empirical knowledge which is the 'outcome' of methods used to generate knowledge; and secondly as a 'process' which relates to the logical and systematic methods used to generate knowledge. According to Suppe and Jacox (1985) the problem central to the philosophy of science is understanding the nature of scientific knowledge. The following brief overview will illustrate how this has changed over time.

Historical aspects of the philosophy of science

Aristotle, the Greek philosopher and a pupil of Plato, lived during the period 384–322 BC. He studied the whole field of knowledge and considered that knowledge was derived from deductive logic. He considered that 'the scientist was primarily a passive observer of what was' (Fitzpatrick, 1989). This view about knowledge continued until the sixteenth century when Francis Bacon, the famous English philosopher and a

INDUCTION

Statement of observations made
'I have observed that all patients that I have admitted for elective surgery have appeared anxious.'

Generalisation by induction
All patients admitted for elective surgery will be anxious.

DEDUCTION

General theory
Stressors, be they biological, psychological or social, produce specific physiological changes.

Logical deduction
John has stated that he is in constant pain, and he is worried about his wife visiting him after dark.
John is experiencing multiple stressors.
John will exhibit specific physiological changes.

Figure 3.2 Examples to demonstrate inductive and deductive approaches in nursing

founder of modern science, rejected Aristotle's view of knowledge generation in favour of the inductive method. Bacon considered that the purpose of science was to improve 'man's lot on earth' and 'if we wanted to understand nature then we must consult nature and not the writings of Artistole' (Chalmers, 1982). This could only be achieved by inductive methods. Such methods involve producing universal statements by generalising from repeating organised and careful observations of specific situations or phenomena (i.e. induction is defined as an approach which produces generalisations from specific situations, and deduction the reverse; the application of general principles to specific situations through the use of logical argument). To clarify induction and deduction Figure 3.2 provides an example of both.

Empiricism is an approach that considers all knowledge to be derived from experience via pure observation and collection of facts through the senses. This approach was strongly supported by the English philosopher John Locke in the seventeenth century. Rationalism is an opposing view of how knowledge about the world could be generated. It can be defined as an approach to generating knowledge through the application of reason and was pioneered in the seventeenth century by the French mathematician René Descartes who was concerned with the finding out as to why anything can be said to be true.

Auguste Comte founded positivism in the nineteenth century. Positivism considered that only data which was arrived at by experiment and objective observation was 'positive' truth. Empirical methods for generating knowledge therefore involve 'the collection of "facts" by means of careful observation and experiment and the subsequent derivation of laws and theories from those facts by some logical progression' (Chalmers, 1982).

From the 1920s through to the 1960s philosophy of science has been dominated by 'logical positivism' (later to be renamed logical empiricism). This approach is considered to be an extreme form of empiricism and was postulated by a group of philosophers subsequently named the 'Vienna Circle'. This view is encapsulated by the 'received view' or 'the scientific method'. The focus of this view of science is the 'justification' of discovery and resulted from 'an amalgamation of logic with the goals of empiricism in the development of scientific theories' (Meleis, 1985). The key features of logical positivism are:

- Only statements confirmed by sensory data, through sensory experience are valid.
- True statements are only those based on experience and known through experience.
- Rejection of abstraction as a method of generating theory, and any ethical considerations.
- Science is value-free and scientific method is the only method for generating knowledge.
- Scientific method is characterised by 'reductionism, quantifiability, objectivity and operationalization' (Watson, 1981).

The approach outlined above has been criticised because it takes for granted 'cause', and rejects the effects of context on discovery. As a result, the use of the scientific method is no longer seen to be the predominant approach to knowledge generation by many disciplines, although nursing has based much of its early theory building efforts on this approach even though such reductionist ideas are incompatible with the holistic values embodied in nursing models. Problems in developing nursing's knowledge base, according to Meleis (1985), have therefore occurred because nursing has used this outdated approach to develop knowledge about aspects of nursing which 'are neither reducible, quantifiable, nor objective'. Benner (1984) and Rogers (1989) also purport that nursing cannot be separated from the context of care, and suggest that many aspects of nursing cannot therefore be reduced to the minutest detail and examined. It is Meleis's view that nurse theorists have not followed the 'received view', but that they have generated their conceptual frameworks from their experiences, and include ideas that are 'subjective, intuitive, humanistic, integrative and in many instances not based on sense-data' (Meleis, 1985).

Sir Karl Popper, the British philosopher of science, has, since the 1950s, rejected the doctrine that all knowledge starts from perception and sensation, and proposes instead that it is developed through guesswork and refutation. He suggests that propositions are only valid if they have repeatedly and exhaustibly survived attempts to falsify them, although it has been found that it is as difficult to falsify theories as it is to confirm them (Suppe and Jacox, 1985).

Pragmatism is an American school of philosophy which is concerned with the usefulness of knowledge. It was first proposed by Charles Peirce supported by his friend William James but not really acknowledged until later into the twentieth century. Pragmatists consider that truth, and therefore knowledge, is validated by whether it can be put to good use, rather than whether there is evidence to support it.

Figure 3.3 outlines chronologically famous philosophers of science and their main contribution to the understanding of scientific knowledge.

Today, there are constant changes in views as to how philosophy of science describes knowledge and although the positivists have been discredited there is no one view that has displaced it. The main concern in nursing is identified by Suppe and Jacox (1985), who state that nursing literature continues to reflect the discredited ideas of the logical positivists, and that nurses interested in developing and testing theory must become aware of issues within the philosophy of science. In their conclusion they state that

Date	Person/founders	Ideas
384–322 BC	Aristotle	Deductive logic
1561–1626	Bacon	Inductive method
1596–1650	Descartes	Rationalism
1632–1704	Locke	Empiricism
1798–1857	Comte	Positivism
1920s	'The Vienna Circle' of philosophers	Logical positivism/ logical empiricism
1930s	Peirce/William James/ Dewey/Kaplan	Pragmatism
1950s	Popper	Falsification

Figure 3.3 Important people and their ideas in philosophy of science

'Multiple approaches to theory development and testing should be encouraged', therefore identifying the need for greater diversity and tolerance in theory testing than was previously permitted by the logical empiricist. They finally consider that 'Debates about inductive versus deductive and qualitative versus quantitative approaches to theory development and testing are useful insofar as they make clear that alternatives exist'.

References

Benner, P. (1984) *From Novice to Expert: Excellence and Power in Clinical Nursing Practice.* Addison-Wesley, Wokingham.

Bergendahl, G. (1983) Higher Education and Knowledge Policies. *Journal of Higher Education*, **54**(6): 599–628.

Bevis, E.M. (1992) *Curriculum Building in Nursing: a Process*, 3rd Edition. Mosby, St Louis.

Chalmers, A.F. (1982) *What is This Thing Called Science?* 2nd Edition. Open University Press, Milton Keynes.

Chinn, P.L. and Jacobs, M.K. (1987) *Theory and Nursing*, 2nd Edition. Mosby, St Louis.

Fitzpatrick, J. (1989) The Empirical Approach to the Development of Nursing Science. *In Conceptual Models of Nursing*, 2nd Edition. J. Fitzpatrick and A. Whall (Eds.) Appleton and Lange, Norwalk.

Meleis, A. (1985) *Theoretical Nursing: Development and Progress.* Lippincott, Philadelphia.

Rogers, M.E. (1989) Nursing: a Science of Unitary Human Beings. *In Conceptual Models for Nursing Practice*, J.P. Riehl-Sisca (Ed.) 181–95. Appleton and Lange, Norwalk.

Sarter, B. (1988) Philosophical sources of nursing theory. *Nursing Science Quarterly*, **1**(2): 52–9.

Suppe, F. and Jacox, A.K. (1985) Philosophy of Science and the Development of Nursing Theory. *Annual Review of Nursing Research*, **3**: 241–67.

Watson, J. (1981) Nursing's Scientific Quest. *Nursing Outlook*, **29**(7): 413–16.

4

Research—What It Is and What It Is Not*

J. CHAPMAN

The place of nursing research (or why bother with the subject?)

Tradition and custom dictate much of what nurses do. Henderson (1969) summarises tradition and custom as 'what we all know to be true . . . nursing develops by role modelling, being handed down, usually going unchallenged because we have always done it that way . . .'. In this situation the applicability or usefulness of the action is not generally questioned. The taking of temperatures four hourly, or the starving of patients from twelve midnight for operation during the morning session, which may be any time from seven in the morning to twelve midday, are examples of such practice. This source of decision making is often coupled with authority, either from the Ward Sister, for example 'Sister likes us to use this particular treatment for wounds', 'Sister likes the beds made in this way'; or from higher up the management structure through policies and procedures, such as medicine administration policies and catheterisation routines. In these cases because someone else has made the decision as to the course of action to take there is, perhaps, no need to understand, or even explore, the rationale for the practice.

Trial and error can also be the source of decision making for practice. When faced with an unfamiliar situation the care delivered can often be the result of trial and error, which is generally unsystematic and haphazard, but may be successful in solving individual problems. By working through a random scheme of trying method (a) then (b) and then (c) and so on the 'right' treatment might eventually be found, or the patient may recover despite the treatment offered. This is analogous to trying to find a way to stop a baby crying in the middle of the night by adopting a succession of different strategies such as rocking, feeding, ignoring, and so on. When success is achieved the situation is not generally analysed and lessons learned for next time; the triumphant person tends just to creep away relieved. The consequence of this route of decision making is that whilst success may ultimately be achieved, the reason why (the rationale) is obscure and therefore one is not in a position to be able to predict with confidence whether the same method would work again in the future.

---

*This is an abridged version of a chapter in A. Perry and M. Jolley (1991) *Nursing: a knowledge base for practice*, Edward Arnold, Sevenoaks, pp. 28–51.

It must be said that in certain situations both these decision making pathways are acceptable, however research as an aid for the decision making offers certain features not to be found in these other methods. Research, when properly conducted, can provide unbiased, objective evidence on which to base a decision. It can supply a description of the 'reality' of the current situation for example, rather than a 'rose tinted' picture of what is thought to be happening. It can provide predictive information in which an analysis of past events can be used to accurately predict future trends such as recruitment and retention issues, outbreak of certain infectious diseases, or uptake of further education courses. Research can provide objective evaluation of two methods of treatment, or choices of nursing action, and this evidence can be used to make a professional judgement in the clinical situation, thus tradition, custom, authority and trial and error can be superceded by the delivery of nursing care based on sound scientific evidence of its efficacy.

To illustrate the contribution that research has to make to nursing three situations will be described.

Research can provide scientifically defensible reasons for nursing actions. Perhaps it is not possible to provide a firm theoretical basis for all nursing actions, however many clinical practices have now been examined under research conditions and effective, and efficient, courses of action have been scientifically identified. For example research conducted by Norton *et al.* (1962), Barton and Barton (1981) and others has determined appropriate action to be taken if pressure sores are to be avoided (regular relief of pressure, the use of pressure reducing beds and mattresses and so on). Hayward (1975) and Boore (1978) have conducted widely accepted research which demonstrates that the provision of pre-operative information is a beneficial aid to post-operative recovery.

Research can increase cost effectiveness of nursing activities. Nurses, in common with other health care professionals, are being put under ever increasing pressure to provide a value for money service, whilst at the same time having to make cuts in the service to constantly strive to keep within target spending levels. With the advent of ward accounting and the responsibility for ward budgets being increasingly invested in the ward sister research has an important role to play in the provision of sound evidence to help to guide the most prudent use of available funds. Reliance on systematically collected research findings can, where available, save wards and departments considerable amounts of money by reducing poor 'trial and error' spending. In management circles it is often argued that, at times of economic constraints, research is a luxury which cannot be financially supported. The author would argue that it is at these times that research is most valuable. A simple survey of bath additives conducted by Sleep and Grant (1988) clearly demonstrates the savings that can result from the implementation of research findings. Sleep and Grant conducted an experimental study of bath additives used by post-natal mothers for the first 10 days post delivery. The sample of 1800 mothers were each assigned to one of three groups: one group added salt to the bath water, another added Savlon solution, and the third group did not use any bath additive. The results indicated that all three groups found the baths soothing and helpful in reducing discomfort, and the midwives concerned reported no significant differences in the rates of healing or the incidence of any complications such as infection. Based on the results of this study Health Authorities and individuals can save considerable amounts of money by following a policy of not using any bath additives for this client group. Romney (1982) conducted a similar trial, also focusing on maternity patients.

She conducted an experiment to examine the rates of infection amongst groups of women who were shaved pre-delivery and groups who were not. As with Sleep and Grant's study no differences were evident between the outcome measure examined, i.e. the rates of infection in the two groups. The study provided a sound scientific basis for not performing pre-delivery shaves. Nursing time and unnecessary expenditure on razors were saved, to say nothing of the increased satisfaction experienced by the future mothers.

What is research—definitions and parameters

Sources of nursing knowledge have been discussed above, including tradition, custom, authority, and trial and error learning. One way of beginning to understand the value of research is to examine the qualities of research as a basis for problem solving and decision making compared with these other sources of knowledge.

Research can provide evidence on which to base selection of appropriate treatment/course of action whereas tradition and trial and error can, at best, provide experience. Research can provide information to explain why a method, a treatment or a course of action actually works (research based rationales). Tradition and trial and error are not generally concerned with rationales. If rationales are provided they tend to be subjective and judgmental rather than objective and scientific. Research, through the use of inferential statistics, can provide parameters as to how far the available evidence may be confidently generalised to a wider population. Experiential evidence cannot, with the same reliability, be used in this way.

How does a researcher set out to discover this evidence or nursing knowledge? Research always starts with a question. Of this rather obvious point Lancaster (1975) said that research '. . . needs people who ask questions, who have "hunches", who want to find a better way of doing things, who refuse to be put off by platitudinous replies to their questions. Without such people research would never get started.' A topic for research may come from practical experience, from reading, through discussion with colleagues, or just as a 'flash of inspiration'. Whatever the source of the problem the same series of steps must be systematically followed if reliable and objective scientific evidence concerning the problem is to be revealed. These steps, referred to as the research process, are listed below.

(i) The topic of study is identified and the research question posed.
(ii) A search of relevant literature is undertaken.
(iii) The research question is refined.
(iv) The investigation is planned and data collection methods developed.
(v) A pilot study is conducted.
(vi) The main data set is gathered.
(vii) The raw data is sorted and analysed.
(viii) Conclusions and generalisations are drawn from the analysed data.
(ix) A report containing the findings is prepared.
(x) This information is disseminated to the appropriate people.
(xi) The findings are utilised/implemented as appropriate.

Posing the question

Posing the question follows directly from identification of a particular problem that you wish to solve, or from an idea or vague hunch you want to explore. There are three main sources of research questions; they can be generated from experience, from other research or from theory.

Experience may lead to the identification of a specific problem, or perhaps just a 'hunch' as to a way in which care could be improved, or maybe a desire to understand the rationale for the success of a particular course of action. Research questions can be developed from all such suggestions. Investigating the question in a scientific way by following the research process may produce evidence which will help to explain the situation and may indicate a proposed change in practice.

Reading reports of completed research can also be a rich source of research questions. Speculation as to whether the evidence generated by a particular study would apply in the reader's own situation may prompt a desire to repeat the study in a different location to test the validity and the reliability of the original study, and also perhaps lead to a wider implementation of the recommendation based on the findings.

A third source of research questions is directly from theory. A nursing theory is a set of assumptions put forward to explain events. The explanation is, or should be, the best available summary of the current knowledge on a specific subject. Research questions can be developed by logical deduction from theories. An hypothesis can be generated to test the theory, and if the hypothesis is confirmed then the theory can be supported.

In reality the nature of the investigation which is undertaken and the actual research question(s) which form the focus of the investigation are determined by a range of external constraining or self limiting factors. These include:

- time available to be devoted to the problem;
- the levels of knowledge and experience of research within the research team;
- the availability of financial and other resources such as access to expert statistical advice and computing facilities.

In the context of all these external constraints the final definition of the research question to be addressed and the methods to be adopted is generally made following the second stage of the research process, i.e. the literature search.

Searching the literature

Searching the literature can be an exciting and illuminating experience or a frustrating and disappointing journey leading nowhere. Keys to successful literature searching include the following.

- A helpful, skilled librarian;
- Familiarity with the layout of the libraries to be used, e.g. how far back do the journals on the shelves go to, is there another location for older journals?
- Knowledge of the principles of literature searching, familiarity with indexes, bibliographies, methods for computer search (use librarians if needed);

- Conscientious indexing of sources investigated—an unrecorded reference source may take many hours to retrace. Index cards or a computerised index of sources examined, including full reference, and comments to remind you of the content should be kept and frequently updated throughout the project.

What should the literature be searched for? In broad terms a literature search is a search for material which provides information on the following aspects of the problem under investigation—the size of the problem; any commentators identifying the problem; have other research studies investigated the problem; or does it seem to be unique? If the problem has been previously identified can the history of the problem be traced?

The aim of the literature search is to develop a theoretical framework which encompasses the above factors and provides a justification for and the investigation method to be adopted for the project. In practice the following steps may prove useful.

(i) Define the topic in terms of keywords and synonyms which will guide the search through indexes and abstracts.
(ii) Decide how widely you wish to search. For example, are you going to include just United Kingdom research or research from other countries as well? How far is it reasonable to go back to look for material? (The smaller the amount of literature on a topic generally the farther back the search needs to go.) Are any foreign language papers to be considered? If so, can translation be arranged?
(iii) Is it appropriate to search outside recognised nursing literature? For example, should medical, dietetic, or physiotherapy literature be included in the search? The topic and the range of reference obtained from the initial investigation of available nursing literature may guide this decision.

A literature search should not be conducted in isolation but should be coupled with discussion of findings with colleagues, experts, mentors, in fact anyone who is interested in the same problem. A final hint for a student new to the art of literature searching is that time spent discovering the material available from different sources is time well spent. It is useful, for example, to understand what indexes, abstracts, bibliographies, on-line searches and so on can offer. Time spent with a librarian or working through a guided study exercise may prove very useful in terms of developing an ability to search the literature efficiently and effectively in the future.

Refinement of the research question

Following the literature search the researcher is in a position to decide exactly what the purpose of the study is to be. This involves developing the initial question or idea into a form that is suitable for investigation by the research process. This stage generally consists of defining precisely what you are interested in and narrowing the original question down into a very specific question for which a clear cut answer is obtainable. For example a general hunch that some nurses assess wounds in rather different ways can be developed into several widely different research studies. Amongst many alternatives it could lead to:

(i) a study of documented records of wounds kept by nurses;

(ii) a descriptive account of the criteria used by nurses when deciding how to manage a wound; or
(iii) an observational study of whether nurses change their practice following a wound care study day.

In each case the researcher has focused from the initial topic into a particular, more specific direction. But in each situation further clear definition of the specific aspects to be studied is required before the research can proceed. The research question should contain a single idea and not several. The final format of the research focus can be in the form of a statement or a hypothesis. A hypothesis is a specific form of research question that states a predicted relationship between variables, in such a way that it can be directly tested.

Planning the investigation

At this stage the research method selected is developed into a reality for the topic of study. In essence this involves choosing the appropriate research method, seeking permission and, where appropriate, ethical approval for carrying out the investigation, the development of the data collection method(s) to be used, the planning and preparation necessary for calculating, identifying and incorporating the sample to be studied, and the training of data collectors where appropriate.

Within the context of this chapter it is not possible to discuss all the aspects of the range of research methods available. The following brief description of some of the main methods and terms used will, it is hoped, allay some of the confusion often encountered at the early stages of becoming familiar with research and stimulate further study of a range of these methods.

Descriptive method

In a descriptive study the researcher does not change any aspect of the area or subjects being studied. The study aims to describe the current situation. The area to be investigated is generally presented in the form of a research question. Many descriptive studies take the form of surveys, for example David *et al.* (1983) surveyed current treatments across England for patients with established pressure sores. A total of 737 wards in 20 health districts were surveyed, and a total of 961 patients with one or more pressure sores, seen by the research team. Descriptive information relating to the (then) current practice of nursing care of patients with pressure sores was collected.

It may be thought that descriptive information of this nature cannot have a direct effect on practice, however a summary of some of the uses the pressure sore data was put to may quell such an idea. The findings were used to formulate and focus future research ventures, and have enabled managers and others to rationalise and review resource allocation. The research prompted pharmacists and wound care experts to examine the efficacy of the huge range of products found to be in use for the treatment of sores. A total of 98 products were identified during the survey. In addition, the survey findings provided valuable education material which in many instances encouraged ward managers and others to review local practices in respect of pressure sore management.

Experimental method

In an experimental study an attempt is made to reveal the existence of a relationship between two or more factors (variables). In its simplest form this might be establishing whether a particular form of treatment is better than no treatment. The experiment would proceed by giving the treatment to one group of patients and no treatment to another similar group. The effect of the treatment or no treatment would be measured for both groups and the results compared. For example Romney (1982), in addition to conducting a trial of pre-delivery shaving conducted a similar trial on the value, if any, of pre-delivery enemas. Her hypothesis was that there would be no difference in the rates of faecal contamination, duration of labour, and incidence of infection between mothers who did and did not receive an enema prior to delivery. The research evidence generated supported this hypothesis and widespread changes in maternity practice resulted.

Quantitative and qualitative research

Quantitative research refers to research which involves measurements that can be directly recorded and quantified. In essence, quantitative research is concerned with the measurement of 'facts', for example physiological measurements of fluid balance and temperature, tests of knowledge under examination conditions, rates of admission and discharge, rates of recruitment and wastage.

Qualitative research refers to studies which attempt to measure concepts which do not lend themselves to direct measurement, such as pain, anxiety, attitudes, and opinions. Indicators to represent the concepts need to be developed and therefore this approach is more subjective than quantitative research. However it is important to recognise the need for both types of research in nursing, which is concerned with both physiological and psychological dimensions. There is often an inappropriate distinction drawn between these two approaches which supports the belief that quantitative is scientific and reliable in a way that qualitative research can never be. Goodwin and Goodwin (1984) argue that the methods should be seen as opposite ends of the same spectrum and not mutually exclusive methods. They point out that they are in fact just two different approaches to data collection and analysis and not two different philosophies of life. In nursing research it is often appropriate to use both quantitative and qualitative data collection methods in order to obtain a realistic picture of the true situation. For example Boore (1978), when looking at the relationship between the amount of pre-operative information received and the rate of post-operative recovery, collected both physiological (quantitative) and psychological (qualitative) data in order to demonstrate a positive effect between the provision of pre-operative information and the promotion of recovery.

Action research

Action research, a term first used by Kurt Lewin (1948), is a type of applied social research. The main feature of action research is that the researcher and the practitioners collaborate throughout, unlike the majority of other methods where the researcher adopts a 'fly on the wall' role. As evidence becomes available to indicate a possible positive change to practice, practice will be changed during the course of the study. The study continues by investigating the consequences of the change. The advantages of this method for local problem solving are considerable. However, because of the on-going developmental nature of the changes in practice there are limitations to the general application of the findings. Further useful discussions on the method can be found in Greenwood (1984), Towell (1979) and Lathlean and Farnish (1984).

Data collection methods

Data can be collected using a variety of methods which can be grouped together into four major categories: data collection by observation; by questioning; by looking things up; and by concurrent recording. A variety of instruments can be used for each of these approaches. For example, observation data can be recorded on video film or directly on to a simple chart, such as that used for recording observed temperature and blood pressure measurements or on a carefully devised recording sheet which allows a data collector to record a variety of events observed. Data can be obtained by questioning either by the use of a questionnaire which is completed in the absence of the researcher, or by interview when a researcher asks questions face to face. The schedule used needs to be appropriate to the method and to the questions being asked. For example it is possible to offer clarification in a face to face interview but not possible to do this in a postal questionnaire and questions need to be formulated to take account of this. Data can be collected from a wide variety of records which may be patients' care records or management information which is routinely collected. Data may also be collected by asking participants in the study to compile information relating to an aspect of their work/life, for example in the form of an activities or food diary.

Pilot study

A pilot study is a small scale trial of the main data collection methods to be used. During the planning stage many pre-pilot studies may be carried out, but a final 'dry run' should be carried out to ensure that no insoluble problems will be encountered during main data collection. For example the pilot study may reveal problems with recruiting suitable subjects, or may reveal that superfluous data is being generated. Steps can be taken to sort out these problems prior to the collection of the main data set. If major modifications are required then a further pilot study may be necessary. In the event of poor reliability, validity or logistical problems, changes should be made to the data collecting methods prior to collecting the main data set.

A data collection instrument is said to be reliable *if* it is used on two separate occasions and the same results are obtained, providing that the 'who' or 'what' being measured has not changed. For example a ruler made of elastic is clearly not reliable, nor is the following question included on a questionnaire: 'Please list qualifications obtained whilst at school'. This may be interpreted as passes obtained in the General Certificate of Education or the General Certificate of Secondary Education examinations, but is open to interpretation to include for example all ballet, swimming and piano qualifications obtained whilst between the ages of five years and leaving school. The reliability of obtaining the required information can be improved if the question states exactly which type of qualifications are being referred to.

A data collection instrument is valid if it actually measures what it is intended to measure. The researcher must ensure that an abstract concept such as pain is validly reflected in the range of information collected which may include patient report of pain using a numerical indicator (a pain thermometer), timing and nature of analgesia received, reports of previous pain experiences, factors which relate to anxiety status, outcome of definition of the pain (if pain is reported to be low then is discharge an option, if pain is reported to be high does the respondent run the risk of further surgery or painful treatment?). Generally a single question or observation can only be a valid data collection method when collecting information relating to a simple construct for example age, sex, height or current weight. In order to be valid a more complex construct should be operationally defined in such a way as to cover all relevant aspects of the construct.

Problems of reliability and validity must be addressed prior to collecting the main data set.

Collection of the main data set

This is the most tedious part of any project as it involves the performance of many repetitive tasks. Data must be collected from the subjects in a consistent way and researchers must not allow themselves to 'drift' into asking new questions, or applying new knowledge gathered as the project evolves.

Analysis of data

Once data has been collected it needs to be sorted, analysed and presented in such a way that interpretation of the findings is possible. Plans for analysis should be made throughout all preceding stages. The nature of the analysis that can be undertaken depends on the nature of the data collected. Data can be grouped, classified and coded to enable a picture to be built up. Features of the data can be counted and frequencies of responses calculated. Beyond this, more detailed and sophisticated pictures can be established using statistical methods. Expert statistical advice may be required for this.

Conclusions

Once data has been analysed and presented in an easily assimilated form, for example using tables, graphs and histograms, conclusions can be drawn. Conclusions should summarise all that has been learned from the data set and all the inferences and generalisations that can be drawn.

Report

A report should summarise all the stages of the research project. Readers of the report should be able to follow the research process through and to understand how the conclusions were arrived at. The findings then need disseminating by publication, presentation of the report to appropriate groups, and through education channels via seminars, study days and conferences.

Implementation

Nursing research cannot implement itself. Implementation requires that nurses identify the research relevant to their area of work or responsibilities, weigh up the evidence presented and then formulate a plan to best utilise the findings (if appropriate). What is required is truly research minded practitioner nurses who seek out, evaluate, interpret and then utilise the research which is available.

An examination of these four stages of implementation reveals the reality of problems which will be encountered. Finding time to seek out relevant research is not always seen as a priority by many practitioners. Studies such as those conducted by Myco (1980) and Barnett (1981) have shown that nurses tend to read very little in the way of professional material of any kind. In the author's experience, when questioning groups of nurses at the beginning of a research course/lecture as to the professional reading they had undertaken in the preceding week many will admit to having looked at the weekly journals only. On further questioning the respondents tend to identify that, within these journals, the news pages and the job advertisements have received attention and few are able to recount the content or even the subject matter of any research reports contained in the journal. A possible solution to this problem is the establishment of a 'journal club' where a group of nurses agree to review a range of professional journals relevant to their sphere of work. Each member has responsibility to examine just one or two journals to identify any papers which may be relevant to the group. As many professional journals are issued only monthly or bi-monthly the journal club should meet about six times a year. At the meeting each member should report the content of any relevant findings to the group who can together reflect on possible implications of the study; for instance, is it just interesting or does it warrant further consideration, or possible implementation? This can be a very successful venture and many other research related activities may be able to be carried out by and through the group, for example arranging seminars and developing proposals for small scale studies.

Where should nurses be looking for material? In the United Kingdom there are two refereed general journals where researchers may choose to publish their report—the *Journal of Advanced Nursing* and *The International Journal of Nursing Studies*, both of which cover research on all aspects of nursing practice, education and management from the United Kingdom and abroad. Several nursing research journals are produced in the United States of America, including *Nursing Research, Research in Nursing and Health*, and *Western Journal of Nursing Research*.

In addition, most nursing specialities are served by specialist journals, and it is appropriate for many nurses to seek information from journals that are not specifically nursing but are from related disciplines. These journals are not generally found at railway stations or in the newsagents alongside the weekly publications and their price is too prohibitive to recommend the purchase of individual copies. Hence the visiting of professional libraries will be required in order that the available material can be reviewed. Knowing about relevant research demands an interest and a willingness to seek out the information. The feeling that 'somebody else' will keep one up to date does not bode well for progress. Teaching from a research-based curriculum which encourages questioning and examination of available evidence for the theories and practices being taught may go some way to alleviate the apathy and encourage individuals to see that keeping up to date with relevant research is the responsibility of all practitioner nurses.

The second step towards successful implementation is an ability to weigh up the evidence in an informed way. Hunt (1981) argues that one of the inhibitory factors to successful implementation is that nurses do not believe research findings. It could be argued that, in order not to believe research findings, such findings need to have been critically read and understood, and the evidence weighed up in such a way as to be in a position not to believe findings. In reality this is not often the case. Unwillingness to accept research findings which directly challenge traditionally held beliefs and practice is not uncommon. The disbelief of the findings is a defence for the accepted practice. For example a traditional approach to wound care was to keep the wound clean and dry and therefore nurses may be unwilling to accept research findings which support the idea that a moist wound environment will encourage more rapid healing than a dry wound environment.

One way of overcoming this scepticism is to encourage nurses to accept research for what it is, namely evidence, and to ask them to be prepared to objectively weigh up the strengths and weaknesses of the evidence, as they would if in a position of jury member in a court of law. Nurses need to decide if the results and conclusions appear to be reasonable, formulated from an appropriate sample, and of sufficient statistical significance. At the same time, nurses need to learn to re-examine practices for which they are unable to provide a sound rationale or research basis, and be prepared to examine new evidence, as it becomes available, which may indicate a possible change in practice.

A further component in the process of implementing research findings is the need to understand them. The ability to understand research findings occurs as a result of a sound understanding of the subject under study, a basic knowledge of research theory and methods, a modicum of statistical appreciation and a willingness to read carefully and thoroughly and exercise a professional judgement whilst reading. Understanding does not come easily at first, but, with wide reading, more and more research methods are met and basic knowledge and skills will develop over time. The novice may well be advised to seek more experienced help, for example from a nurse researcher or a statistician.

If implementation is contemplated, the following steps should be observed.

(i) The weight of the evidence for the conclusions of the study should be carefully considered.
(ii) The feasibility and resource implications of the proposed implementation should be identified.
(iii) The desirability and cost effectiveness of the proposed change should be considered, and the reassurance of quality of care as a result of the proposed change—does the proposed implementation have a direct positive effect on the quality of patient care or is it something that just makes for an easier life for the nurses?
(iv) A strategy for implementation needs to be developed which pays particular attention to the education and training needs of the staff who will be involved.
(v) Finally, a review programme should be established to formally evaluate the effectiveness of the change.

Summary

Nurses need research to enable them to identify and demonstrate a rational basis for the care that they give. There must be a move away from tradition and custom as the basis for what nurses do and a striving to develop scientific knowledge for practice. This will serve to improve the care delivered to patients and clients and strengthen the knowledge base on which the profession of nursing is based.

References

Barnett, D.E. (1981) 'Do nurses read?' *Nursing Times*, **77**(50), 2131–3.

Barton, A. and Barton, N. (1981) *The Management and Prevention of Pressure Sores*, Faber and Faber, London.

Boore, J. (1978) *Prescription for Recovery*, Royal College of Nursing, London.

David, J.A., Chapman, R.G., Chapman, E.J., and Lockett, B. (1983) *An Investigation of the Current Methods Used in Nursing for the Care of Patients with Established Pressure Sores*, Nursing Practice Research Unit, Northwick Park Hospital and Clinical Research Centre, Harrow.

Goodwin, L.D. and Goodwin, W.L. (1984) 'Qualitative vs quantitative research or qualitative and quantitative research', *Nursing Research*, **33**(6), 378–80.

Greenwood, J. (1984) 'Nursing research: a position paper', *Journal of Advanced Nursing*, **9**(1), 77–82.

Hayward, J. (1975) *Information – a Prescription against Pain*, Royal College of Nursing, London.

Henderson, V. (1969) *Basic Principles of Nursing Care*, Revised edition, Karger, Basel.

Hunt, J. (1981) 'Indicators for nursing practice: the use of research findings', *Journal of Advanced Nursing*, **6**(3), 189–94.

Lancaster, A. (1975) *Guidelines to Research in Nursing, No. 1: Nursing, Nurses and Research*, 2nd edition, King Edward's Hospital Fund, London.

Lathlean, J. and Farnish, S. (1984) *The Ward Sister Training Project: an Evaluation of a Training Scheme for Ward Sisters*, Nursing Education Research Unit, Department of Nursing Studies, King's College, University of London, London.

Lewin, K. (1948) *Resolving Social Conflict*, Harper & Row, New York.

Myco, F. (1980) 'Nursing research information: are nurse educators and practitioners seeking it out?' *Journal of Advanced Nursing*, **5**(6), 637–46.

Norton, D., McLaren, R., and Exton-Smith, A.N. (1962) *An Investigation of Geriatric Nursing Problems in Hospital*, National Corporation for the Care of Old People, London.

Romney, M.L. (1982) 'Nursing research in obstetrics and gynaecology', *International Journal of Nursing Studies*, **19**(4), 193–203.

Sleep, J. and Grant, A. (1988) Occasional paper. 'Effects of salt and savlon bath concentrate post-partum', *Nursing Times and Nursing Mirror*, **84**(21), 55–7.

Towell, D. (1979) 'A "social systems" approach to research and change in nursing care', *International Journal of Nursing Studies*, **16**(1), 111–21.

5

Fundamentals of Communication*

L. EWLES and I. SIMNETT

Summary

This chapter discusses some fundamentals of relationships with clients, communication barriers and basic communication skills. The application of these skills often will be in one-to-one situations, although they may apply when working in groups and when teaching as well. These skills will help to develop better communication, but they should not be expected to provide a blueprint for every situation, or a quick and easy route to being a good communicator. They are a start, but improving communication is a lifelong developmental process.

Exploring relationships with clients

We begin by asking health promoters to look at some fundamental—and possibly uncomfortable—questions: for example, what is your basic attitude towards the people you work with? Do you accept them on their own terms or do you judge them by your own standards? Do you aim to encourage people to be independent, make their own decisions, take charge of their health, solve their own problems? Or are you actually encouraging dependency, solving their problems for them and thereby decreasing their own ability and confidence to take responsibility for themselves? We suggest that you should work through the following questions, thinking about how you relate to the people you work with.

Accepting or judging

Accepting people means:

- recognising that people's knowledge and beliefs emerge from their life experience, whereas your own have been modified and extended by professional education and experience;

*This is an abridged version of a chapter in L. Ewles and I. Simnett (1992) *Promoting Health—a Practical Guide*, Scutari Press, London, pp. 121–130.

- understanding *your own* knowledge, beliefs, values and standards;
- understanding your clients' knowledge, beliefs, values and standards from their point of view;
- recognising that you and the people you work with may differ in your knowledge, beliefs, values and standards;
- recognising that these differences do not imply that you, the professional health promoter, are a person of greater worth than your clients.

Judging people means:
- equating people's intrinsic worth with their knowledge, beliefs, values, standards and behaviour: for example, saying of someone who drinks 'people who get drunk are stupid' judges (and condemns) that person, and takes no account of life experience and cultural background—'drunkenness can result in people getting hurt' does not judge the person;
- ranking knowledge and behaviour: for example, 'I'm the expert so I know better than you' is judgmental; 'I know more than you about this particular thing' is not—it is a statement of fact: 'my standards are higher than yours' is judgmental, 'my standards are different from yours' is not.

Autonomy or dependency?

There are a number of ways in which you can help clients to take more control over their health.

Autonomy can be helped by:
- encouraging people to make their own decisions, and resisting the urge to 'take over' the decision-making;
- encouraging people to think things out for themselves, even if this takes much longer than simply telling them;
- respecting any unusual ideas they may have.

Autonomy can be hindered if:
- you impose your own solution on your clients' problems;
- you tell them what to do because they are taking too long to think it out for themselves;
- you tell them that their ideas are no good and will not work, without giving an adequate explanation or opportunity to try them out.

We suggest that the appropriate aim is to work towards as much autonomy as possible; by doing this, you are helping people to increase control over their own health, which is a basic aim of health promotion. Obviously, there are times when people are dependent on a health promoter, and rightly so; for example, they may be ill, confused or likely to put themselves or other people in danger. There is also the very real problem that working towards autonomy is time-consuming. However, in the long run it is time that is well spent.

A partnership or a one-way process?

Do you think of yourself as working in partnership with people in pursuit of health promotion aims, or do you see health promotion as your sole responsibility, with yourself as the 'expert'?

A partnership means:
- there is an atmosphere of trust and openness between yourself and your clients, so that they are not intimidated;
- you ask people for their views and opinions, which you accept and respect even if you disagree with them;
- you tell people when you learn something from them (eg. 'I never thought of it that way before');
- you use informal, participative methods when you are involved in health education, drawing on the experience and knowledge which clients bring with them;
- you encourage clients to share their knowledge and experience with each other. People do this all the time, of course—for example, knowledge and experience is discussed between patients in a hospital ward and mothers in a baby clinic—but do you deliberately foster and encourage this?

A one-way process means that:
- you do not encourage clients to ask questions and discuss problems;
- you imply that you do not expect to learn anything from your clients (and if you do, you do not say so);
- you do not find out what people already know and have experienced;
- you do not encourage people to learn from each other, only from you;
- you use formal methods when you are undertaking health education, such as lectures, rather than participative methods.

Clients' feelings—positive or negative?

A change in people's health knowledge, attitudes and actions will be helped if they feel good about themselves. It will rarely be helped if they are full of self-doubt, anxiety or guilt.

Clients will feel better about themselves if:
- you praise their progress, achievements, strengths and efforts, however small;
- the consequences of 'unhealthy' behaviour (eg. smoking) are discussed without implying that the behaviour is morally bad;
- time is spent exploring how to overcome difficulties (eg. practical strategies to help a client stop smoking). This will help to minimise feelings of helplessness.

Clients will feel bad about themselves if:
- you ignore their strengths and concentrate on their weaknesses;
- you ignore or belittle their efforts;
- you attempt to motivate them by raising guilt and anxiety (eg. 'If you don't stop smoking you'll damage your baby' or 'you're killing yourself with what you eat').

To sum up, we suggest that the health promotion aim of enabling people to take control over, and improve, their health is best achieved by working in a non-judgmental partnership. This should seek to build on people's existing knowledge and experience, move them towards autonomy, empower them to take responsibility for their own health and help them to feel positive about themselves.

Communication barriers

As a health promoter, you may encounter numerous difficulties in communicating. Recognising that communication barriers exist is the necessary first stage before work can begin on tackling the problems. There are no easy solutions, but increased awareness and skill can go a long way towards improvement.

Common communication barriers may be categorised as:

Social and cultural gaps

A number of factors can cause gaps, among which are:

- different ethnic background;
- different social class, which may be apparent in dress, language or accent;
- different cultural or religious beliefs, for example, about hygiene, nutrition or contraception;
- different values, reflected in a different emphasis on the importance of health issues;
- different sex, reflected in different approaches, interests or values.

Limited receptiveness

You may want to communicate, but the reverse is not always true: people may not want to be communicated with. They may be unreceptive for many reasons, including:

- mental handicap or confusion;
- illness, tiredness or pain;
- emotional distress;
- being too busy, distracted or preoccupied;
- not valuing themselves, or not believing that their health is important.

Limited understanding and memory

There may be difficulties because people:

- understand and/or speak little or no English;
- have limited intelligence and/or education, and may be illiterate;
- are being confronted with technical words, jargon or medical terminology which they do not understand;

- have poor or failing memories and cannot remember what was discussed previously.

Contradictory messages

Communication barriers are erected when people get different messages from different people. For example:

- individual health professionals give different advice;
- family, friends or neighbours contradict health promoters;
- 'the experts keep changing their minds' as information is updated.

Overcoming language barriers

Language is only one facet of the gulf which may exist between people of different ethnic backgrounds. The root of many communication problems is racism; this is a huge topic, largely outside the scope of this book, but we recommend all health promoters to take time out for racism awareness training, looking at their own attitudes and practices when working with people from different ethnic groups.

However, when we focus solely on the question of language barriers, learning a few key words and phrases may help. Words such as hello, goodbye, hot, cold, food and money may be useful. Help with learning the language may be available from multicultural education centres run by local education authorities.

When faced with a language barrier, there are some useful guidelines which you can follow to help someone with limited English to understand what is being said.

1. Speak clearly and slowly, and resist the temptation to raise your voice in an effort to get through.
2. Repeat a sentence if you have not been understood; repeat it using the *same* words. This gives the listener more time to 'tune in' and understand, whereas if you use different words you are likely to cause more confusion by introducing even more words which are not understood.
3. Keep it simple. Use simple words and sentences. Use active forms of verbs rather than passive forms, so say 'The nurse will see you' rather than 'You will be seen by the nurse'. Do not try to cover too much, and stick to one topic at a time.
4. Say things in a logical sequence: the sequence in which they are going to happen. So say 'Eat first, then take the tablet' rather than 'Take the tablet after you eat'. If the listener does not pick up the word 'after' correctly, he will take the tablet first, because that is the order in which he heard the instruction.
5. Be careful of idioms. Being 'fed up', 'popping out' and 'spending a penny' may be totally incomprehensible.
6. Do not attempt to speak pidgin English. It does not help people to learn correct English, and sounds patronising.
7. Use pictures, mime and simple written instructions which may be read by relatives or friends who understand written English. Be careful of symbols on written material; ticks and crosses, for example, may not convey what you intend.

8 Check to ensure that you have been understood, but avoid asking closed questions that require a one-word answer such as 'Do you understand?' A reply of 'Yes' is no guarantee that your client really *has* understood.

Non-verbal communication

Non-verbal communication includes all the ways by which people communicate with each other other than by using words, and is sometimes called body language. The main categories of non-verbal communication are as follows.

Bodily contact

Bodily contact is people touching each other, how much they touch, and which parts of the body are in contact. Shaking hands, holding hands or putting an arm around someone's shoulders, for example, all convey a meaning from one person to another.

Some health promoters, such as nurses, obviously touch patients frequently in the course of their work, whereas others such as environmental health officers may rarely do so. Touching people is surrounded by 'rules' dictated by cultural expectations and taboos, and by expectations of 'professional distance', which may be barriers to the positive use of touch. For example, a handshake can say 'I'm glad to see you—welcome' and touching a distressed person can say 'I'm here for you'.

Proximity

Proximity is how close people are to each other. Consider the different messages being conveyed to a bedridden patient by someone who talks to him from six feet away at the foot of the bed and someone who comes closer and sits on the bed or a chair. However, people vary in the amount of 'personal space' they need, and may feel uncomfortable when others come too close.

Orientation

How individuals position themselves in relation to other people and objects is known as orientation. A useful example is to consider the messages conveyed by the layout of a room where a small group of people are meeting. Chairs in rows facing one separate chair (perhaps with a table in front of it) imply that one person will dominate and control the meeting, whereas chairs placed in a circle without a table to act as a barrier imply that everyone is encouraged to join in, and that no one individual is expected to dominate.

Level

This refers to differences in height between people. Generally, communication is more comfortable if people are on the same level; so it feels better to bend down or sit down to talk to a child or a person in a wheelchair, for example. Talking to someone on a different level can leave one or both parties feeling disadvantaged, and sometimes this is done deliberately; not offering a chair to someone entering an office conveys a message that the visitor is not welcome to stay.

Posture

Posture is how people stand, sit or lie. For example, are they upright or slouched, arms crossed or not? Posture can convey a message of tension and anxiety, for example, by being hunched up with arms crossed, or one of welcome by being upright with arms outstretched.

Physical appearance

All kinds of messages may be conveyed by physical appearance, such as a person's social standing, personality, tidy habits or concern with fashion. Physical appearance may be very important to health promoters because of the messages it conveys. A uniform may convey an impression of professional competence, but it may also convey an unwelcome image of authority. Casual dress in a formal committee may convey the impression (perhaps a false one) that the committee's work is not being taken seriously.

Facial expression

Facial expression can obviously indicate feelings, such as sadness, happiness, anger, surprise or puzzlement.

Hand movements and head movements

Movements of the hands and head can be very revealing. Nods and shakes of the head obviously convey agreement and disagreement without the need for words. (But beware of the fact that movements of the head may not convey the same meaning in different cultures.) Clenched fists, fidgeting hands (and sometimes tapping feet) reveal stress and tension, whereas still, open hands usually denote a relaxed frame of mind. Mental discomfort, such as confusion or worry, is often shown by putting hands to the head and playing with hair, stroking a beard or rubbing the forehead.

Direction of gaze and eye contact

Whether people are 'looking each other straight in the eye' is significant. As a general rule, a speaker looks away from the listener for most of the time when talking (because she is concentrating on what she is saying), and she looks directly at the listener when she wants a response. For the listener, the general rule is that she will look the speaker straight in the eye while she is paying attention to what the speaker says, but will look elsewhere if her attention has wandered.

This is particularly important if you work with people on a one-to-one basis: a person who is talking to you will infer that you are not listening if you are looking anywhere other than at the speaker. This is most relevant when counselling someone in distress; the counsellor needs to be giving the client full attention, and if the client looks up and sees the counsellor gazing elsewhere, the implication is that the counsellor is not listening.

Non-verbal aspects of speech

Consider how many ways a word like 'no' can be said. How it is said can convey meanings such as anger, doubt or surprise. Tone and timing are two non-verbal aspects of speech which convey messages to the listener.

Raised awareness of non-verbal communication can help you to improve communication between yourself and the people you work with. For example, a person who says 'Yes, I understand' in a doubtful tone of voice, with a puzzled frown or with clenched fists clearly requires further help. Words alone are only part of a message, and can be misleading. Non-verbal communication is an area worth further study.

Listening

As a health promoter, you need to develop skills of effective listening, so that you can help people to talk and identify their needs.

Listening is an *active* process. It is not the same as merely hearing words. It involves a conscious effort to listen to words, to the way they are said, to be aware of the feelings shown and of attempts to hide feelings. It means taking note of the non-verbal communication as well as the spoken words. The listener needs to concentrate on giving the speaker full attention, being on the same level as the speaker and adopting a non-threatening posture.

It is easy to allow attention to wander. Some of the things you may find yourself doing instead of listening are planning what to say next, thinking about a similar experience, interrupting, agreeing or disagreeing, judging, blaming or criticising, interpreting what the speaker says, thinking about the next job to be done or just plain day-dreaming.

The task of a listener is to help people to talk about their situation unhurriedly and without interruption, to help them to express their feelings, views and opinions, and to explore their knowledge, values and attitudes. This reinforces the speakers' responsibility for themselves and is essential for helping them towards greater responsibility for their own health choices.

6

The Quality of Community Nursing Services: Report of an Exploratory Study in a UK Health Authority*

MARJORIE GOTT and HESTER PACKHAM

Introduction

While there is currently much interest in quality as a concept in nursing and health care, there remains debate about its interpretation and measurement. This study seeks to clarify the debate in relation to quality of nursing service.

> The lack of consensus on what is meant by quality is shown to support the argument that an individual embarking on a quality improvement programme must define it in their own forms, concentrating on local circumstances and the needs and views of consumers.[1]

Literature searches identified that quality measurement of the type undertaken in this study is fairly unique. Most surveys of consumer satisfaction have sampled hospital in-patients—very few studies have been undertaken in the community.[2]

Aim and background

The project commissioned by Community Health, a part of North Staffordshire Health Authority and funded by Regional Quality Funds, was designed to measure quality of specific services as perceived by the consumer.

Three quality dimensions have been identified by Donabedian.[3] These are:

1 *Technical aspects*: concerned with fitness for purpose, i.e. does the service do what it is supposed to do? Does it do it efficiently and effectively? And is what is offered appropriate?

*This is an abridged version of an article first published in *International Journal of Health Care Quality Assurance*, Vol. 6, No. 1, pp. 24–31, 1993.

2 *Interface aspects*: about how the service is delivered and perceived. Interpersonal relationships between workers and users are important here, as is evidence of team working . . . consumers need to have confidence that workers know what each worker is doing and why, i.e. that there is a coherent, defensible, shared vision for service delivery.
3 *Environment aspects*: concerned with the physical and social ethos in which service delivery occurs and its conduciveness to participatory relationships between workers and users, i.e. is the perception that the service is run for the service, or for the people? . . . and for all of the people, or some of the people? (equity).

Nurses were drawn from three disciplines: district nursing, health visiting and school nursing. The sample was service users, naturally selected at point of contact with the service, over a given period of time. In addition to direct users, parents and teachers, as well as older schoolchildren, were included.

Three different locales were selected for collection of main study data and these were different from the locale selected for the pilot study.

Methodology

A research schedule was drawn up. However, before research instruments could be developed, the project director (first named author) spent some time getting a feel for the pertinent issues. This included background reading and a day spent out in the field, taking an ethnographic stance and allowing random perceptions to occur. Following this, instruments were developed. These included a postal questionnaire, a semi-structured interview schedule and field notes guidance forms. In designing the instruments the three quality dimensions identified earlier were used.

Because nurses have many roles, not one, and because their roles are changing by both evolution and mandate, five nursing roles were identified (from nursing and quality literature) and 'sort' cards used with individual participants who were asked to rank them in order of 'most important' to 'least important'. People at interview and by questionnaire were also offered a free response category in which to record their views about the role of the nurse.

The five nursing roles which were identified from the aforementioned sources were:

1 giving care to sick people;
2 screening and immunizing to prevent disease;
3 checking that people are progressing/developing normally;
4 teaching people how to live a healthy lifestyle;
5 influencing local businesses, councillors, shopkeepers, etc. for healthy public places.

The three research workers (nurses working within the unit) received training in order to:

- orientate them into 'quality issues';
- review and build on the communication and interviewing skills necessary for data collection;

- familiarize them with the research methods to be used;
- offer them the opportunity to use some research instruments and roles.

The instruments were tested with a small sample of all three subject groups and, following the pilot study, minor adjustments were made to the questionnaire and semi-structured interview schedule.

Main study

Each research nurse worked in a different discipline and area from that in which she was trained/normally worked. They then were assigned to and 'tracked' a community nurse in each discipline in each study district selected, and worked from her case load. There were four interviews for each discipline case load. Interviewees were systematically selected from the visiting list (i.e. every third person) and interviewed in their homes by the research worker after permission had been obtained.

Thirty questionnaires were randomly distributed by the community nurse (each district). She/he used her/his judgement about who to leave them with (lucidity, mobility). The carer instead of the patient sometimes participated.

Field notes were made on half-day visits with community nurses and during clinics.

The same instruments, process and sample were used for school nurses with the following additions. Parents were captured by use of a 'tear off' reply letter of invitation. Four parents per district were interviewed, four teachers per district were also interviewed and group interviews were conducted with senior secondary schoolchildren in each district.

As raw data this yielded:

49 questionnaires (53 per cent response rate)
48 interviews
12 sets of field notes
3 group interviews

} 100 per cent response rate (bracketing 48 interviews, 12 sets of field notes and 3 group interviews)

Findings

Interview data: district nurses

The interview sample was predominantly female (9) and over 65 years of age (10).

The role of the district nurse was seen overwhelmingly as looking after sick people at home (13). Most mentioned the fact (and the value which they placed on it) that the district nursing service allowed people to be cared for in their own homes:

> The nurse's job is to look after people who can't go to the doctors, who are ill but who don't want to go into hospital.
> (*Lady, under 65 years*)
>
> If they didn't come in to me I would have to go into a home.
> (*Lady, 65 years*)

Three users said that the nurse also assessed people's health, and one mentioned a role in advising about health. Two said that she also dealt with other problems.

When asked whether they thought the role should change, users were vociferous in their praise for the service which they had experienced. The few changes which were suggested were to do with getting more of the existing service, i.e. increasing the number of visits was mentioned twice, as was the need for more resources. Ranking of roles showed 'giving care to sick people' as the most frequent first choice (10) and 'screening and immunizing' and 'checking progress/development' trying in second place. 'Influencing for healthy public places' came last more frequently (9) with 'teaching about healthy lifestyles' falling in a mid- to low-ranking.

It was believed that nurses worked more with older people than any other group (7) and the view was sometimes offered that older people needed more help (4).

The consumer's voice in service delivery was believed to exist (9), although three people commented that people did not necessarily know what was needed and one felt that assertiveness was necessary.

> Those who speak up for themselves . . . I firmly but politely told one nurse to mind her own business when she was making remarks about my clothes. (*Lady, 67 years*)

Technical aspects of the service were very highly regarded, both effectiveness and efficiency being praised by all respondents. Two mentioned having to wait because of shortage of staff. They did not blame nurses for this but 'high-ups':

> You can always contact them, but they have a job to do. (*Man, 76 years*)

Questionnaire data: district nursing

An attitude scale was used to measure opinion in the three quality areas under study. The scale ranged from '*strongly agree*' to '*strongly disagree*' with a '*don't know*' category at mid-point. Sixteen from a possible sample of 30 responded.

The answers to the questionnaire in general mirrored the responses obtained in the interview setting.

The consumer's voice in service delivery was thought to be accommodated in service provision by two-thirds of respondents. However, when asked again, in a different way almost half (7) agreed that 'ordinary people don't have a say in the way the service is run'.

Communication with their own district nurse was satisfactory. However, in terms of the health service in general there was a less positive response.

Technical aspects were rated highly, only one disagreeing that the nurse always seems to know what she is doing. Five strongly agreed that she always did. Two would like the nurse to become aware of their problems.

District nurses' field notes

Researchers had been asked to relate their observations to the three quality dimensions already discussed. Three district nurse treatment sessions were observed.

All three nurses observed were described as having good interpersonal skills, being able to relate well to new and established patients alike. The clinic was regarded as a 'social event' by some patients and was therefore well received. In general there were no complaints about the physical aspects of the clinic, although access in winter was an issue for two patients.

One regular patient said that he enjoyed coming to the clinic, because he could have 'a laugh and a bit of a joke with the nurses'.

For another patient the best thing about the clinic was that, because of being a regular, he had got to know several other patients, so he could have a bit of a chat. He also thought that the nursing staff were 'kind and made you feel at home'. One lady, when asked if she would prefer someone to go to her home every week to give her the injection she needed, replied: 'No, it gets me out a bit and I enjoy a change of scenery'.

Standards of nursing care were assessed to be high in two of the clinics. However, in the third clinic some procedures witnessed seemed to be informed more by habit and ritual than good practice.

Quotes which typified the patients' views of the district nursing service include:

> Anyone who needs a nurse can have one.
>
> They go all over the area day and night.
>
> I feel I am not alone in caring for my husband.
>
> No one is available between 7 a.m. and 9 a.m.

Interview data: health visitors

The interview sample comprised 12 mothers under the age of 40 years.

The role of the health visitor was seen as checking and advising on the normal development and progress of infants (10). Over half the sample (7) also mentioned that she advises on problems connected with childbearing. Some were unsure of her background:

> I didn't know she was a nurse, I thought she was a social worker. I found out at the ante natal class.

Her role in giving personal advice and support was highly valued:

> She is a guide and mentor, someone at the end of the phone.
>
> Her job is about calming you down when you leave hospital, having had your baby. Health visitors who aren't married and do not have children talk to you as if you don't know anything . . . ones who've had children have had the experience and that is far better than doing it through the books.

However, one client had a view of the health visitor as a sort of social policewoman. This may reflect the profession's origins (lady visitors) or the current social climate in which child abuse is a high profile public issue.

Ranking of health visitor roles showed almost equal weighting to screening and immunizing, checking progress development and giving care as first choices. All three roles always fell within the mid- to top point range, whereas teaching people about a healthy life ranked low (in fourth position ten times, last twice). Influencing local policy was ranked last all but twice.

Despite being in contact with the health visiting service there was still some confusion on the part of some mothers as to the actual role of the health visitor.

The consumer's voice in service delivery was thought by almost half (5) to be ignored. Others, however, were well satisfied with what was on offer and one mother recognized the element of choice in taking advice which was being offered.

Technical aspects of the service were most frequently linked with efficiency (seen as health visitors calling when they had said they would). Five, however, mentioned difficulties of access to the service, commenting that it was overloaded, and therefore slow.

Access was also often linked with information, four wanting more information about what was available.

Effectiveness was spoken about in relation to supporting first-time mothers. This role was highly valued (9) but seen as very under-resourced (5).

Questionnaire data

There were 18 from a possible 30 respondents in this group. The role of the health visitor was seen as primarily work with individuals.

Ranking of roles was interesting because respondents did not score highly influencing healthy public policy although 'teaching people how to live a healthy lifestyle' did rank first in a third of the responses. Also, despite the health visitor's role with young children, 'checking normal progress and development' scored low.

Answers to the questionnaire ran along similar lines to those obtained in the interview setting in respect of health problems, consumer's voice, and communication and technical aspects of the service.

Field notes: health visitors

Interface quality was reported as being high in all the three clinics observed, with the exception of the interpersonal style of one health visitor, which was described as cold, efficient and giving the attitude of getting the job done (weighing the baby).

Environment was generally unsatisfactory. Although bright, cheerful and adequate resources were offered in all clinics, in one clinic there was nowhere for mothers to talk privately with the health visitor, and in another two there were no safe play areas for older toddlers:

> I get so anxious because X wanders about and could easily run on the road outside.

Technical quality of the service was rated as very high in two clinics, but not in the one where the interpersonal problem had been noted earlier.

Quotes which typified the mothers' views of the health visiting service include:

> HVs who aren't married talk to you as if you don't know anything.

> Her job is to check your house and your family.
>
> People are not generally asked what they need.
>
> You don't always have to take their advice.
>
> Between me and the health visitor it is good.
>
> They should listen to mums more.

Interview data: school nurses

Responses from both parents and secondary school teachers were required. Parent responses will be discussed first in each category. The parent sample comprised 12 mothers, 11 of whom were under 40 years of age, and 12 teachers, mostly 40 plus.

Mothers in general saw the role of the school nurse as assessing normal progress and development, although her role in screening also ranked fairly high.

Teachers also recognized the role of the school nurse in preventive work and health education. They had a greater awareness of the role. Both groups consistently placed influencing healthy public policy last. Three others felt that the role should be extended to offer counselling to parents.

The consumer's voice, in the view of the mothers, was unanimously felt to be lacking. However, teachers generally felt that they had a say in the service but were less sure as to whether parents had a say.

Communication was sometimes problematic for the parents, and teachers endorsed this view, though only in respect of parents. As with other groups of nurses, school nurse clients spoke about lack of information regarding services, saying that they did not know what was available and how to go about getting it:

> The teachers might know what the nurse does but parents probably don't know . . . a lot think she just inspects heads.

Some teachers (4) endorsed this view, saying that they didn't believe parents knew what school nurses did.

As with other groups of nurses, school nurse clients spoke about lack of information regarding services, saying that they did not know what was available, and how to go about getting it (4).

Regarding technical aspects, not surprisingly, given the above comments, there was a lot of discussion about resources. Generally, people stated that they did not know what was available to them as parents and to their children as service consumers. Five people said that the service should advertise what was available. These comments arose in relation to a question about the universal accessibility of the service. A fairly frequent comment was:

> I think the service is open to everybody, but I don't think everybody knows about it.
>
> I think so, but I wouldn't know who to contact.

Two people mentioned that the service would be more accessible, if it was held out of school hours.

Efficiency was, as with other nurses, seen as frequent or correctly timed visits.

Group interviews with schoolchildren

In addition to interviewing parents and teachers it was considered important to gain the views of the youngsters themselves. Three senior secondary school classes were therefore interviewed.

The role of the school nurse was thought to be about checking normal progress, immunizing, and health education.

In ranking the role, giving care and checking progress were generally high, while influencing healthy public policy was seen as a low priority.

With regard to changes in role, all three groups wanted more time with a nurse in school, who would be available to listen to their problems.

Like their parents, they did not think the consumer view was well represented.

Communications were seen as poor and technical aspects were seen as a lack of resources.

Questionnaire data: school nurse

Fifteen from a possible 30 responses were collected. The role of the school nurse was seen as principally working with individual children.

Ranking of nursing roles reflected a very traditional view with almost equal weighting being given to screening, checking progress and giving care. Health education came above the mid-rank only twice.

All respondents felt that people should take health problems to the nurse. Answers to the questionnaire again followed similar lines to the interviews with parents. In general their respect for the service being provided by the school nurse was reflected in a number of respondents seeing her as an adequate substitute for the doctor:

> The excellent care and concern you receive and the understanding of your problems. The school nurse has been so helpful to me. She is also very kind.

School nursing field notes

Interface quality was generally thought to be good, though, in one, a screening session, this was less evident. Children were, however, offered a chance to discuss any problems, etc. with the nurse.

Technical quality was always reported as high; nurses carrying out efficient and effective procedures. A high level of communication skill was also reported.

Environmental factors varied from being warm and friendly, to being inadequate for the activity being undertaken. A selective medical session for 13 year-old boys evoked very conflicting views from the children. Some felt very relaxed about seeing the nurse, while one in particular would have preferred to see the doctor and would not think of telling his problems to the nurse.

Quotes which typified the consumers' view of the school nursing service include:

> They are needed when new intakes start.

Nurses should be based in school.

People don't take kindly to being told of problems.

Most people are not aware of what is there.

(Teacher) Nurse is valued.

Review of findings

District nursing

District nursing is a highly valued service which allows people to be nursed in their own homes. This is not only more cost-effective than caring for sick elderly people in institutions, it is also in line with their own wishes.

District nurses are perceived as working with families as well as individual patients and this is probably reflective of the support and advice given to carers.

Consumers were generally satisfied with their communications with district nurses, but less so with communications in the health service as a whole. It was often felt that people did not have a say in the way services were run. They also wanted more information about what services were available and how to get them. They expected this information to come from district nurses.

Although there was overwhelming satisfaction with the service which was provided, there was also a broadly based call for more of it.

This finding is in line with other studies in other health districts.[4–6]

For many patients the personal qualities of the nurse are as highly valued as her technical abilities. Patient/nurse relationships allow for free discussion of problems, initiated by either party. Visits are valued socially as well as functionally. Clinic treatment sessions are valued for the same reason.

Health visiting

There was a degree of confusion surrounding the role of the health visitor and, when the clients' view of the role is contrasted with that of the health visitors, there is a clear mismatch. If the service is to be effective, either the health visitors must alter their role to meet client expectations or they must publicize their role in order to provide the client with a greater understanding of what the health visitor can offer. Probably a combination of both these approaches would ensure a more effective service to the clients.

What is evident from the data is that the majority of clients valued their relationship with the health visitor and that they put a lot of faith in her advice and support, although this did not always extend to lifestyle issues. Parents were particularly looking for help with issues and challenges of everyday living. It may be that such advice could be available from other sources, as demonstrated by the Community Mothers Scheme currently being offered in the Republic of Ireland.[7]

Such a scheme would not replace the health visiting service but act to enhance it at a time when, as identified by the data, the service is seen by the consumer to be under-resourced. Other data indicated a need to review and reorganize some child health clinics, which tended to lack privacy for consultation, and safe play areas for toddlers.

School nursing

Knowledge about the school nurse's role was better than for health visitors, although parents were less well informed than teachers or children. Lifestyle issues were not seen as important despite the growing emphasis on health education and health promotion with school nursing.

The role of the school nurse in counselling and advice was seen as more important and this was an area which many people wished to see developed. The need for more information and greater emphasis on consumer issues was highlighted. The need to balance the technical role and the interpersonal role was noted, particularly within screening sessions. Time for personal interviews would raise the quality of the overall service.

Summary and conclusions

Although perceptions about all three services varied, certain key issues emerged and common findings were reflected in the three instruments used for the data collection.

The pivotal quality feature, which was highlighted throughout the study, was the value placed on personal relationships developed with the professional.

However, it was generally noted that services were under-resourced with all three groups of staff working hard to meet the constant demand for services. Clients deeply valued what they were receiving but felt in a number of cases that they were not getting enough. Communications were considered to be a problem, not in general between client and nurse, but certainly within the organization and the NHS as a whole.

Throughout the study the importance of information was stressed and the lack of it in some areas noted. Poor facilities within the clinic setting were identified particularly for child health clinics, although facilities in schools were also not always seen as adequate.

One strategy for meeting the quality demand which clients have so clearly articulated is to identify and use other skilled sources of support for some nursing functions. With the advent of the NHS reforms dealing with efficiency and effectiveness in service delivery, role prioritization is inevitable, and can be seen as an opportunity, rather than a threat.[8] Project 2000[9] and PREPP[10] reforms recognize the importance of community nursing and are giving it greater precedence in basic and post basic training. Advanced practitioners of community nursing are advocated who will, as well as giving care and practising preventive medicine, provide leadership to teams (skill mix). Teams are likely to comprise (in addition to trained community nurses) registered nurses, support workers and lay and voluntary helpers.

Notes

1. Hadfield, L. 'In Search of excellence in accident and emergency', *Nursing Standard*, Vol. **3**, No. 25, March 1989, pp. 19–22.

2. King's Fund. *Quality Assurance Readings Lists*, Nos. 2, 7, 8, King's Fund Centre, Albert Street, London, 1991.

3. Donabedian, A. *Explorations in Quality Assessment and Monitoring*, Vols 1, 2 and 3, Health Administration Press, Ann Arbor, Michigan, 1980, 1982, 1985.

4. CHC. *A Report on Health and Women in Central Birmingham*, Central Birmingham Community Health Council, 1990.

5. CHC. *The Health and Health Needs of Women in Wakefield*, Wakefield Community Health Council, 1990.

6. CHC. *A Survey of Health Care Facilities*, Purbeck District, East Dorset Community Health Council, 1990.

7. Godinho, J., Rathwell, T., Gott, M. and Daley, J. *Tipping the Balance Towards Primary Health Care*, Final Report, European Commission, Brussels, October 1991.

8. James, E. 'Future Uncertain', *Primary Health Care*, March 1991, pp. 29–30.

9. UKCC. *Project 2000: A New Preparation for Practice*, United Kingdom Central Council for Nursing, Midwifery and Health Visiting, 23 Portland Place, London, 1986.

10. UKCC. *Report on the Post-registration and Practice Project*, United Kingdom Central Council for Nursing, Midwifery and Health Visiting, 23 Portland Place, London, 1991.

SECTION 2

Child Development

Introduction

A major area of controversy in the field of child development is the so-called 'nature versus nurture' debate. To what extent are developmental processes driven by genetics and how is this modified by the child's physical and social environment? The papers collected for this section offer insight into this debate.

The family represents the immediate social environment for most children, although the nature of that environment is determined to an extent by the parents' perceptions of their own role, and by the style of parenting that they adopt. The family unit, whatever form it takes, exists within a wider social context and is deeply embedded in a set of cultural values and beliefs. These values are not consistent across society, they vary between social classes and with other factors such as ethnic origin. Social and political change in society is constantly redefining how parents are able to nurture their children and what is considered acceptable behaviour. In the first paper in this section Mussen *et al.* look at the well established psychological process of conditioning, and demonstrate how a great deal of learning in early life is dependent on both classical and instrumental conditioning.

The second paper explores the concept of play for both adults and children, and shows how the development of play is inextricably linked to other aspects of development. The way that the nature of play changes as the child moves through developmental stages is elucidated and is used to illustrate the universality of play.

The context of development is the general theme which links the following papers by Mussen *et al.*, Mares, Henley and Baxter, and Bamford. Families which appear very similar may have quite different internal dynamics. Mussen *et al.* examine the most widely accepted classification of parenting styles, and discuss the effects of these on children.

Mares, Henley and Baxter, in an extract from their well known text, look at the way family systems vary in Britain between different ethnic groups. The emphasis of the paper is that Britain is a multicultural society and that health care workers need to be able to adapt to different cultural norms, particularly in relation to the rearing of children.

In a wide ranging, specially commissioned, paper, Bamford looks at an area which has received little publicity or research attention: the effect of parental employment on children's health. Reproductive health is discussed, and a section on work patterns examines the impact of modern work pressures on family health.

In the final paper we hear in children's own words how they perceive illness, hospitals and the staff who work in them. Moloney argues for a move towards a more individual assessment of children's level of understanding, away from the accepted models based on stages theories of child development.

7

Learning Through Conditioning*

P. MUSSEN *et al.*

Changes in the motor and cognitive capabilities of the infant are summarized in Table 7.1. Many of them undoubtedly have a maturational basis—they depend at least partly on changes in the neurological system and on other aspects of physical maturation. As we have already noted, however, complex human behavior is almost always influenced both by the biological attributes of the individual and by experience. One framework used by psychologists to study the changes produced by experience is learning theory, particularly the basic concept of conditioning. We will discuss conditioning in this

Table 7.1 Developmental milestones during the first year

Area	Age in months					
	0–2	3–4	5–6	7–8	9–10	11–12
Motor	Turns head; lifts chin when lying on stomach	Lifts chest; holds head erect; reaches for an object	Holds head steady; transfers an object from one hand to another	Sits with support	Stands with help; crawls	Pulls self to standing position; walks with support
Cognitive		Recognition of the past; controlled scanning of stimuli	Selected imitation	Retrieval memory; object permanence	Comprehension of language	Symbolic play; first meaningful words
Emotion		Distress to discrepancy; smile to assimilation		Stranger and separation anxiety begin; facial signs of anger to frustration		Sadness to loss of an attachment figure

*This is an abridged version of a chapter in P. Mussen *et al.* (1984) *Child development and personality*, 6th edn, Harper and Row, New York, pp. 107–109.

section as it applies to infants, but the concepts presented apply more generally to learning by humans at all ages and by many animals as well.

Infants learn new habits and emotional reactions through two types of conditioning, classical and instrumental. *Conditioning* refers to the creation of a new association between a feeling, physiological state, or action on the one hand and a stimulus event on the other.

The most famous example of classical conditioning (sometimes called respondent conditioning) is Pavlov's pioneering set of experiments with the salivation response in dogs. Pavlov showed that a dog could be conditioned to salivate to the stimulus of a buzzer. This was accomplished by pairing the presentation of the sound of the buzzer (called the *conditioned stimulus*) with the presentation of food (called the *unconditioned stimulus*). Food in an animal's mouth innately elicits the salivation response, while salivation does not ordinarily occur to the sound of a buzzer. As a result of repeated pairing of the buzzer and the food, the buzzer alone came to elicit the salivation response. The dog had learned a new association between the buzzer and salivation.

An *unconditioned stimulus* is an event that produces a certain response (the *unconditioned response*) automatically, that is, without learning. The *unconditioned response* to food is the production of saliva; to thunder it is an increase in heart rate. If the unconditioned stimulus is repeatedly associated in time or space with a neutral stimulus that does not ordinarily produce the response, a link is formed between the neutral stimulus and the response. Soon the neutral stimulus alone (now called the *conditioned stimulus*) will elicit the response (now called the *conditioned response*).

A child looking out a window at a passing bus hears an unexpected clap of thunder and cries. The next time he sees a bus pass the house, he may experience the feeling of fear. The association of the sight of the bus (the conditioned stimulus) and the fear reaction to the thunder (the unconditioned stimulus) changes the child. The sight of the bus now has the capacity to elicit the conditioned response. It is likely that many feeling states are classically conditioned in children. Fear of lightning and fear of dogs are two obvious candidates.

Despite almost three-quarters of a century of research, we still do not know how classically conditioned associations are established. Psychologists assume that infants (and older people as well) are prepared, by their biology, to associate certain events with certain internal reactions or overt responses. Not all stimuli are capable of becoming conditioned stimuli for a particular response, and conditioned associations do not occur every time two events occur close together in time. A nursing baby, for example, is prepared to associate the fragrance of the mother's perfume with the feeling state that accompanies feeding but is less prepared to associate the temperature of the room or color of the walls with that feeling state.

There is another form of conditioning, called instrumental or operant conditioning, which differs from classical conditioning in many respects. A 1-year-old cries when his mother tucks him into bed, turns out the light, and begins to leave the room. The child's cry provokes the mother to reenter the room, turn on the light, and return to the infant's side. That sequence increases the probability that the child will cry when put to bed the next day, because the mother's return is a reinforcing event. Another 1-year-old picks up her glass of milk by the top, causing it to spill. When she picks up the second glass and holds it by the side, it does not spill, and she drinks the contents. The successful outcome is called the reinforcing event. Because the reinforcement—the return of the mother or being able to drink the milk—was attained by crying or holding the glass on the side, those responses have a higher probability of occurring again in response to those specific conditions.

The exact form of a young infant's sucking response can be modified by presenting or withholding milk, and babies can be instrumentally conditioned to turn their heads to certain sounds. They learn to *discriminate* cues in the environment that signal when they will be reinforced or which of several behaviors will be reinforced. One scientist (Papousek, 1967), presented 6-week-old infants with either a bell or a buzzer. When the bell sounded, the baby would receive milk only from the nipple on the left, not from the one on the right. When the buzzer sounded, milk was available only on the right and not on the left. After about 30 days of such experiences, the infants learned to turn to the left when they heard the bell and to the right when they heard the buzzer. Papousek was even able to condition 4-month-old infants to make two consecutive turns to one side or to alternate turns to the left with turns to the right.

Reinforcement increases the probability of the recurrence of the instrumentally conditioned response in a particular context. When the reinforcing event reduces a biological drive like hunger or thirst, it is called a *primary reinforcer*. Any objects or people who were present when the biological drive was reduced may acquire reinforcing value and are called *secondary reinforcers*.

In the past, it seemed that the important thing about a reinforcement was its ability to provide pleasure. But this definition is too simple. We do not feel pleasure every time we engage in instrumental behavior—that is, in actions that attain a goal. Getting in a car to commute to school or work, for instance, is an instrumental behavior that may be performed daily even though it produces little if any pleasure.

Some psychologists argue, therefore, that any change in experience can be reinforcing if it increases the probability that a response will recur. But changes in experience do not always increase the likelihood of a response. In addition, with repetition, an event that is initially reinforcing seems to lose its reinforcing qualities. Consider an example of a baby who strikes a balloon full of plastic beads, causing it to move and make a noise. The baby laughs and repeats the action, and the baby smiles. The movement and interesting noise appear to be reinforcing. This sequence seems to be a nice example of the principle of instrumental conditioning, implying that the baby should repeat the act again and again. But after only a few minutes the baby stops, as if bored. This remarkably common phenomenon—boredom following attainment of what appears to be a desirable goal—suggests that the child's state changes after he experiences reinforcements, and as a result the child's motivation for the reinforcing event is altered. This process is described in learning theory as *satiation*.

Instrumental conditioning has proved to be extremely useful in changing human behavior. For example, it has been used to help retarded children learn basic skills, such as how to tie their shoes or eat with silverware. Both primary reinforcers like cake and candy, and secondary reinforcers, like money, tokens, and gold stars have been used effectively.

Reference

Paponsek, H. (1967) Experimental studies of appetitional behaviour in human newborns and infants. In H.W. Stevenson, E.H. Hess and H.L. Reingolds (Eds), *Early Behavior*. New York: Wiley.

8

Play*

KATHY SYLVA and PAM CZERNIEWSKA

1 What is play?

> Once upon a time, at a conference of psychologists, we happened to fall into conversation with a prominent government scientist and his wife, as we were strolling back from lunch. One of us happened to mention that our psychology department had just acquired its own small but nonetheless very expensive computer installation, and went on to remark that this would provide a beautiful new toy which a lot of people in our department would enjoy playing with. The scientist's wife was clearly shocked at the levity of this remark, and at the thought of the abuse of a very large sum of taxpayers' money, and she said as much. But her husband quickly stepped in with the reassurance that the word 'play' had obviously been used jokingly, and continued to the effect that academic psychologists were highly responsible people who only used such expressions as a modest cover for their earnest dedication to the pursuit of important scientific questions. Not being able to decide, on the spur of the moment, which of these attitudes misunderstood our meaning most thoroughly, we let the matter drop; but the incident brought home to us that not everyone automatically shares the developmental psychologist's view of the nature of play: which can be expressed in the paradoxical statement that play is perhaps the most serious and significant of all human activities.
> (Newson and Newson, 1979, p. 11)

When adults 'play' there will be different views about its function. Some will see it as a way of relaxing; others as something slightly frivolous, and a few will regard it as an important activity for learning. What would have happened if in the above anecdote the psychologists had said they had just bought a new toy for a child? The

---

*This is an abridged version of a chapter in K. Sylva and P. Czerniewkska (1985) *Personality development and learning*, Open University Press, Milton Keynes, pp. 7–14.

reactions would undoubtedly be different. Most people think that it's very natural for a child to play and probably most would agree that play is important for the child's development rather than being just an enjoyable, time-consuming activity.

Behind such views lie a number of assumptions about what play is, what function play serves and at what age play ceases to be significant. It is to questions such as these that many psychologists have addressed themselves in the hope that their answers will be able to contribute both to theories of development and to the provision of valuable environments for the young.

Defining play

Many psychological concepts seem strange to the non-psychologist. The word *play* seems pleasantly familiar, it's instantly recognized and, you may think, easily defined. But is it? Consider the following examples.

(a) A young mother nibbles the toes of her four-month-old baby while changing his nappy. The mother announces 'I'm going to get you . . . I'm going to eat you all up' and the child laughs with delight, swinging his legs in the air. The mother laughs too.
(b) Two five-year-olds are playing in a preschool group. One is the 'nurse' and the other the ailing 'baby'. The nurse upbraids the other child, who is the younger of the two, scolding and bossing. 'Be quiet. Lie still. Here's your medicine.' The younger child begins to sob and hides his head under the pillow.
(c) A four-year-old walks alone down the garden path, stepping carefully on the largest stones and avoiding the smaller ones. He smiles as he goes.
(d) Two ten-year-old girls are engrossed in chess. The dark-haired one ponders her next move for more than a minute, frowning all the time. The fairer partner stares intently at the board, fidgeting with her hair and biting her lower lip.
(e) Two teams of professional footballers meet in a cup final. Each individual shows determination and tension during the game knowing that the final outcome involves a great deal of money for the winning team.

In fact, psychologists have argued for decades about the precise definition of play; they don't disagree about what might be called quintessential play—merry games of pretence or tumbling down slides into wading pools below. But these are stereotypes that spring to mind. To delve deeper into the topic you will have to collect behavioural descriptions of your own, including 'borderline' cases to help you draw firm distinctions.

Most psychologists shy away from a one-sentence definition of play, preferring instead to list characteristics common to its varied forms. Catherine Garvey, for example, has drawn up such a list which you should compare with your own definition:

(a) Play is pleasurable, enjoyable. Even when not actually accompanied by signs of mirth, it is still positively valued by the player.
(b) Play has no extrinsic goals. Its motivations are intrinsic and serve no other objectives. In fact, it is more an enjoyment of means than an effort devoted to some particular end.

(c) Play is spontaneous and voluntary. It is not obligatory but is freely chosen by the player.
(d) Play involves some active engagement on the part of the player.
(e) Play has certain systematic relations to what is not play.
(Garvey, 1977, p. 10)

The first characteristic, that play is for pleasure, seems uncontroversial though how one decides, when laughter is not present, what is 'positively valued' is almost impossible. Is a two-year-old, with furrowed brow, trying to fit rings onto a stick positively valuing the task? And what of the many non-play activities which are pleasurable, like eating and drinking. Should they be called play?

The second characteristic refers to a lack of extrinsic goals. Play is characterized here as something done for its own sake not because of some reward such as prize-money. Often it's difficult to tell whether an activity is extrinsically or intrinsically motivated. For instance, playing a game may appear to be extrinsically motivated by the promise of a prize and yet, if the prize were removed, play may not necessarily stop. Another difficulty with this characteristic is that it includes some activities which would not seem to be play, for example thumb-sucking.

Thirdly, 'spontaneity' describes much play activity, though in a structured nursery class or in organized games how much play is voluntary and spontaneous is not always clear. Similarly, 'active engagement' in characteristic (d) is a slippery phrase. Should this include intellectual as well as physical activity? If so, how can one judge whether the child staring into space is busy creatively playing 'in her head' or whether she is doing nothing?

The last characteristic, (e), is an important one and needs further explanation. For Garvey (and many others) play is a 'non-literal' activity which can be recognized by its contrasts with 'literal' activities. For example, if you hit somebody over the head you may be charged with grievous bodily harm. But if you rain light blows and say cheerfully, 'I'll kill you', you are merely playing at attack; you are adopting a non-literal mode which can be recognized by its contrast with the literal attack: reduced strength, a wink or a smile. Young children soon learn to signal when it's real and when it's play:

X: I've got to go potty
Y: (turns to him) Really?
X: (grins) No, pretend
Y: (smiles and watches X)
(Garvey, 1972, p. 576)

This relative definition of play—play is what is not non-play—relies on the correct interpretation by both participants and observers of play of the other person's motives and intentions. And such interpretations are prone to error.

A four-year-old girl, playing with her wooden horse as with a doll, whispered:

'The horsie put on a tail and went for a walk.'
Her mother interrupted her play, saying:
'Horses' tails are not tied to them—they cannot be put on and taken off.'

'How silly you are, Mommie! I am just playing!'
(Chukovsky, 1963, 1968 ed., p. 26)

While Garvey's list of characteristics seems to identify *some* features of *some* play, they will not always, on their own, allow us to say of one piece of behaviour 'that is play' and 'that is non-play'. This does not seem a very satisfactory beginning, and yet it reflects a fundamental problem facing psychology and other human sciences. Human behaviour does not generally fall into neat packages ready for psychological exploration and explanation. For example, consider such practical educational questions as: What is play? What good is play? or What kind of play is good? You're bound to face categories of behaviour with fuzzy edges, and find it hard to agree on definitions. Furthermore, you're likely to find that each person attempting to answer the questions will have identified different aspects of play for analysis, without necessarily recognizing another's boundaries.

This opening section should have demonstrated the complex nature of play, the range of activities to be encompassed under the word *play* and the difficulties of classifying and defining play. In the next section we will continue the attempt to describe play, this time looking at play from a developmental perspective. We will attempt to outline the major types of play that children engage in during their first five years.

2 The development of play

How does play develop? Clearly, at different ages children engage in different types of play. Development of play will of course depend, to some extent, on the child's physical, intellectual and social development: playing hopscotch cannot occur until the child has learnt to walk and to hop; constructing a model plane requires fine motor control and playing 'Ring-a-roses' will depend on motor and language abilities as well as social abilities.

Play must be viewed as dependent on the cultural context as well as the developmental context. Not all children in all cultures will exhibit similar play patterns, and our evaluation of play will change over time, as the following quote demonstrates:

> The mother of 1914 was told: 'The rule that parents should not play with the baby may seem hard, but it is without doubt a safe one. A young, delicate and nervous baby needs rest and quiet, and however robust the child much of the play that is indulged in is more or less harmful. It is a great pleasure to hear the baby laugh and crow in apparent delight, but often the means used to produce the laughter, such as tickling, punching, or tossing, makes him irritable and restless. It is a regrettable fact that the few minutes' play that the father has when he gets home at night, may result in nervous disturbance of the baby and upset his regular habits. It is relevant to note that at this time 'playthings . . . such as rocking horses, swings, teeter boards, and the like' are cited in connection with masturbation, as means by which 'this habit is learned.' The dangerousness of play is related to that of the ever present sensual impulses which must be constantly

> guarded against. (In 1929–38, play becomes less taboo, but must be strictly confined to certain times of the day. In this period the impulse to dominate replaces erotic impulses as the main hazard in the child's nature, and the corresponding danger is that he may get the mother to play with him whenever he likes.)
>
> In the recent period, play becomes associated with harmless and healthful motor and exploratory activities. It assumes the aspect of diffuse innocuousness which the child's impulse life now presents. Play is derived from the baby's developing motor activities, which are now increasingly stressed. 'A baby needs to be able to move all parts of his body. He needs to exercise . . . At a very early age the baby moves his arms and legs aimlessly . . . As he gets older and stronger and his movements become more vigorous and he is better able to control them he begins to play.' Thus play has been successfully dissociated from unhealthy excitement and nervous debilitation and has become associated with muscular development, necessary exercise, strength, and control. This is in keeping with the changed conception of the baby, in which motor activities rather than libidinal urges are stressed. For the baby who is concerned with exploring his world rather than with sucking and masturbating, play becomes safe and good.
>
> Play is now to be fused with all the activities of life. 'Play and singing make both mother and baby enjoy the routine of life.' This mingling of play with necessary routines is consonant with the view that the good and pleasant coincide. Also, as the mother is urged to make play an aspect of every activity, play assumes a new obligatory quality. Mothers are told that 'a mother usually enjoys entering into her baby's play. Both of them enjoy the little games that mothers and babies have always played from time immemorial.' (This harking back to time immemorial is a way of skipping over the more recent past.) 'Daily tasks can be done with a little play and singing thrown in.' Thus it is now not adequate for the mother to perform efficiently the necessary routines for her baby; she must also see that these are fun for both of them. It seems difficult here for anything to become permissible without becoming compulsory. Play, having ceased to be wicked, having become harmless and good, now becomes a new duty.
> (Wolfenstein, 1955, pp. 172–3)

With the provisos that our views of play are influenced by our views of childhood and child-rearing, a few play 'milestones' can be identified.

From coos to skipping

During the first two years there is much exploratory and repetitive play, such as pulling, shaking, throwing and grabbing objects, as well as filling, emptying, building and destroying anything which can be grasped. During these first years, language is developing and play with sounds is evident beginning with coos and gurgles but later turning into language practice such as that recorded by Johnson (1972) of a two-year-old:

> Nolly, lolly, nolly, lolly, nilly, lolly, sillie, Billie, nolly, lolly . . .
> (quoted in Cazden, 1973, p. 606)

Much play involves motor movements. At first there is jumping and bouncing to which will later be added skipping and hopping. The practice of motor skills, which develop so rapidly during the early years, seems to dominate children's play and it is easy to speculate that such play allows children to develop muscular control and perhaps also to gain information about the world. Some would go further than this, saying that children's play allows them to achieve a sense of *mastery* and to realize that they are effective actors in the world.

Let's play pretend

Some time around the end of the first year, a particular form of play emerges which will last for at least five years. This is *symbolic* play which at first mainly involves using an object or person to represent something else. Either an object is transformed into something else (a bath towel becomes Batman's cape) or a person is transformed into someone else (the little girl becomes a shopkeeper). Fein (1975) has charted a developmental sequence in symbolic play which becomes increasingly complex between one and five years:

> At about 12 months of age, pretending involves a familiar and well-practised behaviour detached from its customary context: the child tilts his head back as he drinks out of an empty cup, or closes his eyes pretending to sleep without actually doing so. In these early forms, the materials are typically ordinary household objects, while the behaviours are notable because the child enacts eating or sleeping in the absence of any apparent desire for food or sleep. By 18 months of age, pretend play begins to acquire two new characteristics. First, the focus shifts from self to other: the child might pretend to feed his mother, a doll or a toy animal . . . Second, between 20 and 26 months, pretending becomes increasingly dependent on the features of the immediate situation: an inanimate object (doll or stick) might be treated as if it were animate, and a great many things might be treated as cups, spoons or beds . . . (Fein, 1975, p. 291)

Around three years of age, children begin to adopt *roles* in their symbolic play. Garvey (1977), from her observations of preschool children, describes how central are family roles in play:

> Of great importance were family roles. They usually came in pairs. One could generally predict, for example, that when a 'Mommy' appeared, she would instantly be joined by a 'Daddy' or 'Baby'. These roles were treated by the children as if they were always potentially

> available. They were 'there' and needed only to be matched to self or partner or be invoked to be effectively present. These were, of course, Mother, Father, Wife, Husband, Baby, Child (Daughter or Son), Brother, Sister, and much more rarely Grandfather and Grandmother; only one Uncle was mentioned. A parent, not specifically marked for sex, was sometimes enacted. To be included here is Pet, who was sometimes treated as a Child. The stuffed animals were usually drafted for this role. (Garvey, 1977, p. 90).

To be able to engage in such symbolic play children must have distinguished play from reality, the non-literal from the literal mode, to use Garvey's phrase. They must also have learned some general rules for interaction, such as turn-taking, and also some specific rules for behaviour in a particular context. Garvey (1972) gives an example of children's play in which one child has to remind the play partner about the rules of play:

> (*X*, preparing to speak on telephone addresses *Y*):
> *X*: Pretend you're sick.
> *Y*: OK.
> *X*: (Speaks into phone) Hey, Dr Wren, do you got any medicine?
> *Y*: Yes, I have some medicine.
> *X*: (to *Y*) No, you aren't the doctor, remember?
> *Y*: OK.
> *X*: (speaks into phone) I need some medicine for the kids. Bye. (turns to *Y*) He hasn't got any medicine.
> *Y*: No? Oh, dear.
> (Garvey, 1972, p. 578)

Eeny, meeny, miney, mo

During the preschool years, children derive hilarious pleasure from language play. Like symbolic play, such as doctors and nurses, playing with language seems to involve the recognition that there are rules that can be played around with. This kind of play is really an informal 'game with rules' preceding formal games like chess or football.

Language play may involve rhyming games, often turning senseless syllables: *trunk-munk-lunk*, or combining these into nonsense chants. Chukovsky, a Russian poet, collected many examples of language play. For example, rhymed monologues:

> Five-year-old Vova was the author of the following soliloquy:
> Is this a spoon?
> No—it's a balloon.
> Is this a fork?
> No—it's a stork.
> Is this a stove?
> No—it's a 'Vov'.
>
> And so on—for a long time. And this is what three-and-a-half-year-old Tania did with the word milk:
> Ilk, silk, tilk,

I eat kasha with milk.
Ilks, silks, tilks,
I eat kashas with milks.
(Chukovsky, 1963, 1968 ed., p. 63)

Such language play later progresses to jokes playing on the structure and meanings of words:

Q: What do you call a dark horse?
A: A night mare.

These types of symbolic and language play, while played 'just for fun', may also be helping children by preparing them for future combinations. For example, children's play with language such as their use of rhymes may help them, when they begin to read, to see how sounds are combined in words. Whether the play itself *helps* the learning process or whether such play is simply the outward expression of what has been learned is difficult to decide.

Play with rules

From about seven years, and reaching into adulthood, 'play with rules' emerges. There is much rule-governed play at younger ages but formal games like 'tag' or football seem later in occurring. Piaget claims that children cannot understand formal rules until they have reached the period of concrete operations. Before that, they 'play at' games by, for instance, kicking a football around a pitch, but they do not really understand the systematic properties of rules or their artificial nature. Many psychologists would disagree with Piaget, claiming that even babies join in rule-governed play such as peek-a-boo and must understand the basic rules. Given these reservations, it does seem that the amount of cooperation needed between groups of players about what is and what is not allowed in many formal games requires the abilities of a school-aged child.

Looking at the overall nature of the development of play, we can recognize a gradual shift from the context-embedded to the disembedded. Contrast the eleven-month-old child playing with a rattle with the eleven-year-old playing chess. In the former the motor activity *is* the play. (Piaget would say that the structure of sensorimotor thoughts is not different from the sensory-motor movements that it guides.) But in chess the motor movements are astoundingly simple compared with the cognitive structures that guide the movement of, say, the rook from one square to the next. Chess players consider the immediate past in their game, they think about several alternative moves, then evaluate the likely outcome of each. The essence of play has shifted from the act itself, embedded in the present, to an abstract bit of strategy that is carefully placed in a temporal sequence that includes realities as well as possibilities. The strategy of war has become ritualized and formalized in chess and herein lies the fun. Jerome Bruner has pointed out that every chess player knows that you can capture the opponent's queen by reaching across the table and putting it in your pocket! What makes it a game is the understanding on the part of both players that this would be the most boring way imaginable of 'winning' the match.

Although the developmental sketches describe the dominant forms of play seen during each age, remember that these are not the only ones, and that earlier forms continue through life. The dominant forms seem to be pretty much universal: one-year-olds of all nationalities are likely to play with pebbles (or their equivalent) and to jump and bounce; three-year-olds almost everywhere will play at mothers and fathers and most four and five-year-olds will play with their language and explore elaborate make-believe.

This apparent universality of play has prompted parents, teachers, philosophers and psychologists to attempt to explain why it occurs and what role it plays in development. Play is not, of course, just restricted to young humans. Play can be observed in many species, from the stickleback performing a play courtship dance when alone in a tank, to the rough-and-tumble play of baboons and children.

References

Cazden, C. (1973) *Play with language and meta-linguistic awareness*. In J.S. Bruner, A. Jolly, K. Sylva (eds) (1976), *Play: Its role in development and evolution*. Harmondsworth: Penguin Books.

Chukovsky, K. (1963, revised edition 1968) *From Two to Five*. Berkley, University of California Press (translated by Miriam Morton).

Fein, G. (1975) *A transformational analysis of pretending*. *Developmental Psychology*, 3, p. 291.

Garvey, C. (1972) *Some properties of social play*. In J.S. Bruner, A. Jolly, K. Sylva (eds) (1976), *Play: Its role in development and evolution*. Harmondsworth: Penguin Books.

Garvey, C. (1977) *Play*. London Fontana/Open Books.

Johnson, H.M. (1972) *Children in Nursery School*. New York: Agathon Press (first published 1928).

Newson J. and Newson E. (1979) *Toys and Playthings*. Harmondsworth: Penguin Books.

Wolfenstein, M. (1955) *Fun Morality: Analysis of Recent American Child-Training Literature*. In M. Mead and M. Wolfenstein (eds), *Childhood in Contemporary Cultures*. Chicago: University of Chicago Press.

9

Dimensions of Parent Behaviour*

P. MUSSEN *et al.*

All parents have an implicit or explicit ideal of what their children should be like—what knowledge, moral values, and behavioral standards they should acquire as they grow. Parents try many strategies designed to move the child toward that goal. They reinforce and punish the child, they use themselves as role models, they explain their beliefs and expectations, and they try to choose neighborhoods, peer groups, and schools that support their values and goals.

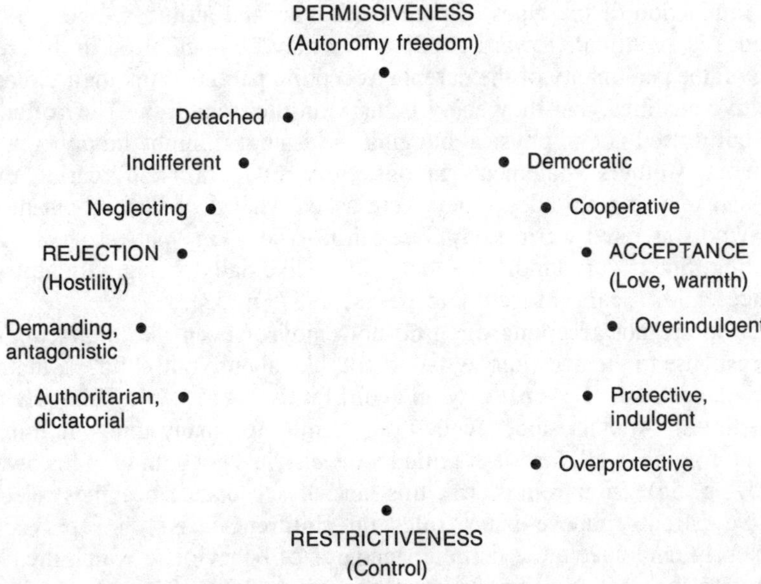

Figure 9.1 An illustration of the types of child rearing that can be described by classifying parents' behavior on acceptance-rejection (the horizontal axis) and restrictiveness-permissiveness (the vertical axis). The labeled points show where parents might fall on the two dimensions. For instance, a parent who is very restrictive and slightly rejecting is described as authoritarian, dictatorial. (Adapted from E.S. Schaefer. A circumplex model for maternal behavior.)

*This is an abridged version of a chapter in P. Mussen *et al.* (1984) *Child development and personality*, Harper and Row, New York, pp. 382–385.

The 'ideal child' varies from culture to culture, however. Most of the information we will discuss here applies to contemporary American culture because that is where data have been gathered. Some goals of socialization shared by many people in our culture are academic achievement, independence, control of aggression, and skill in social relationships with peers. Therefore, these become the focus of many investigations of socialization. Other cultures may value different socialization goals or endorse different family patterns.

Psychologists have studied parents' behavior with a variety of methods: direct observation, interviews with parents or with children, ratings by observers and questionnaires. When different methods produce similar results, we generally have more confidence in the conclusions than when only one method is used. Two dimensions describing important qualities of parenting emerge consistently from different methods: acceptance-rejection and restrictiveness-permissiveness.

In Figure 9.1 the dimensions of acceptance and restrictiveness are shown as they combine to form different patterns of parent behavior. The labels in each quadrant of the figure describe how a parent might behave when showing different combinations of acceptance and restrictiveness. For example, a parent who is both accepting and restrictive might be called protective and indulgent. A parent who is rejecting and restrictive might be labeled demanding and antagonistic. A permissive, rejecting parent could be considered indifferent, and a permissive, accepting parent might be described as democratic. The meanings of these rather abstract terms can best be garnered from a closer examination of the types of parent behavior and attitudes involved.

Acceptance is an attitude toward children that may be manifested in different ways depending on the personality of the parent. Accepting parents think their children have many positive qualities, and they enjoy being with their children. They often express affection, but it need not be physical hugging or kissing; it might simply be a smile or a proud look. Mothers' statements in one early study of child rearing exemplify accepting and rejecting attitudes. They were asked what they liked about their child. A mother who was rated warm said, 'Everything—how very patient she is, and how understanding. She is very kind.' Another said, 'I like Sally, being with her, she is an awfully nice child' (Sears, Maccoby & Levin, 1957, p. 53).

Parents who are not accepting often do not enjoy or even like their children very much. In response to the question 'What do you like about your child?' a mother rated low in acceptance said, 'He's naughty an awful lot, . . . but I enjoy him. He talks too much sometimes.' Another said, 'Well, I don't enjoy too many things in him because at the rate he's going, well, he doesn't mind too well; he's got a mind of his own' (Sears *et al.*, 1957, p. 55). In extreme form, this lack of acceptance becomes rejection.

Restrictive parents impose many rules on children, insist on supervising their children closely, and have quite definite standards of behavior to which their children are expected to conform, but they do not necessarily punish often or severely. In fact, a successful restrictive parent has a child who usually complies with rules and does not require frequent punishment. The kinds of rules and restrictions that parents impose depend, of course, on the age of the child. In the preschool years, parents make rules about noise, neatness, play on furniture, obedience, aggressive behavior, nudity, masturbation, and how far from home the child can go alone. Restrictive parents also make demands for mature behavior, good school performance, table manners, and cleanliness. As children get older, parents make rules about being informed where the child is, sexual and aggressive behavior, leisure activities, and friends. They demand good school performance, responsibility in carrying out household jobs, and self-control (Baumrind, 1973; Martin, 1975).

Although parents who are restrictive about one area, such as not hitting adults, also tend to be restrictive about other types of behavior, there are differences in what parents restrict. An example of restrictiveness about aggression appears in a mother's response to a question about what she does when her children get in a fight. 'I don't like to see them quarrel. There is no need for it. I don't let it get too bad. I just reprimand them right away' (Sears *et al.*, 1957, p. 242). The same mother may not be restrictive about children's table manners or about how far they can go from home without an adult.

At the other extreme are permissive parents. These parents generally have few rules and make few demands on their children. They do not emphasize learning table manners; they make relatively few demands for mature behavior; they do not restrict noise or play that might damage furniture and household objects; they are not concerned about neatness or obedience; they tend to view aggression, nudity, and masturbation as natural; and they allow their children considerable freedom to play without adult supervision or intervention. A parent rated permissive said she would intervene in a fight between her children 'if they're making a terrible amount of noise, or if they're going to do bodily harm to each other. And I don't mean slapping—that doesn't bother me. If one of them picks up a shovel or something, then I'd stop it. Otherwise, I have found that if I sit back and watch without their knowing it, they work it out themselves' (Sears *et al.*, 1957, p. 242).

Although many early studies included attempts to learn about the effects of acceptance or control as children, very few simple associations have been found between these global child-rearing dimensions and children's behaviour. Warmth or acceptance is important because it provides a background for parents' efforts to discipline their children and teach them values. In general, warm, accepting parents are more effective than others in transmitting their own values and goals to their children. Extreme rejection is often associated with problem behavior among children (Martin, 1975).

The effects of parental control or restrictiveness vary with the methods that parents use to enforce restrictions. Three broad categories of disciplinary techniques have been studied extensively: power assertion or coercion, inductive techniques such as explanations, and love withdrawal. *Power-assertive* discipline includes physical punishment, shouting, depriving the child of privileges, and using tangible rewards. In general, such techniques rely on the parent's control over things the child wants or on the parent's superior physical strength. *Inductive* techniques, by contrast, include reasoning, praise, and explaining the consequences of the child's actions for other people. Such techniques rely on the communication between the parent and child and on the child's ability to internalize and understand the basis for the parent's demands. *Love withdrawal* includes isolation, expressing disappointment, and shaming or ignoring the child. These techniques are based on the child's need for the parent's love and approval; they threaten the child with loss of love, at least temporarily.

The effects of these methods of discipline are complex for several reasons. First, efforts to discipline children are most effective when the child and parent have a warm, supportive relationship. Second, most parents use a combination of methods; families differ in how much they rely, for instance, on power assertion versus induction, but it is a rare family that does not use some of each. Third, the type of discipline used depends partly on the child's response to initial attempts. In general, parents use mild reprimands and explanations initially. If the child is unresponsive, they gradually escalate to more intense and power-assertive methods. Consider the following example.

> Deborah and Sharon are playing, and both want to ride the one available bicycle. Their mother tells Sharon, who is riding the bicycle, that she should take turns. Mother explains that it is fair to share the bicycle and that Deborah will feel bad if she does not get a turn (induction). If Sharon gives Deborah a turn, no further discipline is necessary. If Sharon does not give Deborah a turn, then Mother may repeat her instructions. If Sharon continues to ride the bicycle after Mother's inductive attempts, however, Mother will probably resort to power assertion by telling her to get off the bike, or else. If Sharon still refuses, Mother will probably punish her.

References

Baumrind, D. (1973) The development of instrumental competence through socialization. In D.A. Pick (Ed.), *Minnesota symposia on child psychology (Vol. 7)*, Minneapolis: University of Minnesota Press.

Martin, B. (1975) Parent–child relations. In F.D. Horowitz, E.M. Hetherington, S. Scarr-Salapatek and G.M. Siegel (Eds), *Review of child development research (Vol. 4)*. Chicago: University of Chicago Press.

Sears, R.R., Maccoby, E.E. & Levin H. (1957) *Patterns of child rearing*. New York: Harper and Row.

10

Different Family Systems*

P. MARES, A. HENLEY and C. BAXTER

> I just went to that—what do you call it—social welfare or something, but I don't want to go there again. It's a strange place. I get the feeling they don't want to see me. I had to wait a long time. Then they took me to this tiny room where an English officer—a boy young enough to be my son—spoke to me. I couldn't explain myself properly. I don't think he understood—you know us women, we have such different problems, our family ways, only our own people can understand.
>
> Asian woman
> (Amin 1977)

The way in which the Western nuclear family is organised and is developing is only one of many possible ways. It is the result of a multiplicity of interlinked factors: economic, historical, political, religious, climatic, cultural and so forth.

Although no two British families are completely alike, certain values are generally accepted, and certain assumptions form part of majority British cultural and social norms. These then define and influence the way that health and other services are organised in Britain, and the way that most health workers approach individuals and families. If such norms are not compared with other family systems during professional training, health workers' expectations of 'normal' family relationships may be based on very culture-specific values.

As a result families in Britain with different structures and different cultural norms and assumptions may find that health and other services are offered in such a way that they cannot use them or are alienated by them. The assessments that health workers make of minority group families and their needs, and the service they offer, may be wrong or irrelevant.

This does not only affect ethnic minority families. The barriers between professionals and clients from different classes in Britain have long been acknowledged, but those faced by people of minority cultures are often greater. Most professionals are sensitive to cultural differences between classes and recognise a responsibility to make professional practice appropriate to the lifestyle and needs of working-class families.

---

*This is an abridged version of a chapter in Mares, P., Henley, A. and Baxter, C. (1985) *Health Care in Multiracial Britain*, London, Health Education Council/National Extension College, pp. 80–93.

There has been less willingness to recognise the needs and rights of ethnic minority communities in this respect. Some people still feel that ethnic minority ('immigrant') communities must adapt to the services offered in Britain or do without. If the Health Service is to fulfil its intended role, that of enabling, supporting, caring for and helping, it must respond sensitively and positively to all its clients or patients as they are. The way services are organised must not cut out, intentionally or unintentionally, families and individuals who do not present themselves in a predefined way because their way of life is different from the majority norm. Health workers must *work with* families of different kinds, making use of their strengths and taking care not to ignore or undercut a family's chosen way of doing things. They must *work with* individuals, respecting the priorities and values they live by, not imposing additional pressures of rejection and ignorance. For most people their family provides a vital and lifelong source of support and security. This must be sustained, not undermined.

Working within other family systems

Each of us has a personal set of beliefs about families and the way they should be: about, for example, the size and shape of a 'normal' family, the emotional relationships it should contain, and the kind of support our family can be expected to give; the rights and responsibilities of different family members; how much independence and freedom of action family members normally have, and how much they must abide by other people's decisions.

We are not always aware of our own beliefs until we encounter people whose family systems and values differ sharply from our own. We tend to regard our own values as universal and to expect other people to see things in roughly the same way. There is however a danger that we will regard other systems as deviant rather than just different, or as flawed versions of our own system rather than as independent systems with their own internal logic. There is a danger that we will see them as problems, and work against or despite them rather than with them.

Because our views are to a large extent defined for each of us by the culture and society in which we grow up it is difficult or impossible to detach ourselves from them.

- What are your own beliefs about families and how they should be? What kind of family did you grow up in?
- What do you think a family is for?
- What does it consist of? How many people?
- How many people do you define as your immediate family? What kinds of relatives do you include? How many people in your family do you feel a responsibility for?
- Is there a chain of authority within your family? How important and firm is it?
- Who has authority over whom in your family? Until what age? Why? How far does anyone have the right to enforce their authority?
- Does anyone have ultimate authority over you?

- Which is the most important relationship in a family? Husband and wife? Parent and child? Brother and sister?
- At what age do you think a young person should be independent of his or her family? What do you mean by 'independent'? In what decisions should older family members still be allowed to have a say?
- How important is your family's reputation to you? What would harm it? Do you avoid doing certain things to protect its reputation?
- How close would you want to live to your parents?
- When you are old do you expect to live with your children? With other relatives? Alone at home? With other people of your age? Or go into an old people's home?

The family is the unit through which values and priorities are learnt and handed down and through which we learn most of our deeply felt ideas about our roles and duties in life. People brought up in different family systems are therefore likely to have very different expectations of acceptable family behaviour, and different values and priorities. For instance, it is not true that 'a mother is a mother all over the world'. Mothers in different cultures have different roles and practical responsibilities and different ideas about what makes a 'good' mother, what are desirable motherly qualities and behaviour, and what a mother's duties are.

To work effectively, therefore, in a multi-cultural society, we first have to be aware of and analyse our own preconceptions and deeply held cultural beliefs about how families and individuals should behave. It is important that we do not impose them inappropriately on other people who believe in and live their lives according to a different system.

Views about the relationships between families and individuals are bound to vary between communities. There may be some striking differences between the expectations of minority communities in Britain and those of the majority.

- **The centre of the family** may be the mother; the grandmother; the biological parents; the grandparents; or the wider extended family.
- **Family members and the family unit may be far more important** in people's lives.
- **People may have far greater family responsibilities**: their priorities and values may be closely tried up with those of their family. Decisions may be made by the whole family rather than by individuals. The welfare of one member may be seen as dependent on the welfare of the whole family and all its members.
- **There may be a formal hierarchy of responsibilities and authority**. It may be the duty and responsibility of older family members to make all major and many minor decisions. If older family members are living elsewhere they may still be referred to for most important decisions, many of which might be considered entirely personal and individual in British cultures.

> Even though my parents are back in Pakistan we always ask them and discuss it with them if we are going to take any big step, or about the children. Like when we bought this house, or even, you know, about my daughter's school. If it's any big decision, anything big, we'd always ask them. The only problem is, so far away you know, it takes a long time, and also it's difficult to discuss it properly in letters.
>
> Muslim man

- **People may consider themselves to be a part of a large family network all their lives**. Marriage, for example, may not necessarily mean the setting up of a new and independent unit, in which a young couple moves finally out and away from the authority of their own parents. A married couple may remain physically and emotionally very much part of the extended family unit. They may still regard older family members as having ultimate responsibility for decisions affecting their welfare.
- **Individual freedom or self-interest may not be a goal to be aimed for**. Individualism may be seen as undesirable, or selfish, as a sign of coldness and lack of proper human feeling. Children may not be brought up to see individualism as a desirable goal; they may grow up with the view that self-interest and self-reliance at the expense of caring about the family are not moral virtues. Adults may not see their interests as autonomous or independent from the family's interests. In many families nobody is 'independent', everyone has a responsibility towards other family members; everyone always has the right to look to older members for emotional and physical support; everyone always has the duty to give emotional and physical support to anyone who is younger or in need. Obligations to other family members may be expected to override personal self-interest.

> You bring up your children. We live with ours.
>
> Asian mother

- **The family unit may be large**. It may contain three or four generations and several adult married couples. Children may be brought up by all the adults together, and particularly by the elderly women. They may regard all the adult members of their family as parents. Older family members may have final authority over them rather than their biological parents.

> 'I have many mothers,' said a Ghanaian doctor during a discussion on family relationships, crystallising in a few words the difference between the western style, closed, nuclear family, where the concentration of relationships is between husband, wife and children, and the far more open, traditional, extended family, still the norm in West Africa in spite of inevitable changes resulting from the pressures of modern urban living and the impact of western technology.
>
> (Ellis 1978)

Within the same generation of adults there may be a clearly defined structure of family responsibilities. Older brothers and their wives may have responsibility for younger brothers and their wives and children. Men may have responsibility for women. Respect for the advice and authority of older adults or of men within the family may be very important. Older children may have authority over and expect respect from younger brothers, sisters and cousins.

Even when the family is split up into nuclear units, close bonds of support, love and responsibility may be maintained between the units. In some families it is a normal alternative for children to be brought up by other relatives, uncles and aunts, or by grandparents instead of by their parents.

> A very basic illustration of the kind of misunderstanding that arises can be seen if one looks at the concept of fostering. Although the same term is used in Britain and West Africa, the meanings ascribed to it are very different. In our society, fostering is resorted to reluctantly when there is some kind of breakdown in the normal family arrangements—it is definitely second best. In West Africa, it is a normal part of extended family life; relationships with wider family members are very important and children may move around a great deal during childhood. Fostering is usually kin-fostering but children also go to stay with friends, perhaps so that their education can be furthered. West Africans come to Britain thinking of fostering as a perfectly usual and acceptable practice. They often do not realise that being fostered in a British nuclear family represents a very different set of experiences for the child than being fostered at home in West Africa and that it can have profoundly different consequences for that child's development.
>
> (Ellis 1981)

- **The roles and ambitions of men and women may be the same or may be very different**. Men and women within a family may have different responsibilities and areas of authority. They may have different and separate spheres of interest and influence.

  In some communities the women may take most of the responsibility for children and bring them up alone. They may value and take pride in their own strength and independence and turn mainly to their own mothers and to other women for support and companionship.

  In some communities men may be responsible for taking decisions; women may not be expected to act on their own, but to seek consent from an appropriate male relative first.
- **The honour and reputation of the family may be a major concern of all its members**. If one member gets a reputation for, for example, meanness, ill temper, bad behaviour, promiscuity, or criminal behaviour, this may affect the reputation of the whole family and the lives and futures of all its members. The family may be very concerned to prevent one member from ruining the lives of all the others. Restricting the self-interest of one individual may seem a small price to pay in overall terms.
- **The maintenance and support of the family may be seen as everybody's most important duty**. The family may be seen as the permanent source of all the love, support, companionship and happiness that anyone will need and as the centre and focus of each person's life.

> At home the family structure is different. You have got mother and father, who maybe have got their mother and father. Grandparents take an interest in the children, and you would no more think of cheeking your grandmother than flying in the air. Here it is totally different, because your family is scattered further apart. The family

> involvement in the West Indies is totally different from family involvement here.
>
> Afro-Caribbean woman
> (Cooper 1977)

- **The position of elderly family members varies a good deal**. In some families old people are the most important people and also the centre of power and authority; in others their needs and wishes are subordinate to those of younger members; they may be given care and attention but have little authority. Some elderly people expect to live with their families and be supported by them; others wish to retain their independence as long as they can.

> There is a widely accepted myth that the Asians in this country are able to care for their old as well as their young under one roof because of the extended family system. This may have been the case elsewhere but here the immigrant Asian population is frequently faced with housing problems and other economic structures which make it impossible for children to shoulder their traditional responsibilities towards their parents.
>
> (Asian Community Action Group 1980)

- **All parents very much want their children to marry someone with whom they will be as happy as possible**. The degree of overt or covert influence and control that parents may exert may vary a good deal. In some communities marriage may be seen as a permanent bond between two families rather than two individuals; it is felt to be essential that the experience of older, wiser members of the family is brought to bear in choosing a suitable partner; in some communities marriage may be seen as an intensely personal exclusive union between two people. In some communities marriage may not be particularly important, or may be a step taken fairly late in life to confirm and celebrate an existing relationship.

How do possible differences like these affect the health worker? Check that you are working with the grain of people's lives and values and not against it.

Your effectiveness as a health worker will be badly flawed if you are imposing views or values on your client that he does not share or agree with. Where you are not sure that you and your patient or client are thinking along the same lines it may be necessary to check by asking an explicit question.

Ethnic minority clients are the most direct source of information, but a source that is usually neglected. Ask people about their wishes and values and experiences. If there are problems to be sorted out, find out how they see them and what solutions they would suggest. Provided that people feel you are genuinely interested and that you respect and will value their wishes, opinions and feelings, they are generally glad to discuss their views with you.

Possible conflicts between client needs and professional practice

- The higher proportion of **single-parent families** and families where parents are not married in the Afro-Caribbean community has its basis in the destruction of the African family system in the West Indies by white slave-owners during the period of slavery, and in the economic problems of the colonial period after the abolition of slavery. The brutal relationships imposed by slave-owners upon their slaves are described in this extract by Dilip Hiro:

> Under slavery, marriage was meaningless because the 'husband' could not protect his 'wife' from the sexual demands of other men. Any attempt to protect his 'wife' from being ravished by the white master meant stiff punishment. By law, the slave had no rights; nor could a free man plead for him. Subject women were the exclusive 'property' of the master for whom they performed three major functions: labour; the breeding of slaves; and his sexual gratification.
>
> There was a popular notion among the masters that a slave woman would breed more and better if she were mated with different men. The male slave's function, therefore, began and ended with being a sexual inseminator. As the slave children too were the master's property and could be separated from their mothers at his whim, there was no such thing as a 'slave family'. The end-result was the total destruction of the conventional family system.
>
> (Hiro 1973)

After slavery ended many men were forced to go overseas to find work; either to other Caribbean islands or to Panama and North America. In a situation where men were unable to get work, women and girls could not afford to rely on men for their security. In most Afro-Caribbean families, therefore, girls are traditionally brought up to be self-sufficient and independent.

> In a white man's world black women have it easier than black men. In white capitalist Britain the black man is still at the lower end of the social scale. He is more likely to be unemployed, more likely to be in low-paid work or shift work. White employers often see black men as a physical threat, aggressive, violent, etc. They won't employ them. So black women often find it easier to get work and to support themselves. In a way the slavery and neocolonial patterns are being re-enacted in Britain, with the same effects on relationships and on how men and women see their roles and opportunities.
>
> Afro-Caribbean health worker

Marriage in West Indian society is generally highly respected as a serious responsible step and the confirmation of a lifelong association. As in traditional British culture, a husband is considered responsible for the support of his wife and children. Marriage may therefore be entered into only when the couple know each other thoroughly and often only after they have lived together for several years. They may already have children. Marriage is also traditionally a large and expensive celebration and is therefore a major expense for which a couple may save for several years.

As in British society, class also influences people's view on this issue. Middle-class Afro-Caribbean couples may be more likely to share the values of white British middle-class couples with regard to marriage and children born outside marriage.

Like an increasing number of white British couples, most Afro-Caribbean couples who live together have a stable relationship and are married in all but name. They accept shared responsibility for children. Within some sections of the Afro-Caribbean community the social stigma and reputation for instability, traditionally attached by white British society to cohabiting couples with children, generally do not apply.

Young people of Afro-Caribbean origin in Britain will obviously be influenced by the values of both their parents and the West Indies, and by those of majority British society. In Britain the proportion of young Afro-Caribbean men and women who get married is increasing and is higher than in the West Indies. Nevertheless girls are still generally regarded as self-sufficient and responsible for their own actions. If an unmarried girl has a child she will expect and be expected to take some responsibility for supporting and looking after the child herself. She will also, in most cases, receive help and support from her own parents and from the father of the child.

Bringing up children

> There are few explicitly stated concepts about children or principles of childrearing which would be agreed to by most people in this country.
>
> (Pringle and Naidoo 1979)

> Beliefs about childrearing are usually bound up with beliefs about life itself. They are culturally transmitted and culturally learned. They are held without question.
>
> (Ellis 1978)

Ways of bringing up children, and the values that parents try to instil in them, will depend on the parents' own upbringing, their values, and the circumstances in which they live. What is meant by a 'good child' varies from culture to culture and from class to class.

Socio-economic factors

Culture is of course partly the product of economic and other circumstances. In white middle-class families, for example, with a fair amount of living space and money for books and toys, a 'good' child may be energetic, enquiring, active, voluble and outgoing. In low-income white working-class families living in smaller, noisier accommodation with little space and parents under stress, a 'good' child may be the quiet one in the corner who causes no trouble and is hardly noticed. Economic circumstances, housing and environment all have a major influence on culture, and affect the way that children are brought up as much as they affect the lives and values of the whole family.

For some ethnic minority families the constraints of an unfamiliar industrial inner-city environment and poor housing may seriously restrict their ability to bring up their children as they would wish.

The kind of open-air rural childhood they may have had, for example, is no longer possible, and their children may miss out on the space and natural playthings that they took for granted.

> Over there we'd leave all the doors open and our friends would just walk in and out as they wanted. But here in England people keep their doors shut all the time.
>
> The one thing we really miss here is the space. Just the other day I was saying to the children, 'Are you going to pull the house apart?' They don't have enough room to play about. We children used to spend most of our time outside.
>
> Afro-Caribbean woman
> (Crossfield Family 1978)

Parents may be afraid to let their children play outside in concrete areas littered with glass and dirt, or on streets where cars rush past. They may worry that their children will be harassed by young white racists. Racial harassment has been suggested as a contributory factor to rickets in young Asian children; their mothers are afraid to let them play outside in the sun.

For families where children and childcare are usually shared between several adults the loss of the extended family may cause real difficulties for a mother on her own. A young first-time mother may never have expected to have to cope with a baby or a toddler alone. She may have grown up knowing that her own mother, her mother-in-law or her sisters-in-law would look after it and that when there were problems she would be able to turn to them for help and support. Without family support in Britain she may be isolated and desperate, unaccustomed to looking outside the family for help and support, possibly cut off by language from health workers and other caring professionals, and with small children totally dependent on her.

Although the options open to parents will often have been drastically reduced by their economic circumstances in Britain, each family will still try to bring up its children according to its own beliefs and values. Families from different cultures may therefore differ a good deal in what they consider desirable and right. This places a responsibility on health workers, whose role is primarily to support and help families in the way they wish to bring up their children and organise their lives.

The health worker's influence

Ethnic minority mothers in Britain are often aware that some health workers disapprove of and disagree with their ways of bringing up their children. This may affect their confidence in themselves as capable mothers. Any mother will welcome discussion about her family and her children, but this must be in the context of support of her own views and wishes. Families have the right to bring up their children in the way they know best. A confident relaxed mother will produce confident relaxed children.

A worried, distressed mother, aware that 'the authorities' disapprove of her as a mother, will too often pass her tensions and worries on to her children.

> It's funny you know. Because you know they are watching you all the time, they don't really trust the way you are looking after your kids, you start to get really worried yourself. You start to think, well, maybe they're right to be worried, maybe our way of bringing up kids is wrong, maybe I *am* a no-good mother. It's funny what it does to you.
>
> Middle-aged Afro-Caribbean mother

For many families the intervention of the state and its institutions in intimate family matters, such as the bringing up of children, is threatening. What role does each of the caring professionals who visit their home have? How far are they friends and confidantes? How far are they an arm of the law? On what criteria is the family being judged? Visiting health workers and other 'officials' may need to give a clear explanation of their role and functions. They will certainly need to work at developing a relationship of mutual trust, and to show mothers very clearly that their judgement and childrearing methods are supported and respected, not judged as deficient or inferior.

Racism and bringing up black children in Britain

Children pick up the attitudes of the society in which they grow up. Research in Britain and in America has shown that children distinguish racial groups from an early age (two or three years old) and within the next four or five years have learnt the racial values of the society in which they are growing up. In Britain this means that black children often pick up negative white attitudes towards black people, such as the prejudiced belief that whites are 'intellectually superior', 'more civilised' or 'cleaner'.

Children find it very difficult to identify with a socially rejected group. Some black children have been shown to exhibit a strong preference for the dominant white group, and a tendency to devalue their own group. There is well documented experimental evidence of black children rejecting black dolls because they are 'ugly' or 'bad'; and of choosing a white rather than a black doll when asked which doll looked most like them. There are cases of black children trying to bleach or scrub themselves white because again they wish to reject their black skin and identity.

These attitudes are likely to be reinforced as children get older, by the messages they receive in the media, by racist gibes at school or in the street, by negative or embarrassed references to their parents, origin, culture and backgrounds in the classroom.

> I had a discussion with a small group of Gujarati women about the problems they were having with their teenage children. Much of what the women said showed how their children had picked up the negative attitudes of white society towards them and their community. For example, some of the children were embarrassed and refused to go shopping with their mothers because their mothers did not speak very good English; there was a girl who kept forgetting the lunch her mother prepared for her to take to school because it was Indian food

> and who finally lied to her mother that she was not allowed to take food to school; there were children of 14 and 15 refusing to bring their English friends to their homes but going often to their English friends' houses; there were Asian girls in home economics classes who told their teacher that they never ate Asian food at home; and children who brought English friends home but behaved very strangely and only spoke English while their friends were there, pretending not to understand a word of Gujarati.
>
> Asian community worker

To counteract this, black families and communities are increasingly making moves to reassert their own identity. There are, for example, a growing number of groups set up to teach and maintain aspects of minority group culture, such as black dance and music groups and cultural workshops; there has been, in the past few years, an increase in Afro-Caribbean and Asian youth clubs and schemes, and black women's groups. Young people are also demonstrating their sense of pride and identity in their dress; Sikh boys grow their hair and wear turbans; Afro-Caribbean women wear plaited African hairstyles and African-style jewellery and clothes; young men wear red, gold and green Rasta tams and dreadlocks; Jewish men re-adopt the yamulka. Young British-born Afro-Caribbeans have evolved a dialect of their own that combines elements of the patois of the West Indies with local English dialects.

Many black children have a strong sense of self-esteem and pride in themselves, their families, and their blackness. But some go through a period of rejection and dislike of themselves, their parents and anything that reminds them that they are not part of the dominant and 'superior' white group.

One thing is sure, that race and colour are never *not* issues for black children. As soon as children learn to distinguish colour and to identify themselves as part of a particular racial group, they begin to receive messages about the relative worth of their own and other groups. The messages conveyed, consciously or unconsciously, by authority figures such as health workers in their relationship with a child or its parents form a crucial part of the child's learning process and of his or her way of seeing and approaching the world.

Health workers need to be aware of the attitudes and values they communicate, consciously or unconsciously, towards black people and minority group cultures. No one is ever *not* communicating.

Race, and the experience of racism, should be acknowledged and discussed whenever appropriate. Racism is a central feature of the life of most black people in Britain. To ignore or choose to deny the existence of racism may give the impression of condoning it.

References

Amin, G. (1977) *Some Aspects of Social Policy Affecting Asian Women in Britain*, unpublished paper.

Ellis, J. (ed) (1978) *West African Families in Britain*. Routledge.

Ellis, J. (1981) *Foster Kids in the Culture Gap*. In Cheetham *et al.* (eds), *Social and Community Work in a Multi-Racial Society*. Harper and Row.

Cooper, J.M. (1977) *Elderly West Indians in Leicester*. Unpublished dissertation for M.A. in Social Service Planning, Department of Sociology, University of Essex.

Asian Community Action Group (1980) *Asians Sheltered Residential Accommodation*. Quoted in Glendenning (ed), *The Ethnic Elderly: Cause for Concern*. Unit 16:3 Ethnic Minorities and Social Community Work, E354, Open University, 1982.

Hiro, D. (1973) *Black British, White British*. Penguin.

Pringle, M.K. and Naidoo, S. (1979) *Early Child Care in Britain*. Gordon and Breach.

Crossfield Family (1978) *Seven of Us*. A and C Black.

11

The Effects of Working on Child Health

MARGARET BAMFORD

Children's health and well-being can be seriously affected by the work that their parents do, as much as by their parents being unemployed. This paper addresses the effects of employment. There are approximately 3 million people unemployed in the UK; the effects of this deprivation are more well documented than the effects of work (Townsend and Davidson, 1988; Whitehouse, 1988).

There are 12 million people in employment in the UK, doing a range of jobs which potentially can have an effect on the whole family, especially children.

Reproductive health

The effects of work on health can begin even before conception. Some substances are known to be both teratogenic, that is having an effect on the foetus, and mutagenic, that is having the ability to alter the genetic material of a cell; this alteration can affect subsequent generations of cells. Substances which are thought to be teratogenic are: cadmium, lead, mercury, organic solvents, carbon monoxide, anaesthetic gases, oestrogenic compounds, ionising radiation and carbon disulphide. Substances which are also mutagenic include: chloroplene, perchloroethylene and vinyl chloride, which are halogenated hydrocarbons, anaesthetic gases, some pesticides, ionising radiation and ethylene oxide. So in some occupations it is important that people receive preconceptual advice and counselling. It is important to remember that men and women can be equally affected by these substances. Therefore, people who are working in operating theatres or recovery rooms may need to think about the work they do if they are thinking of starting their family.

Work patterns

Changing work patterns can have an effect on children's health. More young mothers are returning to work following the birth of their children. This does not necessarily mean that children are neglected, but it could mean that mothers have many roles to fill. This could be not only as a wife and mother, but having to fit in with the people at work, who, during her absence, have developed new relationships, have moved on, or may now have new procedures and techniques. This can be a particularly challenging time and a time where confusion and anxiety are evident. This could mean that additional demands are made on health workers, because in some cases children's health concerns are not acknowledged and help sought.

In some families, where the father works shifts, difficulties can occur. It is very difficult to keep children quiet during the day, so that people who are working at night can get their rest and sleep. If there is more than one child then this is even more difficult. There is also the issue in some families that the meals are prepared to suit the major wage earner, this could result in children having to wait long periods between meals or eating inappropriate food, but at the right times. The effects of shift work on an individual's health have been studied insofar as they affect the person (Harrington, 1978; Tasto, 1978; Harma, 1992), but the effects of shift working on families have not been a major research concern.

There is a continuing move in industry and commerce to get maximum return on investment; this has resulted in greater demands being made on people at work, including working longer hours. In some occupations this is extended by 'on call' arrangements. Some people would be described as 'workaholics', always working. These people make a choice; difficulties occur when the demands of work are imposed on family life. Both parents may not be there to share in bringing up the children, or, if they are there, they are too tired to participate fully. This can create tension in relationships and stress in the family. Working long hours can bring financial rewards to the family; however, it *may* only bring the bare necessities, depending on the work done and the wage paid for that work.

Hazards of work

Hazards of work can be categorised into: chemical, physical, mechanical, biological and psychosocial (WHO, 1975). Mention has already been made of some chemical substances which can have an effect on the unborn child, and we have briefly explored some psychosocial aspects of work, such as work patterns.

Chemical substances can be in the form of dusts, gases, vapours, liquids or mists, which are fine particles in the air. Children at home could possibly come into contact with chemicals from the workplace if their parents bring those substances home. An example of this could be if a person at work, in contact with lead, did not go through a proper hygiene routine on finishing work and brought lead dust home on protective clothing, inside shoes or in trouser turn-ups. This dust then transfers to the home floor coverings, and children playing on the floor could become contaminated. This is not a common occurrence, just an illustration of a possible source of contamination.

Physical hazards in the workplace have in many instances been reduced by mechanisation and technology. However, in some instances this mechanisation has created other problems. A fairly common condition occurring in relation to work is repetitive strain injury. This is caused, as its title implies, from repeated strain on some joint or muscle group. It can result in back pain or wrist pain; an old description which most people will be familiar with is housemaid's knee. The condition, when it occurs, is painful and disabling. It could result in some permanent handicap which could prevent parents from taking the full responsibility in caring for their children, such as the inability to lift children, or the inability to cuddle or hold a child of any weight. Also, if the parent is in constant pain, then that can affect their equilibrium and their ability to cope with 'normal' childhood behaviours and play.

Examples of mechanical and biological hazards can be illustrated by thinking of children who live on farms, and the dreadful burden that is placed on families when accidents occur to children in these settings. This is home and workplace combined, and this can sometimes lead to complacency. The regulations governing activities of children in the workplace are very strict, and particular guidance is given on children and agriculture, but accidents continue to happen. For a long time child fatalities in agriculture have been a cause for concern. In 1972 the then Chief Agricultural Inspector made reference to the issue in his annual report, stressing the responsibility that adults had to look after children in this hazardous environment. In 1986 the Health and Safety Executive published a report highlighting fatal accidents in agriculture (HSE, 1986). That report identified 38 children under the age of 16 who were killed during the years 1981–1984: 17 children were playing; 12 children were working or helping an adult, or merely watching an adult at work; five children were passengers on machinery; and four children were horse riding or partaking in other recreational activities.

In many incidents, lack of adult supervision was identified as being the main cause of the accident (HSE, 1986, p. 33).

These figures do not identify children who received other injuries which may have caused permanent handicap or disability.

It is important that health professionals caring for children take a wider view of children's lives, look at the factors impinging on the family, and the possible consequences for the child. Family care can only be offered if all aspects of the family's life and activities are considered. This consideration will need to be reflected in the care and support offered to individual families and the children of those families.

References

Harma, M. (1992) 'The hard day's night for shift workers', *Work Health Safety*, Finland, Institute of Occupational Health.

Harrington, J.M. (1978) *Shift Work and Health: A Critical Review of the Literature*. London, HMSO.

HSE (1986) *Agricultural Black Spot. A Study of Fatal Accidents*. London, HMSO.

Tatso, D.L., *et al*. (1978) *Health Consequences of Shift Work*. CA, Stanford Research Institute.

Townsend, P. and Davidson, N. (1988) 'The Black Report', in *Inequalities in Health*. London, Penguin Books.

Whitehead, M. (1988) 'The Health Divide', in *Inequalities in Health*. London, Penguin Books.

WHO (1975) *Environmental and Health Monitoring in Occupational Health*. Technical Report No. 535, WHO, Geneva.

12

Children's Stories

BOB MOLONEY

Children's perceptions of illness and hospital

It is a generally accepted view that children's knowledge and understanding of health, illness and disease changes with age. As part of the process of cognitive development, children's ideas become more accurate and sophisticated as they progress through the various stages of intellectual maturation, as described by Piaget. For example it is argued that children under 7 years of age often believe that illnesses are a punishment for something that they have done wrong. In the age group 7 to 11 years children are said to focus on contagious processes to explain disease, while older children are likely to explain illness in physiological terms.

This view is beginning to be challenged. Christine Eiser (1990) pointed out that research concerned with children's understanding of disease has become entrenched in a stages model of development. This has happened despite the growing criticism of stages models and the fact that there is less empirical evidence for stage bound behaviour than was previously thought.

One of the effects of the Children Act (1989) has been to encourage health care workers to take more notice of what children are saying about their experiences, feelings and understanding of the world around them. It seems appropriate then that we should be focusing some of our research effort on documenting the views of children on questions related to their perception of illness and hospitals. In so doing we can begin to move beyond the stages approach when dealing with children's anxieties, to more sophisticated, individual and effective communication strategies. Those who have conducted this type of research point to the enormously variable ability of children in any particular age group to understand illness and treatment. Critically important is the belief of these researchers that children's level of understanding of these concepts is determined as much by their personal experience as by maturational process (Eiser, 1990).

Kim Ford (unpublished report, 1991) surveyed 72 children aged 5–10 years, asking them a number of questions about their perceptions of illness and hospital. Her work with children in hospitals over a period of several years prompted her to make these observations of children's reaction to hospital admission:

> A child of three could approach the experience with the same confidence as a child of thirteen and similarly a child of thirteen could be

> as distraught and frightened as a child of three. Their reactions appeared to be dependent, not on age, but on the child's experiences and expectations of hospital.

The children in her study, when asked why people go to hospital, gave 25 different plausible reasons, including this from a boy aged 6 years with no personal experience of hospital:

> Some people they got stomach ache. Some people are bad, some have broken bones and have bandages taken off. Some people have an accident when you cut your arm or leg you have to go to hospital.

And from a girl aged 7 years who had asthma, 'People go to hospital, cos they're ill, my friend had to go to hospital cos she had asthma, like me.' Others made these comments: 10-year old, 'When somebody's got appendicitis or they're got something wrong with their kidneys'; 6-year old, 'When you've burst your eardrum'; 10-year old, 'If they've broken a bone they might need X-rays'; 10-year old, 'To have babies'; 10-year old, 'If they're dying they have to rush them to hospital.'

Eiser (1991) concurs with this impression that children have well ordered ideas about why someone might require hospital treatment. This information is clearly not all derived from personal experience, with books, TV and friends' experiences providing a rich source of data.

Asked what happens in hospitals, a wide range of ideas emerged. Generally those without experience had a more negative image of hospital than those who had first hand knowledge. Some of the descriptions were probably taken from television dramas, such as this graphic sentence (by a 7-year old) which probably represents the trace of a cardiac monitor: 'They sometimes put a breathing thing on you and if its a triangle it means you're alright and if its a line that means you could die!'

A 10-year old boy remembers in some detail his visit to a casualty department, emphasising the excessive waiting for things to happen:

> When I went to hospital I split my head open on a council plant pot. When I got to the hospital they put me in a room with all curtains round it and I had to wait for about an hour. They took me out and they were gonna X-ray me, I was waiting there for ages but then they X-rayed me. A doctor came out and asked me some questions and he done reflexes on my ankles and knees and then . . . he went away and I waited a long while . . . .

Some of those with personal experiences were unclear about what had happened to them, such as this 7-year old: 'When I went to the hospital my legs were kinda, they were the wrong way round. They got a hammer and pushed it on my leg and it hurted so I started to cry.'

This lucid account was given by a 10-year old of her experiences of a tonsillectomy; interestingly she offers an unusual description of the nurse providing postoperative care, possibly because it was a man rather than an expected female.

> I used to suffer from this . . . umm . . . throat infection and I went to the Doctor's and has to keep on going for check ups and one time

> it really was bad and I stayed in there for a few days and the next day this lady came and said I had to go to this room on my bed, this big room on my bed. So the doctors took me up to this big room and lie on this other and I was really scared at what was going to happen to make a butterfly stitch in my hand and what happened is I just went to sleep. Then they just took out by tonsils, then I went back to where I was before. I woke up and I was being really ill and sick and everytime the kitchenman had to change me and everytime they changed me I was sick again and again.

Injections were often mentioned and represented one of the most unpleasant memories of all; a 5-year old girl recalls her frightening experience: 'I went to hoskible cos I broke my arm. I had injections, it was horrible, I had all needles coming out, one there, one there (points to hand), now they've gone.'

Loneliness and separation from family featured high amongst children's fears if they were to be admitted to hospital: 7-year old, 'You miss your family sometimes when they are not there to kiss you, you miss you family'; 10-year old, 'I'd be scared cos I'd never been in hospital and I'd be scared that no-one would talk to me, I'd be all alone.'

Others anticipated making friends and thoroughly enjoying themselves: 7-year old 'I would like it cos if there were some boys and girls there I could make friends and play with the toys there!'

Descriptions of what is an operation provided a marvellous mixture of personal experiences, television images, and pure invention: 7-year old, 'An operation means that you got in this special room and then they take . . . split your back up to see whats inside so if you've got rubbish in there, like tissues, they take it out and sew it back up'; 8-year old, 'I haven't really had one but I think I would be really, really scared'; 9-year old, 'I think it's horrible because what they do they get this blade thing, put a little mark on you and start cutting up; cos on telly I saw this lady having an operation on her nose. They got this hammer, they took this bone out and the nose went flat and all this blood was leaking out, it was so horrible it made me sick'; 10-year old, 'Like if you've got a bad eye or something they might take out your eye and operate on it and if its better they might exchange it for a better eye!'

In these accounts many children thought that having an injection was an 'operation', perhaps indicating how serious they regarded any invasive treatment. Kim Ford noted that a large proportion of children in her study had watched television programmes about hospitals designed for adult viewers so that, instead of giving them better understanding, the images had merely provided fuel for their fertile imaginations. Increasing children's knowledge in this unstructured way may be counterproductive and give rise to unnecessary anxieties and stress when illness or hospital admission is experienced.

In relation to those with chronic illness Christine Eiser (1991) believes that increasing children's knowledge is not necessarily a good thing and that making children more knowledgeable about their illness must be supported by a readiness to intervene and to deal with the social and emotional consequences of the knowledge.

In addition to a strange environment, painful procedures and unknown events, children face a barrage of strangers in a variety of uniforms. Of these, nurses and doctors have apparently ambiguous roles in 'making them better' but perhaps inflicting pain and discomfort on them. Kim Ford asked the children in her study what the role of those two groups of health workers was.

A third of the children had a negative view of the nurse's role, often related to the giving of injections: girl aged 9, 'They give you injections to help you get better'; girl aged 7, 'They put needles in your baby through the belly button'; boy aged 7, 'They have to put a breathing thing on, they have to put a tube on their mouth if they've got asthma or they've been drowned and they have to breath out in this machine'; girl 10 years, 'They make people happy and help each other and make them feel glad and not be miserable from their injuries that they have'; girl 7 years, 'They check the little boards at the end of the bed'; boy 10 years, 'Sometimes if someone has just had a baby they go out to see how the baby is'; girl 10 years, 'If you want to go to the playroom and you can't walk properly they help you'.

Generally the children had an accurate picture of the nurse's ambiguous role as carer and sometimes inflictor of pain. They view doctors in quite different ways. Many were uncertain what their role was and saw them as unhelpful in some instances: boy aged 8 years, 'They call you into a room and tell you to come back tomorrow or the next day'; boy aged 9 years; 'They're a little bit rough 'cos you know when they have injections they don't take no time, they just dig it in; that what they did to me'; boy 10 years, 'They walk around and have little clipboards and papers'; girl 9 years, 'They have this telescope and when they put it to your cheek, right, or your tummy, it feels cold and you feel ticklish. When you laugh and they start laughing too and they are kind to you'.

Denise Jago (1987) describes a 9-year old's experience of a ward round after being admitted following a fall in a playground: 'I don't know why I can't get out of bed. If I ask the nurses they just say, doctor's orders. The doctor never comes round; and when he does; he doesn't talk to me. There's others with him. They all stare at you.'

We need to look more carefully at how information is given to children and avoid situations where they overhear themselves being discussed by doctors, parents and nurses. There should always be adult support on hand to allow children to discuss ideas when new information is being given so that their concepts are clarified and not confused by the new data. This seems to be particularly true of television programmes which can be an extremely useful educational tool but which can increase fears if unsuitable or unstructured viewing is allowed.

Children's views represent a rich course of data which is largely untapped. A great deal of further research is necessary in order to develop a fuller understanding of how children integrate knowledge from various sources. This can assist child health workers to develop more flexible theories which recognise the highly individual nature of children's perceptions and consequent fears and anxieties of illness and hospitals.

References

Eiser, C. (1990) *Chronic Childhood Disease*, Cambridge, Cambridge University Press.

Eiser, C. (1991) 'What children think about hospitals and illness', in A. Glasper (ed.), *Childcare*. London, Wolfe.

Ford, K. (1991) 'Understanding hospital', unpublished study. The Children's Hospital, Birmingham.

Jago, D. (1987) 'Communicating with children', *Maternal and Child Health*, June 1987, pp. 186–188.

SECTION 3

Health Policy

Introduction

An awareness of health policy decisions, and their implications for protecting and promoting health, are necessary criteria for all those who currently work in the health care field. As nurses form the largest group of health service employees, and as they are placed at the 'sharp end' of health service delivery (working with patients and managing resources), a good understanding of health policy is particularly crucial.

The 1980s and the early 1990s has been a time of major change and upheaval in health service provision. The introduction of accountability and of market forces into health care has meant that health service decision-making has become a public (rather than a hidden) activity, thus drawing much comment from health professionals and the public alike. It is no longer possible to 'keep politics out of nursing'; indeed there have been strong active moves by the professional bodies to make nurses more politically aware and active (*see* Guide to Parliamentary Lobbying, in the last section of this book).

In this section we begin with a very broad and egalitarian policy perspective, and invite you to think about the future of health in Europe. We place this paper at the beginning of this section because European integration is now a reality for British health workers, and because the values identified in the paper (equity, participation, social justice) are those on which the World Health Organization (WHO) Health For All and UK Project 2000 reforms are based.

Equity in health care is a major issue for health service providers. In the second reading in this section we identify trends in health inequalities, and recognize the association between a number of sociological variables and ill health.

Like the WHO, the UK government has set targets for health. The extracts from *The Health of the Nation* identify these targets and also indicate how various government departments might work more closely together to promote health and reduce ill health.

The need for broad rather than narrow vision in setting health targets is part of what has become known as 'the new public health'. This recognizes, and places centre stage, the social conditions and contexts within which people live and experience health threats and opportunities. Ashton and Seymour make a strong case for adoption of the new public health as a philosophy for health service planning, and advocate re-orientating health service towards primary health care. Primary health care in the UK began to be revalued towards the end of the 1980s and early 1990s when a number of policy documents were issued. Extracts from one of these, '*Primary Health Care in England*' are reproduced here.

We close the section with a reading that explores issues in health care policy with regard to children, and the value society places on them. In a wide ranging paper, Kurtz and Tomlinson examine concepts of health and childhood, review current policies for children and health care, identify health and illness trends in children in the UK, and conclude by reflecting on opportunities for promoting child health.

13

The Future of Health in Europe*

WORLD HEALTH ORGANIZATION

Since the adoption of the original regional health for all targets in 1984, political developments have had profound effects on the social fabric and the conduct of public affairs in all parts of the Region. The ending of the Cold War and of its sterile ideological divide in the Region means that issues of public policy for health can now be discussed openly and ideas and experience freely exchanged. At the same time, Europe has been going through a phase of economic restructuring, technological innovation and rapid social change, with major health and social consequences. The continuing impetus of political and economic changes in the countries of central and eastern Europe and integration in western and southern Europe will necessitate strong cooperation, openness and flexibility throughout Europe.

Among the possible trends in a future Europe are:

- the increasing importance of transboundary environmental problems, such as acid or toxic rain, food contamination and radiation;
- the rapid development of information technology and support;
- advances in medical technology and a wide range of options for treatment and prevention;
- the further development of intercountry economic cooperation and solidarity, which will create more favourable conditions for economic growth and material well-being;
- widening differences between parts of Europe and between socio-economic groups (although society may evolve to become more responsible and caring);
- increased migration both from outside Europe and within;
- further lengthening of people's life span, combined with slow reproduction patterns and the growth of an active group of the elderly;
- increased demand for user choice and participation in all walks of life and, in response, an improved quality of health care and new professional attitudes towards users of services;
- strengthened, broad partnerships and coalitions for health at local, international and supranational levels.

*This is an abridged version of *Targets for health for all. The health policy for Europe*. Summary of the updated edition, September 1991, WHO Regional Office for Europe, Copenhagen.

In spite of significant changes and new trends in Europe, the fundamentals of the European health for all strategy will remain as relevant in the year 2000 as they are now, and indeed as they were in 1980 when first formulated: to promote health, to prevent the occurrence of disease, to improve people's environment and to improve health services. The regional health for all targets are a reflection of present and anticipated trends, perceived problems and known resources and technology.

We have less knowledge about some trends than about others. There is therefore a need to incorporate further evidence and conclusions and to keep health policy up to date.

To reach these targets, much still has to be done to improve health-related aspects of lifestyles, environmental conditions and health care. Such improvements will not have their full effect, however, if certain prerequisities for health are not met, notably peace and solidarity between the European countries.

Given the magnitude of the task of attaining health for all, strong political will and the mobilization of public support remain of fundamental importance for ensuring that the necessary action is taken. The process of sustaining and mobilizing further support should be seen as a responsibility at the highest level and in all sectors throughout each country.

HEALTH FOR ALL 2000

Target 1. By the year 2000, the differences in health states between countries and between groups within countries should be reduced by at least 25%, by improving the level of health of disadvantaged nations and groups.

Target 2. By the year 2000, all people should have the opportunity to develop and use their own health potential in order to lead socially, economically and mentally fulfilling lives.

Target 3. By the year 2000, people with disabilities should be able to lead socially, economically and mentally fulfilling lives with the support of special arrangements that improve their relative physical, social and economic opportunities.

Target 4. By the year 2000, there should be a sustained and continuing reduction in morbidity and disability due to chronic disease in the Region.

Target 5. By the year 2000, there should be no indigenous cases of poliomyelitis, diphtheria, neonatal tetanus, measles, mumps and congenital rubella in the Region and there should be a sustained and continuing reduction in the incidence and adverse consequences of other communicable diseases, notably HIV infection.

Target 6. By the year 2000, life expectancy at birth in the Region should be at least 75 years and there should be a sustained and continuing improvement in the health of all people aged 65 years and over.

Target 7. By the year 2000, the health of all children and young people should be improved, giving them the opportunity to grow and develop to their full physical, mental and social potential.

Target 8. By the year 2000, there should be sustained and continuing improvement in the health of all women.

Target 9. By the year 2000, mortality from diseases of the circulatory system should be reduced, in the case of people under 65 years by at least 15%, and there should be progress in improving the quality of life of all people suffering from cardiovascular disease.

Target 10. By the year 2000, mortality from cancer in people under 65 years should be reduced by at least 15% and the quality of life of all people with cancer should be significantly improved.

Target 11. By the year 2000, injury, disability and death arising from accidents should be reduced by at least 25%.

Target 12. By the year 2000, there should be a sustained and continuing reduction in the prevalence of mental disorders, an improvement in the quality of life of all people with such disorders, and a reversal of the rising trends in suicide and attempted suicide.

Target 13. By the year 2000, all Member States should have developed, and be implementing, intersectoral policies for the promotion of healthy lifestyles, with systems ensuring public participation in policy-making and implementation.

Target 14. By the year 2000, all settings of social life and activity, such as the city, school, workplace, neighbourhood and home, should provide greater opportunities for promoting health.

Target 15. By the year 2000, accessible and effective education and training in health promotion should be available in all Member States, in order to improve public and professional competence in promoting health and increasing health awareness in other sectors.

Target 16. By the year 2000, there should be continuous efforts in all Member States to actively promote and support healthy patterns of living through balanced nutrition, appropriate physical activity, healthy sexuality, good stress management and other aspects of positive health behaviour.

Target 17. By the year 2000, the health-damaging consumption of dependence-producing substances such as alcohol, tobacco and psychoactive drugs should have been significantly reduced in all Member States.

Target 18. By the year 2000, all Member States should have developed, and be implementing, policies on the environment and health that ensure ecologically sustainable development, effective prevention and control of environmental health risks and equitable access to healthy environments.

Target 19. By the year 2000, there should be effective management systems and resources in all Member States for putting policies on environment and health into practice.

Target 20. By the year 2000, all people should have access to adequate supplies of safe drinking-water and the pollution of groundwater sources, rivers, lakes and seas should no longer pose a threat to health.

Target 21. By the year 2000, air quality in all countries should be improved to a point at which recognized air pollutants do not pose a threat to public health.

Target 22. By the year 2000, health risks due to microorganisms or their toxins, to chemicals and to radioactivity in food should have been significantly reduced in all Member States.

Target 23. By the year 2000, public health risks caused by solid and hazardous wastes and soil pollution should be effectively controlled in all Member States.

Target 24. By the year 2000, cities, towns and rural communities throughout the Region should offer physical and social environments supportive to the health of their inhabitants.

Target 25. By the year 2000, the health of workers in all Member States should be improved by making work environments more healthy, reducing work-related disease and injury and promoting the well-being of people at work.

Target 26. By the year 2000, all Member States should have developed, and be implementing, policies that ensure universal access to health services of quality, based on primary care and supported by secondary and tertiary care.

Target 27. By the year 2000, health service systems in all Member States should be managed cost-effectively, with resources being distributed according to need.

Target 28. By the year 2000, primary health care in all Member States should meet the basic needs of the population by providing a wide range of health-promotive, curative, rehabilitative and supportive services and by actively supporting self-help activities of individuals, families and groups.

Target 29. By the year 2000, hospitals in all Member States should be providing cost-effective secondary and tertiary care and contribute actively to improving health status and patient satisfaction.

Target 30. By the year 2000, people in all Member States needing long-term care and support should have access to appropriate services of a high quality.

Target 31. By the year 2000, there should be structures and processes in all Member States to ensure continuous improvement in the quality of health care and appropriate development and use of health technologies.

Target 32. By the year 2000, health research should strengthen the acquisition and application of knowledge in support of health for all development in all Member States.

Target 33. By the year 2000, all Member States should have developed, and be implementing, policies in line with the concepts and principles of the European health for all policy, balancing lifestyle, environment and health service concerns.

Target 34. By the year 2000, management structures and processes should exist in all Member States to inspire, guide and coordinate health development, in line with HFA principles.

Target 35. By the year 2000, health information systems in all Member States should actively support the formulation, implementation, monitoring and evaluation of health for all policies.

Target 36. By the year 2000, education and training of health and other personnel in all Member States should actively contribute to the achievement of health for all.

Target 37. By the year 2000, in all Member States a wide range of organizations and groups throughout the public, private and voluntary sectors should be actively contributing to the achievement of health for all.

Target 38. By the year 2000, all Member States should have mechanisms in place to strengthen ethical considerations in decisions relating to the health of individuals, groups and populations.

14

Promoting Equal Opportunities for Health*

B. JACOBSON, A. SMITH and M. WHITEHEAD

Social class and health

Almost all health indicators confirm the association between the prevalence of ill health and poor social and economic circumstances.[1,2] In 1981, the death rate was twice as high in the lowest social classes as in the highest. The expectation of life for a child with parents in social class V is over seven years shorter than for a child whose parents are in a social class I.

While there is still an incomplete understanding of this association, recent research has improved the position.

The relative disadvantage of those in the classes comprising the manual workers (classes V, IV and III manual) may be most simply expressed by comparing the actual number of deaths in these classes with the number that would have occurred if they had enjoyed the death rates prevailing among the largely non-manual workers (classes I, II and III non-manual). In 1981:

- men in the manual worker classes had death rates 45 per cent higher than men in the non-manual classes, and women had death rates 43 per cent higher;
- the excess mortality associated with being in the manual worker classes was greater than the total number of deaths from stroke, infectious disease, accidents, lung cancer and other respiratory diseases combined;
- if people in the manual worker classes had enjoyed the same death rates as non-manual classes there would have been 42,000 fewer deaths during the year in the age-range 16–74;
- if mortality at all ages is also considered, the total excess mortality associated with manual work social classes amounts to the equivalent of a major air crash or ship-wreck every day.

What is especially striking is that these socioeconomic differences in mortality experience are not confined to a few diseases in which an excess vulnerability might be

---

*This is an abridged version of B. Jacobson, A. Smith and M. Whitehead (1991) *The Nation's Health: A strategy for the 1990s*. London, King's Fund, pp. 107–19.

associated with specific occupational or social factors. The association between social deprivation and disease is broadly based. Of the 66 'major list' causes of death among men, 62 were more common among social classes IV and V (combined) than among all other men in 1981.[3] Of the 70 major causes of death among women, 64 were more common among women married to men in social classes IV and V.[4]

Trends in health inequalities

Social class differences in death rates have widened almost continuously since 1951.[5–8] While overall death rates have fallen over this period the death rates in the non-manual classes have declined more than those in the manual classes. If this increased social class inequality is expressed in terms of the proportion of deaths among men and women that would need to be redistributed in order to equalise death rates, then that proportion has doubled since the second world war.[8]

A reduction in health inequalities in postneonatal mortality occurred during the 1970s. It was associated with a disproportionate reduction in the number of births in the manual classes during that period. Measuring inequality across *all* classes, however, rather than simply comparing extremes, suggests that this improvement has not continued since the late 1970s.

Inequalities in the mortality experience of the social classes has persisted—and probably increased—at a time when general variation in the life-span has actually decreased.[9] This reduced variation in life-span is predominantly attributable to a reduction in the importance of those causes of death that operate especially at younger ages (the infections and accidents), and a consequently greater influence of diseases that characteristically kill in late middle life or in old age. It is the more remarkable that death rates from these diseases continue to show such striking social inequality.

Inequalities in the experience of illness

Not only are minor ailments more common among the manual classes, there is also evidence that people in manual classes who already have cancers, or heart disease, are less likely to survive.[10] We do not have comprehensive statistics on the occurrence of illness, but interesting data are collected from the General Household Survey which relies on people's own assessments of their health. Although people's assessments of their own health are influenced by varying norms and expectations between classes, reported rates of chronic illness and days of restricted activity in 1986 were twice as high in social class V as in social class I. Differences in the reporting of illnesses which temporarily restricted people's activity were smaller. Surveys of people's perception of their health (as opposed to their sickness) have shown that a sense of wellbeing is also related to social class.[11] While social class differences in height and obesity are small, four times as many people in social class V had no natural teeth, compared with social class I in England and Wales in 1980, and, in 1983, five year olds from manual backgrounds had twice as many decayed teeth as those from professional backgrounds.

Gender, class and health inequality

Mortality patterns for women follow generally similar class gradients to those of men when married women are classified according to their husband's occupation. However, two-thirds of married women are now engaged in paid work of their own. The classification may therefore conceal important occupational influences on women's health. There appears to have been an increase in mortality rates from lung cancer and coronary heart disease among women married to manual workers,[7] and it is important to identify any contribution that women's own jobs may make to these trends. This is especially so in the light of evidence that when working women's smoking patterns are analysed by their *own* class, the familiar class gradient disappears and women in social class I have a smoking prevalence similar to that for classes IV and V.[12]

Health patterns among women may be compared with those of men—irrespective of class. Women seem to have a health advantage over men because they live longer and have lower death rates than men at every stage in life. On the other hand, women are more likely than men to suffer many kinds of ill health—especially mental ill health.[13] They also suffer ill health from sex-specific problems, such as cervical and ovarian cancers which may, in part, explain why young women are heavier users of health services than men. The full explanation, however, is more complex.

While a classification of women by their own occupation would be useful, it would shed no light on that large minority of women (nearly 40 per cent) who fall into the 'economically inactive' group. We have yet to find a satisfactory social classification for women which takes into account both their domestic and paid work. This is likely to be fruitful as we already know that, among women, marital status is not associated with the same patterns of mental ill health as in men.

Health, class and ethnic minorities

There are few studies of the class distribution of health among different ethnic groups in the UK. Studies of immigrants (based on the census classification of people by country of birth) found that only Irish immigrants showed the same social class gradiant in mortality as the rest of the population.[14] The absence of a social class mortality gradient among immigrants from Africa, the Caribbean, Europe or the Indian subcontinent, may reflect selection and the insulating effect of their previous culture and environment. Evidence from other countries shows that these influences tend to diminish with time, and there is evidence that this is already occurring within the Asian community in the UK. Although overall death rates for first generation immigrants from the Indian subcontinent lacked any clear social class gradient, stillbirths and infant mortality rates for subsequent generations of Asian children studied in Bradford showed a steep gradient.[15]

Geographical inequalities

Socioeconomic differences make an important contribution to the marked geographical differences in death rates found in the UK—especially the higher death rates in the north and in Scotland compared with the south and east of the country (*see* Table 14.1). There are climatic, cultural and other natural factors—such as water hardness—which may contribute to this geographical pattern, but we know little about how they may exert their effects. The observed regional differences in death rates cannot be accounted for in terms of differences in the social class composition of the regional populations,[16] for regional mortality differentials are still present after adjustment for social class. The socioeconomic differences between regions tend to reflect differences between the circumstances of people in broadly similar occupational class categories, rather than differences in the proportions of people in different classes. In the more prosperous south east, people in *each* occupational category tend to do better than their counterparts elsewhere (*see* Table 14.1).

At the other end of the geographical scale, health differences between areas as small as electoral wards do reflect the differences in class composition of residential neighbourhoods. Differences in death rates between electoral wards have been studied in several cities. Findings suggest that 60 to 80 per cent of the variation in death rates is related to socioeconomic circumstances.[2,17]

Income and health

Income is clearly associated with health. The evidence is clear that the death rates of old people are affected by changes in the real value of state old age pensions, and also that as occupations move up or down the occupational earnings rankings they show a corresponding and opposite movement in the occupational mortality rate.[18,19] The implication is that income—perhaps the major determinant of standard of living and of life-style—has a direct effect on health. It is also clear that health is more sensitive to small changes in income at lower than at higher income levels.[20]

Unemployment and health

There is strong evidence that the deprivations associated with unemployment are damaging to health.[21] After adjusting for the effects of social class and age, the death rates of unemployed men and their wives are at least 20 per cent higher than expected.[22,23] Unemployment is associated with an estimated 1,500 extra deaths among unemployed men and their wives for each million men unemployed.[24] The two-fold higher death rates from suicide among the unemployed in a given social class, point to the importance of psychosocial factors.[23] The relationship between unemployment and parasuicide and the deterioration and subsequent improvement in mental health following unemployment and re-employment, add weight to the relationship between

Table 14.1 Social class differences in mortality by region

	Standardised Mortality Ratios. Average for Great Britain in 1979–80 and 1982–83 = 100					
Social classes	All	I	II	IIIN	IIIM	IV+V
Scotland						
M	123	74	90	111	137	157
F	124	83	93	100	130	141
North West						
M	114	70	86	105	120	146
F	113	75	88	97	109	135
North						
M	114	72	83	106	115	152
F	112	65	83	92	103	136
Yorkshire and Humberside						
M	104	75	80	100	105	134
F	102	68	79	84	100	120
Wales						
M	104	68	81	99	101	144
F	105	69	81	87	95	125
West Midlands						
M	102	67	76	93	112	127
F	100	67	79	85	105	113
East Midlands						
M	95	69	75	96	92	122
F	95	70	74	80	93	110
South East						
M	89	61	69	87	97	112
F	90	67	72	84	92	100
South West						
M	87	63	70	85	93	108
F	87	66	71	80	88	96
East Anglia						
M	79	65	65	80	80	93
F	81	61	70	72	79	81

Men 20–64, Women 20–59. Married Women classified by husband's occupation, single women by own occupation; N = Non manual; M = Manual.
Source: Office of Population Censuses and Surveys. Occupational mortality 1979–80 and 1982–3, Series D S No 6. London, HMSO, 1986.

unemployment and mental ill health.[21] While unemployment undoubtedly damages a person's sense of self-worth, part of the psychosocial impact of unemployment must arise from the material disadvantages it brings.

Lifestyle and socioeconomic disadvantage

The interrelationships of smoking, alcohol consumption, diet, physical activity and socioeconomic disadvantage are far from straightforward. There is a clear social class gradient in the prevalence of smoking, and those in the non-manual classes are more likely to have stopped smoking. Smoking is particularly prevalent among the unemployed. There is some evidence that smoking is associated with stress[12,25] and that socioeconomic disadvantage is stressful. However, there is also evidence that stress does not impede smoking cessation.[25]

The relationship between socioeconomic disadvantage and alcohol consumption is more complex. The heaviest drinking is concentrated in the manual classes, but there is heavy drinking in all classes.

Dietary differences between rich and poor make a major contribution to global inequalities in health. In a relatively affluent country such as the UK, they are most readily detectable among children born to working class parents, who are shorter than children born to professionals. But interest in diet has shifted more recently from simple undernutrition to malnutrition—the consumption of a diet that contains excessive quantities of fats, salt and unrefined sugars—which is known to contribute to coronary heart disease, and a range of other health problems. The National Food Survey shows that those in the lowest income categories eat—in many, but not all, respects—a less healthy diet than those with higher incomes; the poorest groups eat less fresh fruit, green vegetables and wholemeal bread (which is high in fibre), and more white bread and sugar, which contribute to obesity and tooth decay (see Table 14.2). But there is no equivalent social class gradient in the consumption of fats.

These consumption patterns almost certainly reflect income and cost considerations, as well as differences in culture or education. Research shows that *within* each income group the effect of additional children is to shift the pattern of food consumption nearer to that of poorer families.[26] The nutritional differences between large and small families within each income group are reflected in the tendency for people's height to be related, class for class, to their birth order and family size.[27] Small-scale studies[28,29] suggest that those on a low income may not be able to afford the diet recommended by the National Advisory Committee on Nutrition Education. Although these findings are based on data from highly selected groups, the lack of availability of a healthy range of foods in deprived areas is also an important feature limiting food choices.[30]

People in low income households spend proportionally twice as much of their income on food as those in high income households.[31] There is also evidence of undernutrition among the poor. The diets of many school children leave them below the recommended intake for many nutrients,[32] half of women who are single parents on low incomes cut down on their own food consumption to save money,[33] and 25 per cent of unemployed people do not have enough money for food at the end of the week.[34]

The overall impact of social class differences in nutrition is not yet completely established. But the simultaneous widening of social differences in health and in

Table 14.2 Income group differences in food consumption in 1988

Food	Ratio of average per capita consumption in high income compared with low income households*
Fruit	2.1
Wholemeal and wholewheat bread	1.4
Butter	1.05
Cheese	1.35
Fish	1.35
Vegetables	1.1
Margarine	0.59
Potatoes	0.63
Sugar	0.75

*High income denotes householders where the earners' average weekly income exceeds £375. Low income denotes households where the earners' average weekly income is below £100.
Source: Ministry of Agriculture, Fisheries and Foods. Household food consumption and expenditure 1988. London, HMSO, 1989.

nutrition during the decade following the end of war-time nutritional policy shows that they are important. Social class differences in total fat consumption remained small during the 1950s, immediately after the end of food rationing, but poorer people ate progressively more sugar while the better off ate increasing quantities of wholemeal bread. This period also saw smoking become more common in the manual classes.[35]

The importance of diet is also reflected in statistical relationships between nutrition and health which exist across regions as well as classes.[36] White bread, sugar and potatoes are eaten most by working class people and in the north of the country, while wholemeal bread, fresh fruit and green vegetables are eaten more by the non-manual classes, and those in the south. While the class differences in tooth loss are partly a reflection of differences in sugar consumption, the social distribution of obesity may also be influenced by differences in physical activity, rather than by the comparatively small differences in total calorie intake between classes. Leisure-time exercise is more common among professionals and high income groups, but some of this difference is offset by differences in physical activity between sedentary and manual occupations, and by the effect that car ownership has on people's walking.

Housing and health

The widespread impression that housing is a direct determinant of health originated in the well known association between insanitary conditions, overcrowding and the high rates of infectious (especially respiratory) diseases in the past. While some modern studies have failed to identify any direct effects, most have found that factors such as overcrowding, structural deficiencies and lack of privacy do make a contribution to poor health.[37–39] The location of housing may also have indirect effects on health.

Estates where access to jobs, shops and health services is difficult tend to increase the disadvantage of those who live in them.[40] Two Scottish studies have recently found clear effects of damp housing on the health of children in a deprived area. Respiratory and bronchial symptoms, headaches and diarrhoea were much more common among children living in damp housing, and the effect of damp was independent of the effect of low income or smoking in the household.[41,42]

Although we were hampered by the lack of research, it is clear that much of the modern contribution which substandard housing makes to ill health arises less from its physical impact than from the social and psychological effects of damp, disrepair, inadequate facilities and cramped living accommodation. Housing is almost certainly an important factor in the large social class differences found in mortality from childhood accidents. The lack of indoor playspace and gardens means that young children are more likely to play unsupervised in the street. Another major and growing problem is that of homelessness. In 1990, local authorities accepted 164,000 housing applications from homeless people and families. In addition, estimates of 'concealed homelessness' among young, single people were put at 156,000 by Shelter.

Notes

1. Black, Sir Douglas (chair). *Inequalities in health*. Report of a research working group. London, Department of Health and Social Security, 1980.

2. Whitehead, M. The health divide. In: *Inequalities in health*. London, Penguin, 1988.

3. Office of Population Censuses and Surveys. *Occupational Mortality 1970–2*, Series DS1, London, HMSO, 1978 (with allowances made for wider differentials in 1981).

4. Office of Population Censuses and Surveys. *Occupational Mortality 1970–80 and 1982–83*, Series DS2, London, HMSO, 1986.

5. Preston, S.H. *et al. Effects of industrialisation and urbanisation on mortality in developed countries*. IUSSP Solicited Papers. IUSSP Conference 19. Liege, IUSSP, 1981.

6. Pamuk, E. Social class inequalities in mortality from 1921 to 1972 in England and Wales. *Population Studies*, 1985, **39**: 17–31.

7. Marmot, M.G. Mortality decline and widening social inequalities. *The Lancet*, 1986, **ii**: 274–276.

8. Koskinen, S. *Time trends in cause-specific mortality by occupational class in England and Wales*. Paper presented to IUSSP 20th general conference, Florence, 1985. Unpublished.

9. Le Grand, J. *Inequalities in health: the human capital approach*. Welfare state programme no 1. London, London School of Economics, 1985.

10. Leon, D.A. and Wilkinson, R.G. Inequalities in prognosis: socioeconomic differences in cancer and heart disease survival. In: Fox, J. (ed). *Health inequalities in European countries*. Aldershot, Gower, 1989.

11. Blaxter, M.A. A comparison of measures of inequality in morbidity. In: Fox, J. (ed). *Health inequalities in European countries*. Aldershot, Gower, 1989.

12. Jacobson, B. *Beating the ladykillers. Women and smoking*. London, Gollancz, 1988.

13. McIntyre, S. The patterning of health by social position in contemporary Britain: direction for sociological research. *Social Science and Medicine*, 1986, **23**: 393–415.

14. Marmot, M.G. *et al.* Lessons from the study of immigrant mortality. *The Lancet*, 1984, **i**, 1455–1457.

15. Gillies, D.R.H. *et al.* Analysis of the ethnic influences on still births and infant mortality in Bradford 1975–81. *Journal of Epidemiology and Community Health*, 1984, **58**,3: 214–217.

16. Marmot, M.G. Social inequalities in mortality: the social environment. In: Wilkinson R.G. (ed). *Class and health: research and longitudinal data*. London, Tavistock, 1986.

17. Townsend, P. *The geography of poverty and ill-health*. Paper presented to a meeting of the British Association for the Advancement of Science. University of Bristol, 1986.

18. Wilkinson, R.G. Income and mortality. In: Wilkinson, R.G. (ed). *Class and health: research and longitudinal data*. London, Tavistock, 1986.

19. Wilkinson, R.G. Income distribution and mortality: a 'natural' experiment. *Sociology of Health and Illness*, 1990, **12**: 391–412.

20. Wagstaff, A. The demand for health: theory and implications. *Journal of Epidemiology and Community Health*, 1986, **40**: 1–11.

21. Smith, R. *Unemployment and health*. Oxford, Oxford University Press, 1987.

22. Moser, K.A. *et al.* Unemployment and mortality in the OPCS longitudinal study. In: Wilkinson, R.G. (ed). *Class and health: research and longitudinal data*. London, Tavistock, 1986.

23. Moser, K.A. *Unemployment and mortality 1981–83: follow-up of the 1981 longitudinal study census sample*. Working paper 43. London, Social Statistics Research Unit. City University, 1986.

24. Scott-Samuel, A. Unemployment and health. *The Lancet*, 1984, **ii**: 1464–1465.

25. Marsh, A., Matheson, J. *Smoking attitudes and behaviour*. OPCS Social Survey Division. London, HMSO, 1983.

26. Ministry of Agriculture, Fisheries and Food. *Household food and expenditure*. Report of the National Food Survey Committee. London, HMSO, 1986.

27. Rona, R.J. *et al.* Social factors and height of primary school children in England and Scotland. *Journal of Epidemiology and Community Health*, 1978, **32**: 147–154.

28. Cole-Hamilton, I., Lang, T. *Tightening belts: a report on the impact of poverty on food*. London, London Food Commission, 1986.

29. Haines, F.A., De Looy, A.E. *Can I afford the diet?* Birmingham, British Dietetic Association, 1986.

30. London Food Commission. *Food retailing in London: a pilot study of the three largest retailers and Londoners access to food*. London, LFC, 1985.

31. Department of Health and Social Security. *Family expenditure survey 1985*. London, HMSO, 1986.

32. Wenlock, R.W., Düsselduff, M.M. *The diets of British school-children*. London, DHSS, 1986.

33. Graham, H. *Caring for the family: a short report on the study of the organisation of the health resources and responsibilities of 102 families*. Milton Keynes, Open University, 1985.

34. Lang, T. *et al. Jam tomorrow*. Manchester, Manchester Polytechnic, 1984.

35. Marmot, M.G. *et al.* Changing social class distribution of heart disease. *British Medical Journal*. 1978, **2**: 1109–1112.

36. Wilkinson, R.G. *Socioeconomic factors in mortality differentials*. Mmedsci thesis. Nottingham University, 1976.

37. Duval, D. and Booth, A. The housing environment and women's health. *Journal of Health and Social Behaviour*, 1978, **19**: 410–417.

38. Wilner, D.M. and Walkley, R.P. The effects of housing on health and performance. In: Dahl, L.J. (ed). *The urban condition*. New York, 1963.

39. Booth, A. *Urban crowding and its problems*. New York, Praeger, 1976.

40. Robertson, I. In: Donnison, D. and Middleton, A. (eds). *Renewing the city*. London, Routledge and Kegan Paul, 1987.

41. Martin, C., Platt, S., Hunt, S. Housing conditions and ill-health. *British Medical Journal*. 1987, **294**: 1125–1127.

42. Platt, S. *et al.* Damp housing, mould growth and symptomatic health state. *British Medical Journal*, 1989, **298**: 1673–1678.

15

The Health of the Nation*

SECRETARIES OF STATE FOR HEALTH

Introduction

The achievements of the last 100 years—the scope for improvement—a strategic approach needed

'Nasty, brutish and short.' It is salutary to remember that it is only relatively recently—a matter of a few generations—that Thomas Hobbes' words ceased to be the common experience of life for the majority of people in England. A century ago four out of ten babies did not survive to adulthood. Life expectancy at birth was only 44 years for boys and 47 for girls. As recently as the early 1930s, 2500 women a year died during pregnancy or childbirth.

The transformation, illustrated in Figures 15.1 and 15.2, has been profound. Life expectancy at birth is now 73 years for boys and 78 for girls. Infant mortality—a basic indicator of any nation's health—now stands (1989) at 8.4 deaths for every 1000 live births. During the second half of the 19th and the first half of the 20th centuries death rates from diseases such as tuberculosis, enteric fever, diphtheria, scarlet fever, whooping cough and measles fell to one per cent of their previous levels. Immunisation and the development of effective drug treatments played their part, but the achievement was essentially due to various social and public health changes. Safe water and sewerage, better housing, less overcrowding and better working conditions, greater economic prosperity, more effective methods of family planning, better nutrition and better education lay at the heart of the transformation.

But major health problems remain. People may be living longer but many still die prematurely (Figure 15.3) or have the quality of their lives—especially in their later years—impaired by avoidable ill-health.

The NHS reforms have created significant opportunities—particularly in the change of emphasis in the role of health authorities—for addressing these problems. The Government believes that the time is now right to take a strategic approach to improving health: what needs to be done can best be secured by concerted action within a common strategic framework.

---

*Extracts from Secretaries of State for Health (1991) *The Health of the Nation*, HMSO, London, pp. 1, 2, 78, 21–25, 36 (Consultative Document, enacted 1992).

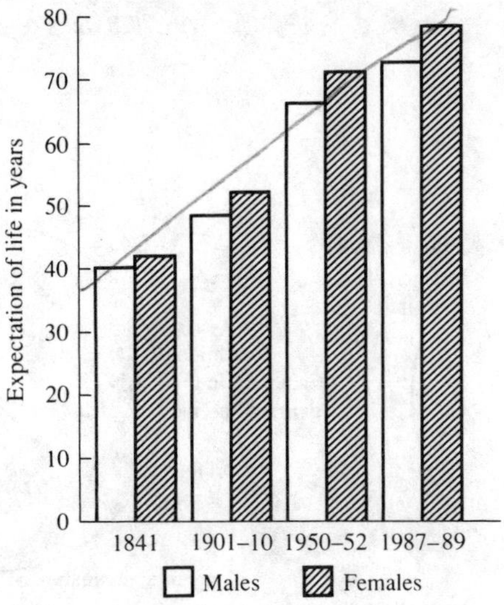

Figure 15.1 Expectation of life at birth: England and Wales 1841–1952; England 1987–1989

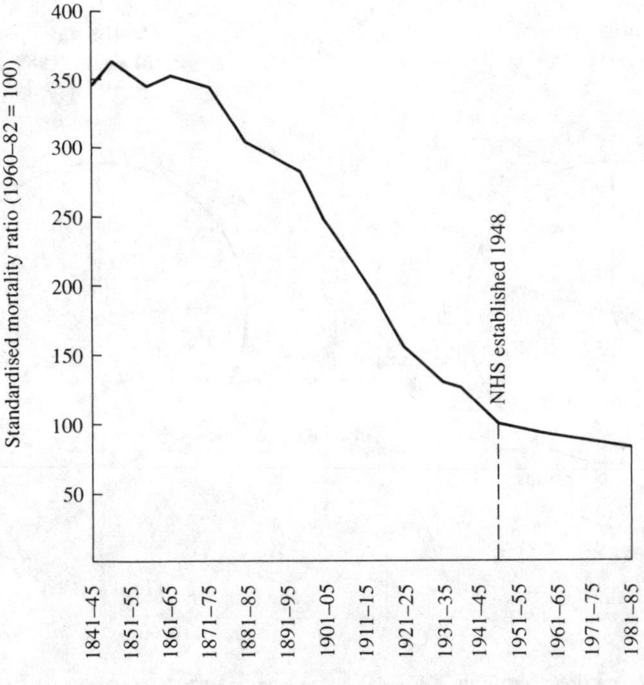

The standardised mortality ratio (SMR) is an index which allows for differences in age structure values. Above 100 indicates higher mortality than in 1950–52 and values below 100 indicate lower mortality. Source: OPCS.

Figure 15.2 Mortality trends 1841–1985: England and Wales, all persons

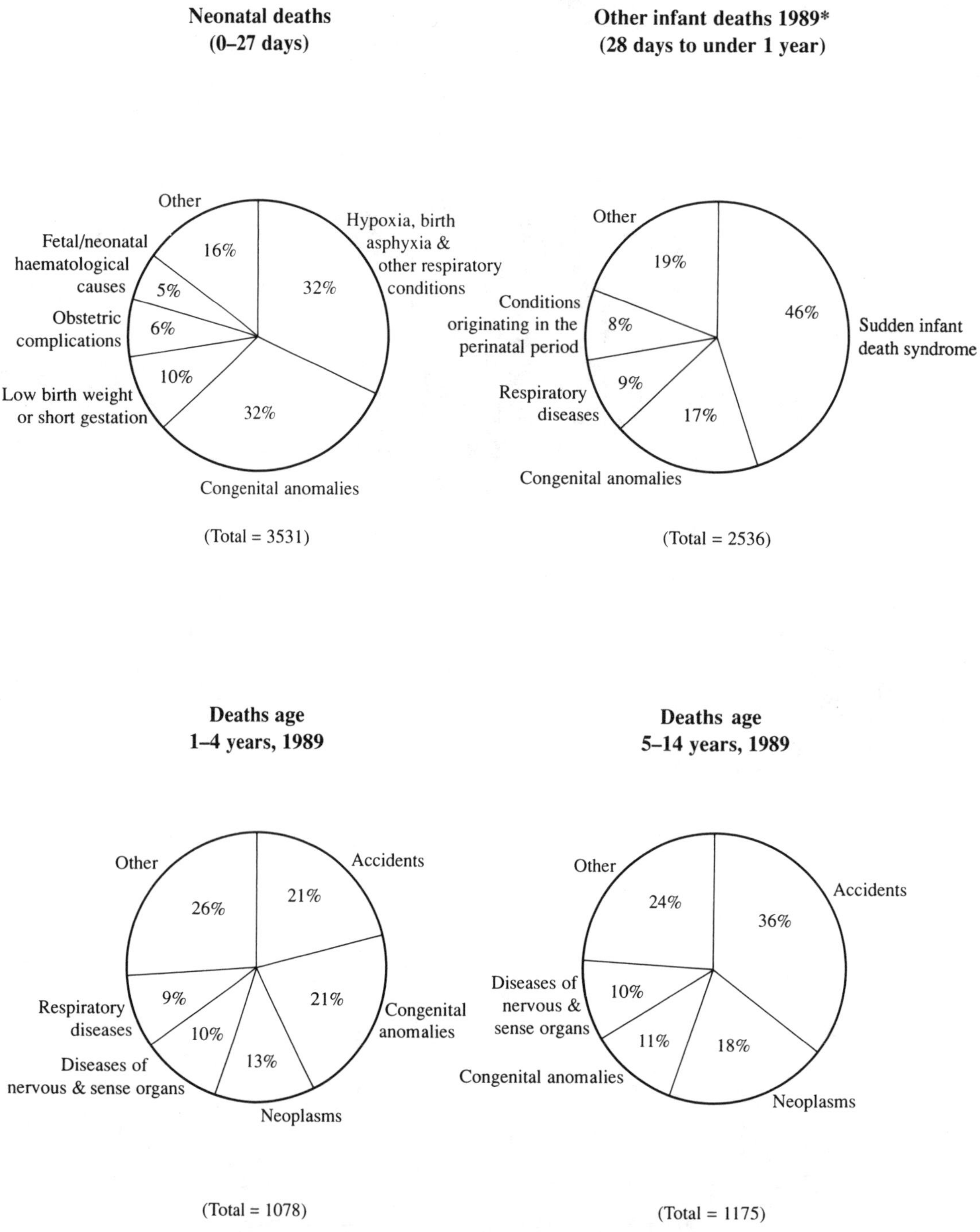

Source: OPCS.

*A new death certificate was introduced in January 1986, from which it is not possible to assign an underlying cause to deaths under 28 days.

Figure 15.3 Distribution of major causes of deaths in children: England and Wales

This consultation document sets out for discussion and comment what the Government hopes to achieve through the development of such a health strategy for England. The overriding aim is that the strategy should genuinely contribute to improvements in people's health by focusing attention and action on the major health problems to be tackled for the rest of this decade and beyond into the 21st century.

This document deals only with England. Separate approaches have been taken in Wales, Scotland and Northern Ireland.

Area	**Criterion 1** **Major cause of concern**	**Criterion 2** **Scope for improvement**	**Criterion 3** **Ability to set targets**
Coronary Heart Disease	Greatest single cause of premature death	Healthy living Effective treatment	YES
Stroke	12% of all deaths 5% of deaths under 65 years	Healthy living Detection and treatment of raised blood pressure Rehabilitation	YES
Cancers	25% of all deaths	Not for all cancers For some – healthy living Screening for breast and cervical cancers	Not for all cancers Screening targets for breast and cervical cancer + see smoking target
Smoking	Largest single preventable cause of death	Not smoking	YES
Eating and Drinking Habits	Contribution to many aspects of health and ill-health	Healthier eating and drinking habits	YES
Physical Activity	Contribution to many aspects of health and ill-health	More people taking regular physical activity	Not at this stage – further information needed
Prevention of Accidents	Most common cause of death under 30	Improvements in engineering, design, environment, etc. Education, awareness Legislation and other controls	YES
Health of Pregnant Women, Infants and Children	Key indicator of the nation's health	Wide subject – scope varies for different aspects	YES
HIV/AIDS	Greatest new threat to public health this century	Safe sexual and intravenous drug using behaviour	Not at this stage – further information needed
Other Communicable Diseases			
(a) preventable by immunisation	Potential for harm should immunisation rates fall	Immunisation	YES
(b) hospital acquired infection	10% of inpatients have an infection acquired in hospital	Good practice	YES

Figure 15.4 Identifying key areas: possible key areas – objectives and targets

Department of Environment

The Department of the Environment helps secure good health by improving the quality of the environment and seeking to ensure that a decent standard of affordable housing is available to all. It coordinates Government policy on environmental protection as set out in the White Paper 'This Common Inheritance'.

Health related action includes:

- **Environmental Protection Act 1990**: introduction of controls by HM Inspectorate of Pollution and local authority environmental health departments to minimise industrial pollution of air, water and land; enhanced noise and litter controls; improved waste disposal and recycling arrangements.
- **Water Act 1989**: establishment of Drinking Water Inspectorate to set and enforce standards for drinking water quality and of National Rivers Authority to control discharges of pollutants into water.
- **Housing**: over the century two million slums cleared and six million subsidised dwellings built; since 1960s two million grants given for home improvement. Nearly £2 billion a year now being spent on renovation to improve the condition of local authority housing; £500 million a year is given in grants—mainly to less well-off owner occupiers—to improve unsatisfactory private houses; the output of housing association subsidised homes is planned to almost double between 1989/90 and 1993/94; and short-term programmes aimed at 11,000 households temporarily housed in bed and breakfast accommodation, and the 3000–5000 people sleeping rough on the streets.
- **Inner cities**: because poor health is often linked to the economic, environmental and social problems in inner cities the Government's inner city policies which aim to improve living conditions will also raise general levels of health. The Urban Programme also funds health promotion and disease prevention, improvements to primary health care, services for homeless mentally ill people and access to health care for ethnic minorities.
- **Sewage treatment**: requirement (implementing EC Directive) to end significant discharges of untreated sewage to inland and coastal waters by 1998 and 2005 and to improve bathing waters.
- **Vehicle pollution**: tight new emission limits for cars and heavy diesels introduced.
- **Toxic metals**: action has reduced human exposure to lead (by, for example, limiting the lead content of drinking water, food, petrol and paint) and other toxic metals, particularly mercury and cadmium; blood lead levels are now half those of the mid-1970s.
- **Radon**: guidance now allows householders in highest risk areas to make informed decisions about risks; free testing of radon levels in affected areas available.

Department of Education and Science

The Department of Education and Science makes a significant contribution to health. The Government's policy is to encourage schools to equip their pupils with the knowledge, skills and attitudes they will need to make well-informed, independent judgements and to safeguard their long-term good health. Health education in schools lays the foundation for the individual's subsequent health-related behaviour and life-style; and sport makes an important contribution to individual health, both at school and in adult life.

The long-term effect of health education on young people is difficult to assess, though there are indications of progress. For example, recent research suggests that despite public concern about drugs, and their availability, the number of school pupils who have experimented with drugs remains very low. There are indications, however, that other forms of unhealthy behaviour are static or increasing—smoking and drinking alcohol are much more prevalent and a greater cause for concern.

The DES also has responsibility, through the overall funding of the university sector and the payment of grant-in-aid to the independent Medical Research Council, for basic medical education and medical and health-related research. In addition the education service is the major provider of initial training for nurses and staff in the professions supplementary to medicine.

Other health related action includes:

- **The school curriculum**: certain health issues are included within the statutory order for National Curriculum science. In addition, the National Curriculum Council identified health education as one of five cross-curricular themes and issued guidance which identifies nine key components for health education—substance use and misuse; sex education; family life education; safety; health-related exercise; food and nutrition; personal hygiene; environmental factors; and psychological aspects.
- **Health education**: Since 1986, DES has funded local education authority initiatives to counter misuse of drugs and, since 1990 to support general health education.
- **Sport**: sport in schools is the foundation to encouraging greater overall participation in sport. Physical education is therefore a compulsory subject for all pupils between five and 16 in maintained schools. DES and DH are jointly examining what can be done to encourage better co-ordination between local health based exercise initiatives and efforts by sports clubs and local authorities to promote greater participation in sport.
- **Sports Council**: Sports Council targets for 1988–1993 include:

  (a) an increase in the percentage of women and young girls taking part in sport from 38% to 42%

  (b) maintenance of the absolute numbers, and therefore an increase in the percentage of young people taking part in sport in the context of the declining number of 18–25 year olds in the population.

Employment Department Group

The Employment Department Group provides help for people with disabilities and long-term health problems who wish to identify appropriate work and prepare for it. The Employment Rehabilitation Service undertakes both these functions, and medical practitioners can make use of its specialist services to seek practical advice for patients.

Disablement Resettlement Officers and the Disablement Advisory Service provide help and guidance to individuals and employers about the integration of people with disabilities into the workforce. The Employment Department Group also helps meet the training needs of people with disabilities or long-term health problems, provides help in training and employment through a variety of special schemes such as loaning equipment to individuals or providing grants to employers to alter premises, and enables people with severe disabilities to work in sheltered accommodation

Health and safety of workpeople and the public affected by work activity is the responsibility of the Health and Safety Commission and Executive. This is carried out through:

- negotiation and definition of standards, which can lead to new legislation;
- issuing guidance on standards and good practice;
- promoting compliance with legislation through inspection, advice and enforcement (170,000 preventive inspection visits were made in 1989–90 with 11,700 improvement and prohibition notices issued and 2200 successful prosecutions);
- promoting better management of health and safety;
- carrying out research and investigations of accidents and ill-health (in 1989–90, more than 11,000 accidents and incidents were investigated and the Employment Medical Advisory Service made 3000 workplace visits to investigate causes of occupational ill-health).

Cancers and lung disease remain the major apparent causes of work-related deaths, often reflecting exposure levels of many years ago which are now better controlled. Overall, there are possibly 2000 premature work-related deaths; 8000 to which work is a contributory factor; and 80,000 new cases of work-related disease each year. There are gaps in information about work-related ill-health and HSC attach high priority to securing improved information on the scale and pattern of industrial ill-health.

Department of Transport

More than 5000 people die on the roads each year, and a further 60,000 are seriously injured and 270,000 slightly injured. The Government has set a target of reducing road casualties by one third by the year 2000 and the Department of Transport is concentrating on three areas to meet the target. First, by raising the level of public awareness so that road safety is seen as an issue for society. Second, by giving special attention to the most vulnerable road users, including children and the elderly. Third, by concentrating on proven and cost effective casualty reduction measures in vehicle and road engineering. In 1990 the Department of Transport, together with the Department of Education and Science and the Department of Health, launched a major child road safety policy initiative, "Children and Roads: A Safer Way", which provides a focus for action to reduce child road casualties.

Ministry of Agriculture, Fisheries and Food

A wholesome and safe diet is integral to good health. In ensuring that food is safe for general consumption, MAFF:

- takes action against diseases transmissible from farm animals (successes include the reduction of tuberculosis and brucellosis to very low levels; efforts are now being made to reduce the incidence of *Salmonella enteritidis* in poultry);
- ensures the milk supply reaches the very highest EC standards (the UK is the only country other than Denmark to do so);
- carries out surveillance and research to identify risks to the food supply and ways of managing them.

MAFF is responsible for ensuring that information is available to allow consumers to choose a healthy diet; action is being taken to encourage better food labelling and more consumer education to underpin consumer choice.

Department of Social Security

Increased prosperity means that those in all income groups have seen real improvements in their living standards during the 1980s. However, the key role that social security benefits play in maintaining health, particularly amongst the more vulnerable in society, is fully recognised. Through the new structure of income-related benefits introduced in 1988, resources are now directed more effectively to those who need them. Additional resources in real terms have been made available to pensioners, sick and disabled people, families with children and lone parents. The priority accorded to lone parents is also reflected in the new initiative on child support which highlights the parental responsibility for providing proper financial support to their children wherever it can reasonably be expected and will facilitate the payment of maintenance without recourse to the courts.

Recent improvements in disability benefits and the new benefits now being considered by Parliament will add up to a more comprehensive and coherent system of support for disabled people than ever before. The Minister of State for Disabled People, who is a Social Security Minister, is responsible for interdepartmental liaison on all issues affecting disabled people.

The Department of Social Security is working especially closely with the Department of Health to ensure a smooth transition to the new community care arrangements in April 1993. In particular, the social security entitlements of those in residential care and nursing homes will be fully protected.

Department of Trade and Industry

The Department of Trade and Industry is concerned with the safety of consumer goods and with valid and analytical measurement, upon which the reliable monitoring of many hazards depends. One of its other responsibilities is prevention of accidents in the home. Every year about 5000 people die and around three million need medical attention, making home accidents the biggest single cause of injury. The Consumer Protection Act 1987 provides a strong legal framework to protect consumers from unsafe consumer goods. DTI also mounts safety campaigns aimed at particular hazards or those most at risk. These have contributed to a fall in deaths from more than 7000 in 1966 to 5000 in 1988 (England and Wales).

Taxes, Duties and Health

The Government levies excise duties on products which can be harmful to health—such as tobacco products, alcoholic drink and leaded petrol. Raising these duties can help reduce consumption, or encourage the use of less harmful alternatives:

- The duty on tobacco products was increased in the 1991 Budget by 15%. The Chancellor of the Exchequer said: "There are strong health arguments for a big duty increase on tobacco. In recent years the duty has fallen in real terms and cigarette consumption, having declined in the early 1980s, has begun to turn up again. Raising the duty will help to counter this unwelcome trend." As a result of the Budget the total real term increase in the specific duty (and VAT) on cigarettes since 1979 is 55%;
- The introduction and widening of the duty differential between leaded and unleaded petrol has encouraged motorists to switch to unleaded and reduced the amount of lead in the atmosphere. Unleaded petrol now accounts for around 39% of the market;
- Since 1988, some low alcohol drinks have been taxed less heavily per unit of alcohol content than higher alcohol drinks in order not to discourage their consumption.

16

The Setting for a New Public Health*

JOHN ASHTON and HOWARD SEYMOUR

In Europe and North America three distinct phases of activity in relation to public health can be identified in the last 150 years.[1] The first phase began in the industrialized cities of Northern Europe in response to the appalling toll of death and disease among the working classes living in abject poverty. The displacement of large numbers of people from the land by their landlords in order to take advantage of the agricultural revolution had combined with the attraction of the growing cities as the result of the industrial revolution to produce a massive change in population patterns and in the physical environments in which people live.[2–6] The predominantly rural ecology of human habitation was ruptured and replaced by one in which a seething mass of humanity was living in squalor.

In Liverpool, in the 1830s one-third of the population was living in the cellars of back-to-back houses with earth floors, no ventilation or sanitation and as many as 16 people to a room. It was not surprising, that epidemics such as tuberculosis, pneumonia, whooping cough, measles and smallpox flourished under such conditions. The response to this situation was the gradual development of a public health movement based on the activities of medical officers of health, sanitary inspectors and their staff, supported by legislation such as the National Public Health Acts of 1848 and 1875 in England.[7]

The focus of this movement was improvements in housing and sanitation standards and the provision of bacteriologically safe water and food.

The Public Health Movement with its emphasis on environmental change lasted until the 1870s and was in time eclipsed by a more individualistic approach ushered in by the development of the germ theory of disease and the possibilities offered by immunization and vaccination. As the most pressing environmental problems were brought under control, action to improve the health of the population moved on first to personal preventive medical services, such as immunization and family planning, and later to a range of other initiatives including the development of community and school nursing and school health services. The second phase also marked the increasing involvement of the State in medical and social welfare through the provision of hospital and clinic services.[8]

---

*This is an abridged version of a chapter in Ashton, J. and Seymour, H. (1988), *The New Public Health*, Milton Keynes, Open University Press, pp. 102–10.

The second phase was in its turn superseded by the therapeutic era, dating from the 1930s, with the advent of insulin and the sulphonamide group of drugs. Until that time there was little of proven efficacy in the therapeutic arsenal.[2] The beginning of this era coincided with the apparent demise of infectious diseases on the one hand and the development of ideas about the welfare state in many developed countries on the other. Historically, it marked a weakening of departments of public health and a shift of power and resources to hospital-based services and particularly those based in teaching hospitals.

Despite the outstanding work of many public health practitioners, in this process the imperative of population coverage which underpins public health rather than concern for individuals who are able to pay for a service has not always been to the fore as evidenced by the continuing and widening inequalities in health.[9–11]

By the early 1970s the therapeutic era was increasingly being challenged. Most countries were experiencing a crisis in health care costs irrespective of their structure of health services; the escalation in costs being in part consequent on technological innovation in treatment methods and an apparently limitless demand for medical care, coupled with the dramatic demographic changes which were taking place with very rapid growth of the elderly population. McKeown's analysis, together with root and branch critiques of medical practice, such as that of Ivan Illich, lent support to the growing interest in a reappraisal of priorities.[2,12]

In 1974, the then Canadian Minister of Health, Marc Lalonde, published a government report entitled *A New Perspective on the Health of Canadians*.[13] It set an agenda for a new era of preventive medicine in Canada; it is arguable that it signalled the turning point in efforts to rediscover public health in developed countries and that it ushered in a new, fourth phase of public health.

What is emerging as the New Public Health is an approach which brings together environmental change and personal preventive measures with appropriate therapeutic interventions especially for the elderly and disabled. However, the New Public Health goes beyond an understanding of human biology and recognizes the importance of those social aspects of health problems which are caused by life-styles. In this way it seeks to avoid the trap of blaming the victim. Many contemporary health problems are therefore seen as being social rather than solely individual problems; underlying them are concrete issues of local and national public policy, and what are needed to address these problems are 'Healthy Public Policies'—policies in many fields which support the promotion of health.[14–19] In the New Public Health the environment is social and psychological as well as physical.

Since 1974, many countries have published similar prevention-orientated documents and there has been an explosion of interest in preventive medicine and health promotion.[18,19] In this growing movement an important lead has been provided by the work of the World Health Organization, in its Health for All by the Year 2000 strategy.

Issues raised by health for all: a conflict between prevention and treatment?

The debate which surrounds the renaissance of public health is often couched in adversarial terms between prevention and treatment. A conflict of sorts between the two approaches has a long history. In the mid-nineteenth century Neumann,[20] arguing for an extended role for the State in public health and the provision of medical care, put it as follows:

> The State argues that its responsibility is to protect people's property rights. For most people the only property which they possess is their health; therefore the State has a responsibility to protect people's health.

In general, this point of view, albeit in what we would now see as a paternalistic form, seems to have triumphed and to this day an inscription above the door of the borough public health department in Southwark, South London proclaims 'the Health of the people is the highest law'. However, in recent years, and coinciding with the revival of public health, there has also been a revival of the argument over the responsibility for health with a modern 'victim-blaming' view attracting considerable support in some quarters. The issue is complicated by a widespread move against paternalistic forms of administration and services, as part of a general move towards participative as opposed to representative democracy. In the ensuing confusion it has been possible for some governments to construe that the public no longer wishes to have public services.

In public health it is customary to divide prevention into three types: primary, secondary and tertiary. Primary prevention together with health promotion has as its aim the prevention of disorders before they occur, either by positive strategies to affect those factors conducive to disorders in an entire, defined population or else in a subgroup of that population who are identified as being at risk.

Such strategies are only possible when causes are known and preventive strategies are feasible. When they are not it is necessary to fall back on secondary prevention, involving early diagnosis and treatment, including screening programmes, with the aim of limiting the course of an illness and reducing the risk of recurrence.

When even that is not possible recourse must be had to tertiary prevention aimed at reducing the burden of disability to the individual and to society and obtaining optimal health under the circumstances. Clearly, with an ageing population and in our current state of knowledge, there is a host of chronic conditions that we do not know how to prevent but where treatment may make all the difference to the quality of life and thus to health. To the extent to which death is itself inevitable sometime, high-quality terminal care is a form of tertiary prevention.

The common theme of all public health strategies of health promotion and prevention is a shift in the direction of health of the entire population, rather than a concern solely with individuals.

The need for comprehensive strategies of health promotion

The need for a broad view which integrates preventive and treatment medicine and acknowledges the wider political and social dimensions of health is not new.

The need was made explicit in the United Kingdom in the Beveridge report of 1942,[21] which makes quite clear the political nature of health problems and particularly of primary prevention. Clearly an interest in health must be a legitimate concern of all members of the community and not solely of doctors and health workers.

Ever since the inception of the British National Health Services (NHS) only a very small proportion of funds has been given over to the promotion of good health and the prevention of disease. In 1976 the Department of Health published *Prevention and Health: Everybody's Business*, which was intended to stimulate discussion about the scope for modern preventive medicine.[19] This was followed up by the DHSS report *Priorities for Health and Personal Social Services in England* (1976) and *The Way Forward* (1977).[22,23] The Royal Commission on the NHS, reporting in 1979, concluded that a 'significant improvement in the health of all people of the U.K. can come through prevention'.[24]

The Black Report (1980) recommended action within the health services and action in other policy areas with a particular emphasis on the need to abolish childhood poverty and to tackle on a multidisciplinary front the toll of death and disability caused by domestic and road traffic accidents.

More recently, the British Government has accepted the need to take active steps to develop primary medical care and has conducted a fundamental review of the Public Health Function in the light of failures of infectious disease control and environmental health monitoring and weakness in the relationship between the medical and other sectors of relevant public policy.[25–27] In Canada, in keeping with its vanguard position, the government has embraced the HFA 2000 Strategy as part of its own commitment to a defined health promotion strategy.[26–28]

Reorientating primary care

The reorientation of medical care towards health promotion, prevention and primary medical care is an essential part of the World Health Organization Strategy.[29,30] This reorientation involves a further shift from primary medical care (a medical concept based on the equitable availability and accessibility of good quality preventive and treatment services from a team of health workers based in the community) to primary health care, which is a social concept going much wider in that it is concerned with populations as well as individuals and that it seeks to involve a range of people other than trained health workers. The implications for training and organization in achieving this paradigm shift are considerable, particularly in respect of the need to achieve real public participation and intersectoral working.

The World Health Organization concept of primary health care incorporates a recognition that health care should be planned to relate to the resources available. It sees primary health care as the most local part of a comprehensive health system and it recognizes that the public should participate both individually and collectively in the planning and implementation of health care.

Primary health care as envisaged by WHO is hard to find. One celebrated example was the Peckham Pioneer Health Centre established in South London in the 1930s.

In planning the new centre it was felt that the population should be essentially healthy and that it should include a cross-section by age. It would be for people to come to the centre rather than for the centre to proselytize, and what happened in the centre would be for the members to decide. It would be continuously available in leisure time and

Table 16.1 The facilities at Peckham Health Centre

Welfare and educational
Antenatal clinic; postnatal clinic; birth control clinic; infant welfare clinic, care of the toddler; nursery school; immunization service; schoolchildren's medical examinations; vocational guidance; sex instruction for adolescents; girls' and boys' clubs; youth centres; sports clubs and recreation clubs of all sorts; keep fit and gymnastic classes; adult cultural education; music, debates, drama, any event desired by members; citizens advice bureau; holiday organizations; outings and expeditions; the bar; billiards; dancing; social gatherings.
Therapeutic
Marriage advice bureau; mothers' clinic; child guidance clinic; poor man's lawyer; social worker; hospital follow-up overhaul; rehabilitation clinic.

its aim was to provide opportunities whenever an opportunity could be taken up (see Table 16.1).

Support for the centre was not forthcoming from the National Health Service, apparently because the ethic was not compatible with the ascendant values of the therapeutic era.

At the present time, within many countries there is an excitement and energy attached to preventive medicine and primary medical care which was not there 20 years ago. Some countries have passed special legislation to assist the shift in emphasis from hospital- to community-based services; several have produced 'National Health for All Strategies' and, perhaps most encouragingly, there is a great deal of interest and activity in developing health promotion, preventive medicine and primary care at the local level. In some countries medical students now actively opt for careers outside hospitals. Yet in England and Wales, for example, where many of the desirable elements for the development of primary health care exist, considerable problems remain, not least in the inner-city areas of the conurbations and on the peripheral public housing estates.[24] In these areas the gap between the health experience of different social classes has continued to increase.

In particular, there is a general lack of what might be called the epidemiological or population view of primary health care as espoused by Tudor Hart and Kark, and there is a great need for the injection of epidemiological skills into the normal functioning of primary health care teams.[31,32] The development of appropriate information systems based on the age-sex register, probably supplemented by intermittent sample surveys of the practice population to assess risk factors and answer specific questions, will be a necessary step in providing the conceptual framework for a rational and comprehensive approach to preventive medicine and health promotion.

However, in British general practice there is little to indicate that doctors as prime movers are ready for primary health as opposed to primary medical care.

When it comes to the kind of community-development linkage with primary health care which is to be found in non-industrial countries and which should be regarded as just as important in, for example, inner-city areas of the United Kingdom, there is nothing to suggest that general practitioners regard this kind of work as having anything to do with them.

Community participation and intersectoral action

The elements of the WHO Ottawa Charter, which focus on the creation of environments which are supportive to health and on the enabling of communities through the development of personal skills and health advocacy, are in a real sense a challenge to professional practice as it is found throughout the world.[33] Professional power and prestige is contingent upon the acquisition of specific knowledge and skills which are exchanged for money in return for a service; the autonomy of the professional in the market is central as is his or her freedom to refuse a client. There is no commitment either to population coverage or to sharing power and demystifying knowledge. In this sense, there is a real conflict between the clinical model based on individual transactions and the public health model based on a social context with entire communities. The consequence of this is that there is a great deal of rhetoric about public participation but a marked unwillingness to really engage in the processes which would bring it about. Most professionals and welfare bureaucracies function only on the lower half of Arnstein's ladder of citizen participation:[34]

Citizen control
Delegated power
Partnership
Placation
Consultation
Informing
Therapy
Manipulation

Yet in wishing for people to take increased responsibility for their own health it is necessary to recognize the close relationship between risk-taking behaviour and lack of empowerment.[35]

Notes

1. Kickbusch, I. (1986) 'Health promotion strategies for action', *Canadian Journal of Public Health*, **77**(5), 321–6.

2. McKeown, T. (1976) *The Role of Medicine—Dream, Mirage or Nemesis*, Nuffield Provincial Hospitals Trust, London.

3. Kaye, T. (1829) *The Stranger in Liverpool*, T. Kaye, Liverpool.

4. Chave, S.P.W. (1984) 'Duncan of Liverpool—and some lessons for today', *Community Medicine*, **6**, 61–71.

5. Kearns, G. (1986) 'Private property and public health reform in England 1830–70', *Social Service and Medicine*, **26**(1), 187–99.

6. Cartwright, F.F. (1977) *A Social History of Medicine*, Longman, London.

7. Fraser, W.M. (1947) *Duncan of Liverpool*, Hamish Hamilton, London.

8. Ashton, J.R. (1979) 'Poverty and health in Britain today', *Public Health*, **93**, 89–94.

9. Gobder, G.E. (1986) 'Medical officers of health and health services', *Community Medicine*, **8**(1), 1–14.

10. Townsend, P. and Davidson, N. (1980) *Inequalities in Health—The Black Report*, Penguin, Harmondsworth.

11. Whitehead, M. (1987) *The Health Divide—Inequalities in Health*, Health Education Council, London.

12. Illich, I. (1975) *Medical Nemesis—The Expropriation of Health*, Calder and Boyars, London.

13. Lalonde, M. (1974) *A New Perspective on the Health of Canadians*, Ministry of Supply and Services.

14. Doyal, L. (1981) *The Political Economy of Health*, Pluto Press, London.

15. Navarro, V. (1976) *Medicine under Capitalism*, Croom Helm, London.

16. Milio, N. (1986) *Promoting Health through Public Policy*, Canadian Public Health Association, Ottawa, Canada.

17. St George, D. and Draper, P. (1981) 'A health policy for Europe', *The Lancet*, **ii**, 463–5.

18. Department of Health Education and Welfare (1979) *Healthy People*, The Surgeon General's report on Health Promotion and Disease Prevention. DHEW Publications, Washington, D.C.

19. HMSO (1976) *Prevention and Health: everybody's business*. A reassessment of public and personal health. HMSO, London.

20. Neumann, S. (1847) *Die Offentliches Gesundeheitstflege und das Eigenthum*, Berlin. Quoted in H. Sigerist op. cit.

21. Beveridge, Sir W. (1942) *Social Insurance and Allied Services*, Cmnd. **6404**, **6405**. HMSO, London.

22. Department of Health and Social Security (1976) *Priorities for Health and Social Service in England*, HMSO, London.

23. Department of Health and Social Security (1977) *The Way Forward—Priorities in the Health and Social Services*, HMSO, London.

24. Merrison, A. (1979) *Royal Commission on the National Health Service*, HMSO, London.

25. Department of Health and Social Security (1987) *Promoting Better Health—The Government Programme for Improving Primary Health Care*, Cmnd. **249**, HMSO, London.

26. Acheson, E.D. (1988) *On the State of the Public Health*, The Fourth Duncan Lecture.

27. The Acheson Report (1988) *Public Health in England*, The Report of the Committee of Enquiry into the future development of the Public Health Function, Cmnd. **289**, HMSO, London.

28. Epp, J. (1986) 'Achieving health for all: A framework for health promotion', *Canadian Journal of Public Health*, **77**(6), 393–424.

29. Vuori, H. (1981) 'Primary health care in industrialized countries'. In *Die Allgemeinpraxix; Das Zentrum der Artzlichen, Grundverorgung Gottleib Duttwierer*—Institut Ruschlikon, Zurich, pp. 83–111.

30. Hellberg, H. (1987) 'Health for all and primary health care in Europe', *Public Health*, **101**, 151–7.

31. Tudor Hart, J. (1981) 'A new kind of doctor', *Journal of the Royal Society of Medicine*, **74**, 871–83.

32. Kark, S.L. (1981) *The Practice of Community Orientated Primary Health Care*, Appleton, Century, Crofts, New York.

33. Chambers, R. (1983) *Rural Development—Putting the Last First*, Longman, London.

34. Arnstein, S. (1969) 'A ladder of public participation'. *Journal of the American Institute of Planners*, Quoted in N. Wates and C. Knevitt (1987) *Community Architecture*, Penguin Books, London.

35. Ashton, J. (1983) 'Risk assessment', *British Medical Journal*, **286**, 1843.

17

Primary Health Care in England*

NHSME

Primary health care services in England are among the most advanced in the world. About 50,000 (whole-time equivalent) nurses work in primary health care, and the presence in the community of such a large and highly skilled nursing workforce is unique. Most of them are district nurses, practice nurses, health visitors, school nurses, and community psychiatric nurses. The number of contacts they make with patients and clients—many in their homes—runs into tens of millions.

Collectively, their work takes in not only care and treatment of people with acute or long-term illness but also health promotion and illness prevention. It includes health surveillance, accident prevention, child protection, health education, family planning and special needs services.

Primary health care offers the first point of contact for people seeking advice, support and treatment. It allows, and encourages, people to participate in the planning, organisation and management of their own health care at home, school, work and in the GP practice. It provides long-term and continuing care. And it is a major force for improvement in the health of communities. A comprehensive primary health care system can prevent over-use of hospital services and thus help to contain costs.

Primary health care defined

The best, if rather elaborate, definition of primary health care has come from the World Health Organisation. The WHO describes primary health care as 'essential care based on practical, scientifically sound and acceptable methods and technology, made universally available to individuals and families in the community through their full participation and at a cost the community and country can afford and maintain at every stage of their development, in the spirit of self-reliance and self-determination'.

The definition goes on to say that primary health care forms 'an integral part both of the country's health system, of which it is the central function and main focus, and of the overall social and economic development of this country. It is the first level of

*This is an abridged version of NHSME (1993) *Nursing in Primary Health Care. New World, New Opportunities*, Leeds, NHS Management Executive, pp. 6–8.

contact for individuals, the family and the community with the national health system, bringing health care as close as possible to where people live and work, and provides promotive, preventive, curative and rehabilitative services accordingly'.

Primary health care is at its most effective when integrated with other health care services—including, of course, hospitals—and when it works in close collaboration with local social, welfare, environmental, and education systems—for example, through 'healthy alliances'.

Cardinal principles

Primary health care is highly professional and intensely personal. People are entitled to expect:

- Safe, effective clinical practice;
- Accessible and appropriate local services;
- Access to 'named' professional practitioners, including 'named nurses';
- Services that can overcome barriers of language, discrimination and deprivation;
- Twenty-four hour cover;
- Confidentiality at all times;
- Continuity, with a minimum number of individuals involved;
- A range of treatment choices and options to meet their health needs;
- Value for money;
- Clarity of provision without confusion over who does what;
- The ability to be involved in decision-making about their care and to be informed about the range of choices available to them;
- Services that work well together and with other agencies.

These expectations can readily be translated into the cardinal principles that should underpin primary health care and give a common focus for the different professions in defining their service and professional objectives.

Fresh impetus

Despite the intrinsic importance of primary health care, it was not until the late 1980s that it began to receive more than fitful policy attention. Until then, it lacked the high profile and 'clout' of the acute hospital sector, both managerially and politically. In spite of major reports related to primary health care—notably *Promoting Better Health*—political debate nearly always focused on acute hospitals, emergency services, waiting lists and life-or-death issues.

Although that is still largely the case, the climate began to change with the introduction of the new contract for GPs and the enhanced role of FHSAs with responsibilities for planning primary health care. The emergence of NHS trusts and the introduction of GP fundholding, together with the development of joint community care plans and new arrangements for supporting people in the community as a result of the NHS and Community Care Act 1990, added fresh and tangible impetus to the development of services.

18

How Do We Value Our Children Today? As Reflected by Children's Health, Health Care and Policy*

ZARRINA KURTZ and JOHN TOMLINSON

Summary

The importance of children in their own right and of their healthy development for the health of society, have been affirmed at an international level by the United Nations Convention on the Rights of the Child in 1989 and by the Children Act 1989 in the United Kingdom. In the UK fifteen years ago, the report of the Court Committee set out a framework for Child Health Services based on the same recognition of the value of children. This paper describes how in spite of the far-reaching recommendations made by the Court Committee, the health of children in this country is far from satisfactory; how health policy and services have failed to meet their health care needs; and how other recent legislation such as the NHS and Community Care Act may well lead to further difficulties in working for the best interests of the child.

Introduction

There are inherent problems in describing the value we give to children in terms of their health because our concepts of both health and childhood change, often independently. However, health is profoundly affected by socio-economic conditions and in this way clearly reflects the values of society. This has not been as fully acknowledged as has the influence of population health on the national economy.

Concepts of health and childhood

Health came to be more highly valued as survival beyond infancy became assured and quality of life, which is included in the broadest definition of health as given by the

*This is an article first published in *Children and Society*, Vol. 5, No. 3, pp. 207–224.

World Health Organisation (WHO, 1946), is increasingly valued as survival into adulthood and old age becomes assured. When we examine children's experience in the light of these ideas about health, it may be seen to what extent we undervalue them or let them down.

Ideas about health are relative over time and at any one time, in different circumstances. If we look back at children's lives in the middle of the last century, there is clear evidence that many suffered severe ill-health and appalling living conditions (Scriven Report in Hoyles, 1979). Over this same period, Dickens spent a lifetime campaigning for improvement in the living conditions and treatment of children but had little regard for what doctors could do (Kosky, 1989). A third of children died before the end of childhood. Survival was the key concern and health was largely taken for granted unless it meant that no contribution could be made to the family income. There was a widespread feeling of indifference towards the fragile childhood that was the chief feature of the demography of the period. But as it became less likely that children would die in infancy, ideas about childhood changed. There was a 'connection between the progress of the concept of childhood and the progress of hygiene, between concern for the child and concern for his health' (Aries, 1973). The health and education of middle class children had already become a prime concern of parents by the end of the eighteenth century. Aries argues that the concept of a long childhood was linked to the success of educational institutions and how, because of their limited opportunities for schooling, the concept of a brief childhood lasted for a long time in the lower classes.

The introduction of compulsory schooling in Britain in the nineteenth century revealed the extent of malnutrition and physical defects for the first time. Voluntary bodies and local education boards responded by providing meals and milk at school. But the spur to the state taking some responsibility for the health of children came when it was found that a high proportion of between 40–60 per cent of men enlisting for the South African War were unfit for service; thus a school medical service was introduced in 1907 to carry out health inspections on all children and later to ensure treatment. Seventy years later, the Court Committee, the only national group ever appointed to review and make recommendations about child health services, published its report, making the following statement in the Introduction:

> In the last two or three generations we have come to realise how precious is our inheritance of children and also to recognise their needs as being different from those of adults. At one time children were dressed in adult clothes, scaled down to size, which seemed to reflect an attitude that they were in a sense retarded adults. Childhood was thought of as an inadequate and incomplete form of the adult state. By contrast we have become increasingly aware of childhood as a separate state, as a period of human experience in its own right. And more important still, we have come to realise the extent to which experience in childhood determines the adult outcome (DHSS, 1976)

Changing social constructs of childhood

The Court Report of 1976 continued its description of our view of childhood:

> It is the mark of the human species that our young are born incomparably more 'immature' than the young of other species. Man is the only species which has gone all-out for general immaturity and open mindness: they are his particular strategies for development. The human baby and child faces a long period of development and dependence during which he develops the fundamental human attributes of speech, thought, self-consciousness and reflection. During these stages the child is a biological organism with biological propensities which needs constant inter-action with his environment, especially the adults around him so that he can learn in innumerable ways and emerge a social as well as an individual being. As the human child grows he is in many important ways literally being created by the slowly forming imprint of experience, the essential tension between the biological and the social, hereditary and environmental influences.

That statement remains a robust account of the modern view of childhood. As a scientific construct, childhood is seen as a biological, psychological and social requirement for adequate development. As a social construct, in any given generation and for any individual, that 'requirement' is subject to necessity, and is more or less realised, distorted or frustrated by contingent realities.

A powerful restatement is given with the perspective of the social historian by Steedman in her biography of Margaret MacMillan (Steedman, 1990, p. 64):

> Developments in scientific thought in the nineteenth century showed that childhood was a stage of growth and development common to all of us, abandoned and left behind, but at the same time a core of the individual's psychic life, always immanent, waiting there to be drawn on in various ways . . . human beings located within time by their own history of personal growth.

The project of health, education and social services in their work with families and individuals is to bring the actualised nearer to the possible. And, because childhood is fundamental, the rearing of the young and the quality and philosophy of the services available to the family, become a focus of civilised concern.

Children represent our investment in the future of our society. Some of the writing of the 1980s has argued that we value children less because we have less confidence in our future, and especially in the values of western society. Other comment points to the way in which the electronic gadgetry of our age, by creating the 'global village', brings the adult world and its images and actions directly to the eyes and minds of children, abbreviating or removing childhood in the process (Somerville, 1982; Suranky, 1982; Postman, 1983). It is all the more necessary therefore that the generation who have been given insight into the essentials of childhood should not betray it. This paper examines the current balance sheet—for there is much to the credit side also—and suggests further steps.

Current policies for children and health care

In the 15 years since the Court Committee received evidence, there have been rapid and far-reaching developments in our understanding of health and knowledge about disease, in therapeutic methods and in medical and allied health services, as well as in the possibilities and problems of children's lives. The underlying ethos of the Court Committee expressed in the passage quoted from the Introduction, has been reinforced in this country by the Children Act (1989) which embodies the view of the child as 'subject' as opposed to 'object' (Freeman, 1987–88). The Children Act 'provides a single consistent statement of the law about caring for, bringing up and protecting children' which up to then 'had been fragmented across the statute book' (DoH, 1989). The Act seeks primarily to support parents, and takes:

> . . . as the fundamental task of parenthood, the duty to care for the child and to raise him to moral, physical and emotional health. The Act seeks to strike a balance between the need to recognise the child as an independent person and to ensure that his views are fully taken into account, and the risk of casting on him the burden of resolving problems caused by his parents or requiring him to choose between them . . . New duties are placed upon local authorities to promote the upbringing of children in need by their families so far as is consistent with their welfare. 'Children in need' covers children who need services to secure a reasonable standard of health and development and includes children who are disabled (DoH, 1989).

Children's health is herein expressed as the outcome of the duty of parents and, if necessary, the state in caring for children. However, there is tension between this clear statement and national policy in other areas, notably in relation to mothers' employment. Social and fiscal policies that have led to the present level and pattern of paid work outside the home among mothers of young children in the UK give rise to difficulties when day care facilities and pre-school education are inadequate, and create greater conflict for parents as more responsibility and involvement in their children's health care is encouraged (Moss, 1990).

There have also been developments along the lines recommended by the Court Committee directly in the field of health care: exemplified by the further specialisation within children's medicine of community paediatrics, by the setting up of multidisciplinary teams, by the increasing involvement of general practitioners in preventive aspects of care, and by projects that increase the participation of parents in the health care of their children. But crucial elements such as a national Children's Committee, needed to lead and support the way forward envisaged by the Court Committee, have been neither sustained nor initiated—demonstrating lack of political will and resulting in the lack of a strategic approach. Children have not been a focus of policy. It is well recognised that in spite of a great deal of well meaning effort, service delivery remains largely fragmented, patchy and uncoordinated (NCB, 1987). The reorganisation of the National Health Service as an internal market following the NHS and Community Care Act (1990) now threatens further serious difficulties, particularly for the delivery of integrated services, for multidisciplinary work, and for the exercise of true parental choice (Woodroffe and Kurtz, 1989). In addition, the Act makes explicit for the first time its basis in a different understanding from that upon which the National Health Service Act 1946 was based: that access to free health care would result in health for all. It is now acknowledged that this has not happened and that it cannot be guaranteed by the health service. By redrawing boundaries between NHS and local authority responsibilities for health care, the NHS and Community Care Act makes a clear distinction between health care and medical care. It remains to be seen whether the contribution of other agencies to health can be brought together more satisfactorily in the new climate created by legislation in the UK, in line with the World Health Organisation statement that the 'realisation of health requires the action of many other social and economic sectors in addition to the health sector' (WHO, 1978). Once again, if policies specifically for health are not developed jointly with policy in other fields at national and local level, we will certainly fail to 'affirm health as a fundamental human right' (WHO, 1978).

At international level, recognition of the needs of children linked firmly to their health has come to the forefront, as exemplified by the UN Convention on the Rights of the Child which came into force in September 1990. The Convention has been ratified so far by 20 countries and the United Kingdom Government has declared its intention to do so. At the same time UNICEF has expressed anxiety that over the last 10 or 15 years the rate of improvement in health of children in industrialised countries has been slowing down and their well-being has possibly even been deteriorating, and that:

> . . . new and subtler forms of deprivation may have been caused by the profound changes occurring over the last forty years in labour markets, in environmental conditions, in family structure, in internal and international migration, in the organisation of society and in other aspects of life.

Because of this, UNICEF commissioned a major review of child deprivation in the industrialised countries, and the results for the United Kingdom (one of eight countries studied in depth) have recently been published (Bradshaw, 1990). Bradshaw discusses the difficulties in defining deprivation and poverty but records that 3.5 million or 28.6 per cent of all children in the UK were living in families with incomes around the supplementary benefit level in 1985—an increase of 49 per cent from 1979. Further, a report published by the European Commission shows that in 1985, Britain was the second poorest of the 12 member states, and that the proportion of children below the poverty line increased from one in five in 1980 to nearly one in four in 1985 (Dillner, 1991).

Health, properly defined, is probably the most valid measure of the sum effect of expression of the values of a society—especially in developed countries where adequate resources are available and where there is choice in how they are deployed. However, health as a measure of value can only be discussed in relative terms; we speak of 'more' or 'less' and how to 'maximise' it (Griffin, 1986). The UK spends a lower proportion of gross national product on health services than the United States and than other European countries at comparable stages of development (Office of Health Economics, personal communication, 1991) (Table 18.1). The way in which NHS resources are distributed according to age group also makes a statement about relative value which

Table 18.1 Proportion of GNP spent on health services in 1988: selected countries

	%
United States	11.2
West Germany	9.2
Sweden	9.2
France	8.0
Switzerland	7.4
Italy	6.7
United Kingdom	5.7

Source: Office of Health Economics

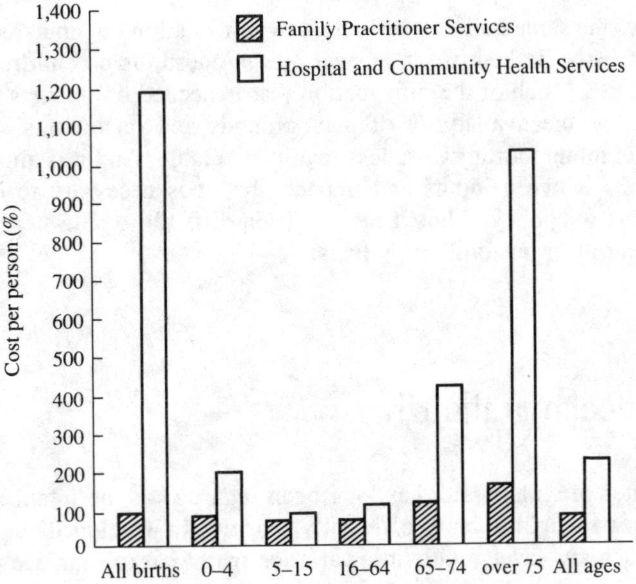

Note – All figures relate to gross current expenditure

Figure 18.1 NHS expenditure by age group, England 1986/87

can be questioned. Significant resources are devoted to the time around birth but children up to the age of 16 who make up 20 per cent of the population, receive disproportionately fewer resources than the elderly, with the over-65s forming 15 per cent of the population (Figure 18.1). It is however, difficult to describe accurately the resources used for child health because of the contribution made by many disciplines and agencies, with separate management arrangements for different services and different groups of children. In addition, information for monitoring the use of and need for health services for children as distinct from other groups, as well as data with which to measure their health status, is poorly developed. This was highlighted in a section on children's health in the report of the Chief Medical Officer in 1988 (DoH, 1989).

Table 18.2 Mortality of male children aged under 16: rates per 100,000 population by age and social class: England and Wales, 1979–80, 1982–83

Social class	Stillbirths	Infant	1–15
I	483	866	25
II	558	964	24
III Non-manual	564	1008	26
III Manual	715	1152	32
IV	847	1510	38
V	919	1814	56
I-V Ratio	1.90	2.09	2.25

Source: OPCS

Bradshaw makes the same point, describing how information on inputs, such as amount of child benefit, is of limited use in answering the questions on children's well-being posed by UNICEF. Much of the information that is needed on impacts such as school enrolment rates or the availability of play grounds and on outputs such as school performance and infant mortality—is less readily available. And it is almost impossible to draw the links between inputs and impacts that it is necessary to do in order to provide the focus for policy. Thus it has not been difficult to side-step attention from much that is central in our children's lives.

Children's health in the UK

The best indicator of child health has long been regarded as the infant mortality rate, although it is now thought to be insufficiently sensitive in developed countries because it has reached such low levels, with little variation from year to year. However, the rate in the United Kingdom has declined more slowly than in some other countries and, with the 1990 figure at 8.4 deaths per thousand live births, is still high in comparison with the latest available figures for France (7.9 in 1986), Italy (8.1 in 1985), Sweden (5.9 in 1986), Hong Kong (7) and Japan (4) (UNICEF, 1991). There are also significant variations in this country between district health authorities, social classes, and ethnic groups. Higher mortality at all ages in childhood is found in the less advantaged social classes IV and V (Table 18.2). Thus comparative infant mortality rates can still usefully draw attention to differences in child health within our own society and in similar groups between societies.

Within the first year of life, mortality at different ages has shown different rates of change. Because these changes can be attributed to particular causes, the contribution made by socio-economic factors and by other factors such as medical care can be identified. Stillbirths and deaths in the first week of life (perinatal mortality) have declined steadily in England and Wales with a 45 per cent reduction between 1950 and 1973, of which about a quarter was associated with shifts in maternal age, parity and

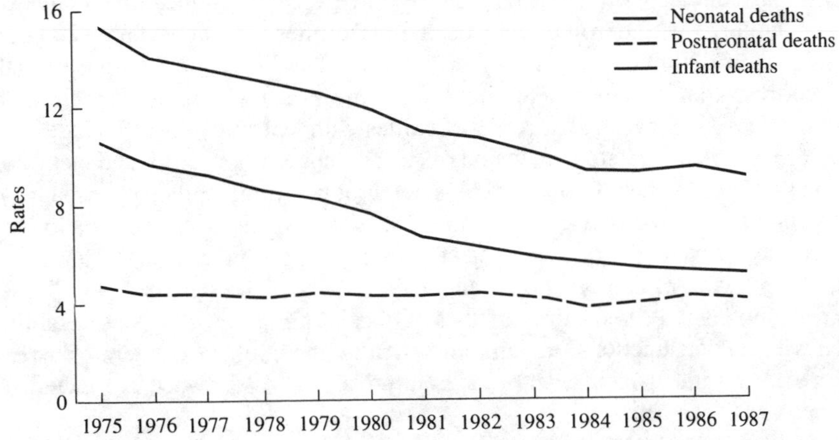

Source: From OPCS SERIES DH 3 no 21. Mortality statistics 1987 Perinatal and Infant: Social and biological factors, England and Wales (p7). HMSO, London: 1990

Figure 18.2 Infant mortality rates, 1975–1987, England and Wales

social class (Pharoah, 1986). Neonatal mortality (deaths between the first and the 27th day) is largely determined by birthweight, and has also shown remarkable falls in all developed countries, particularly since the 1970s (Figure 18.2). This is likely to be chiefly because medicine has put a great deal of effort and resources into special and intensive care for low birthweight babies which has resulted in marked improvement in survival, even of babies with very low birthweights. However, there is now clear evidence that the success in keeping alive ever more tiny and premature babies has led to an increase in conditions such as cerebral palsy in the survivors (Pharoah *et al.*, 1990). Birthweight is closely associated with social class and this probably largely accounts for the differences in neonatal mortality between the social classes. In the early part of the century, postneonatal mortality (28 to 364 day deaths) exceeded neonatal mortality, and because it is far more influenced by social than medical factors, contributed the major proportion of the improvement in overall infant mortality. The rate of fall has flattened out in recent years. In the United States, improvement in postneonatal mortality coincided with the federal 'Great Society' legislation of the 1960s, particularly health programmes for the poor such as Children and Youth projects and the Maternal and Infant Care programmes. There was a simultaneous narrowing of the postneonatal mortality differential between whites and blacks. These unexpected deaths have so far been shown to be more closely linked with social and parental factors than with failures in medical care, and it has been possible to show some improvement in rates through local projects offering special support to mothers who have had a previous unexpected infant death or with a baby known to be particularly vulnerable (Pharoah, 1986). Since funding for these programmes has been cut, improvement in postneonatal mortality has slowed, and there remain marked differences in the rate between whites and blacks (Hogue *et al.*, 1989).

Thus, improved socio-economic conditions have led to lower death rates in children; advances in medical technology and medical care have contributed and have also made possible survival into adulthood of increasing numbers of children with chronic disease, disability and handicap who would formerly have died in infancy. Estimates of the number of children with chronic illnesses and disabilities vary between 2–20 per cent, depending upon definition and the ages included. The Warnock Committee (DHSS, 1978) reported that two per cent of children have a continuing need for special education provision because of severe difficulties with learning. These include children with severe problems related to vision, hearing, speech, physical and neurological function associated with conditions such as cerebral palsy and epilepsy, and to psychological problems. A recent national survey of disability in Great Britain found disabilities likely to have a significant effect on carrying out normal everyday activities in over 3.8 per cent of 5–9 year-olds and 3.5 per cent of 10–15 year-olds (Bone and Meltzer, 1989). Nearly two-thirds of these children had more than one disability. If children with milder functional impairments such as uncomplicated asthma, correctable visual or hearing impairments, and moderate emotional disturbance are included, the prevalence is 20 per cent.

Chronic illness, disability and handicap are key features in the pattern of health of children in Great Britain today. The part played by medicine in the prevention and management of these conditions reveals mixed messages about how we value children. The management of childhood cancer and cerebral palsy offer two examples. Twenty years ago, cure was contemplated for less than a quarter of all children who developed malignant disease. The overall cure rate for childhood cancer in the United Kindom is now over 60 per cent and for some groups more than 90 per cent (Morris-Jones and Craft, 1990), as illustrated by the dramatic improvement in survival for children with acute lymphocytic leukaemia (Figure 18.3). However, long-term follow-up studies have recently shown that many children have significant problems resulting from their successful treatment. These include renal and cardiovascular dysfunction, problems with fertility, secondary tumours, neuropsychological sequelae and social problems. As one in 600 children develop cancer before their 15th birthday, by the year 2000 at least one in 1000 young adults will have been cured of cancer as a child. In addition to longer term sequelae, during the period of treatment the child's immunity is compromised leading to greater risk from infections such as measles. Also, the treatment itself can often hardly be endured. The *British Medical Journal* recently published an account by a 14 year-old girl of the time she underwent chemotherapy two years previously. She wrote of her feelings of isolation and terror each time she went for treatment:

> When that vile yellow toxin was linked to my arm I could make myself sick by just watching it ooze down the tube and into my body . . . . On that table is the only time I can truly say that if I could have stood up I would have killed myself. The feeling of utter hopelessness, frustration, and boredom led to a desperation I never, ever want to experience again.

She also described how simple measures, such as a video to help distract her during the treatment process and attention paid to the special needs of older children in the way the department was run, would have helped enormously (Anonymous, 1990).

Secondly, follow-up of more than 700 children with cerebral palsy born between 1970 and 1979 in the South East Thames Region or resident in the Region at the time

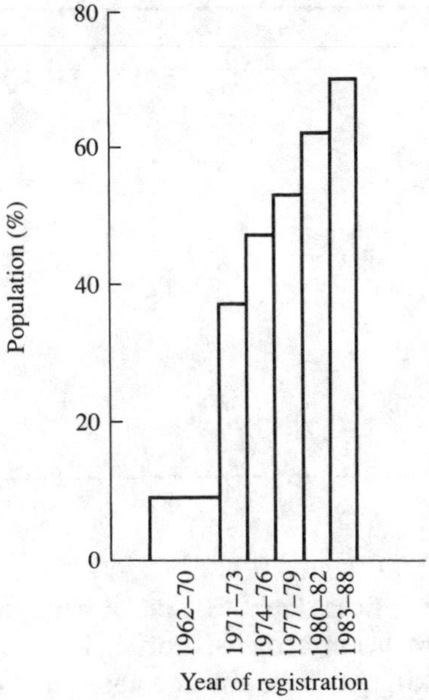

Source: From Cancer research campaign *BMJ* 1990:**300**:1673

Figure 18.3 Five year survival of children under 15 years of age with acute lymphocytic leukaemia by year of registration

of ascertainment, has shown that 90 per cent of the children, now aged between 10 and 20 years old, are still alive (Evans *et al.*, 1990). While acknowledging that the effectiveness of many forms of treatment to improve the quality of life for these children is under review, it was found that some children were not receiving even the most basic treatment—for example, one session per week with a physiotherapist for a child with mobility problems. The authors of this study also acknowledge that further research may not necessarily produce clear financial justification for greater expenditure on treatment programmes, but they make a plea to those responsible for health care planning that appropriate weight to be given to indices of quality of life of the patient and his or her family when assessing both the short and long-term effectiveness and value of treatment.

These aspects are highlighted by the finding that 65 per cent of children with other disabilities had psychological disorders, which were the most common disability found overall (in 2.1% of children) in the National Disability Survey. There has been an increase in prevalence of depression, suicide and attempted suicide in children, and of a number of other conditions such as eating disorders including both obesity and anorexia (Graham, 1986). Accidental injury causes a great deal of morbidity and is responsible for about 50 per cent of deaths in children aged 5–19. Non-accidental injury and child neglect are now more readily and widely recognised. Although existing population data cannot be used to assess trends, the National Society for the Prevention of Cruelty to Children registers indicate a substantial rise in the number of cases (34%

Table 18.3 Trends in the percentage of persons who reported

	1972	1987
Long standing illness		
aged 0–4	4	10
5–15	8	17
Limiting long standing illness		
aged 0–4	2	3
5–15	4	8
Restricted activity		
aged 0–4	6	2
5–15	6	14

Source: General Household Survey

in 1986) (Creighton, 1988). There is little doubt that racial harassment is the cause of a great deal of distress and has now been recognised officially as an issue for schools (Troyna and Hatcher, 1990). Smoking, and the use and abuse of alcohol, solvents and other drugs are now an established part of the lives of many children and this may tell us something about the way in which children and young people value themselves. Furthermore, according to the General Household Survey (OPCS, 1989), levels of self-reported long-standing illness have risen in 5–15 year-olds, as for all other ages since the early 1970s (Table 18.3).

Social deprivation and health

Greater risks to health are found among disadvantaged children; living in crowded and poor quality housing, in homeless families, with a lone parent, and with parents in unskilled occupations, who are poor, or unemployed. Considerable numbers of children live in these situations in the United Kingdom, and the report for UNICEF presents the best available national data. Children living in these situations have higher rates than other children of infant mortality, child abuse, infectious diseases, impaired growth, dental disease, respiratory conditions, accidents, and behaviour and emotional disorders. Families with these health risks tend to be concentrated in inner city districts, where there are also higher proportions from ethnic minority backgrounds who have specific health problems such as tuberculosis and sickle cell disorders. The concentration of multiple deprivation that can be found in inner city districts can be illustrated with data for inner London. Here, 43 per cent of households rent from the local authority in contrast to 27 per cent more generally in the south-east of England; the quality of housing is often poor, and there are more persons to a room with a greater lack of basic amenities such as a bath or shower than in any other urban area. The mobility of families with young children is higher in inner city districts than elsewhere (up to 15% of families moving at least once in a year); the number of families considered to be homeless in London doubled to over 28,000 between 1978 and 1987 (Figure 18.4). Data are available for over a quarter of a million children attending Inner London Education Authority schools in 1988–9 (ILEA, 1989) (Table 18.4). In comparison with national rates, high proportions came from families where there was no wage earner, where the father was in a semi- or un-skilled occupation, from single parent families, and with parents receiving Income Support following the 1986 Social Security Act and thus were eligible for free school meals. Over half the pupils came from a diversity of ethnic backgrounds other than English, Scottish or Welsh, and about 15 per cent were not fluent in English.

In areas such as inner London where children and families with greater risks to health are concentrated, the shortfall between their needs for health care and the type and level of services available is particularly great. The workload in general practice is high and so are the costs of good quality premises and local housing, resulting in greater use of lock-up surgeries and deputising services. Continuity of care is difficult. Many of the homeless or highly mobile families do not register with a GP; records often cannot follow patients quickly enough to ensure satisfactory preventive care; and many depend on the A&E department of the local hospital for primary care. There are in addition, special complexities in delivering satisfactory care to families of different ethnic backgrounds. The health service has failed so far to adapt to the difficulties, particularly in delivering preventive care to children in these situations. This is shown in our national rates for immunisation which still fall short of the 90 per cent target set for this year by the European Region of the World Health Organisation: the latest figures for England and Wales for 1988–89 show that the average proportion of two year-olds with a completed course of immunisation against polio, diphtheria and tetanus was 87 per cent, against whooping cough was 75 per cent, and against measles was 80 per cent (Figure 18.5). These average figures are pulled down by the much lower rates in some districts: in inner London districts comparable average rates were 76, 68 and 67 per cent (DoH Immunisation 'Cover', 1990).

Routinely collected national statistics suggest that children over the age of five are the healthiest age group in the population because of their comparatively low mortality rates, hospital admission rates, and consultation rates in general practice. However, these offer a largely incomplete picture of health status and health problems because the data are mainly based upon the use of services and may be misleading because, for example, deprived families are known to have a different pattern of service use. However, it is clear from information that we now have, some of which is discussed here, that large numbers of children in the United Kingdom today are living lives as painful and difficult in relation to their peers as those of the children for whom Dickens was campaigning 150 years ago. Major advances in medicine and in health care have enabled many diseases to be overcome, but expectations about length of life and quality of life have risen. The types of services available often do not match what we have learned about the causes and likely remedies for the actual health problems of children today.

Certain types of health care for children have little difficulty in attracting resources, as shown by the encouragingly large amount (£54 million) raised in the recent Wishing Well appeal for the rebuilding of Great Ormond Street Hospital. Financing projects that focus on the promotion of health, prevention of disease, and long-term management of chronic conditions, has proved to be more difficult. A Dutch foundation funded the

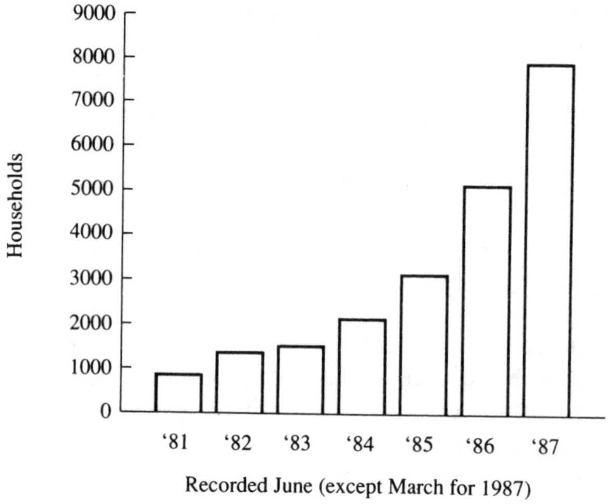

Figure 18.4 Bed and Breakfast in London

Table 18.4 Socio-economic characteristics of children in ILEA schools in 1988–1989

Pupils	Pupils in primary & Secondary Schools n=260,658 %	National figures %	
In families with no wage earner	24.4	8.4	*1
With father in semi-unskilled manual occupation	23.1	16.7	*2
In single parent families	28.7	14.4	*3
Eligible for free school meals	47.6	12.4	*4
From England, Scotland, Wales	48.8	89.9	*5

*
1 Children with an unemployed head of family (Child Poverty Action Group)
2 OPCS Series GHS no 17. General Household Survey 1987 (1989, HMSO)
3 Portion of families with dependent children headed by lone parents (CSO, Social trends 20; 1990, HMSO)
4 School Meals Census, 1988
5 White children aged 0–15 in Great Britain (CSO, Social Trends 20; 1990, HMSO)

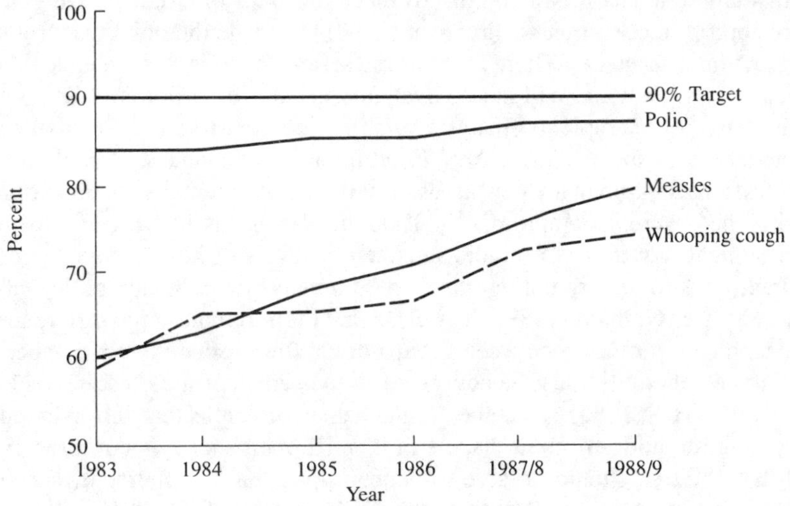

Figure 18.5 Immunisation uptake rate, England, 1983–89

most ambitious project of this nature in this country, the Bristol Child Development Project (Barker and Anderson, 1988). This has shown a number of positive effects including improvements in child nutrition and reduced rates of child abuse, through the use of specially trained health visitors dedicated to working with parents of first children. Funding of other projects such as the Riverside Project in Newcastle (Pearson, 1981), has rarely been continued after the initial development phase. Voluntary organisations frequently undertake the pioneering work, such as suggestions for standards for an acceptable quality of health care services for children, recently published by the National Association for the Welfare of Children in Hospital (Hogg and Rodin, 1989). Lay and voluntary groups also often provide fundamental services such as interpreters and counselling for parents and education for teachers, in particular for children with particular conditions such as sickle cell disorders.

These are indications that policy and legislation in this country are developing in a number of promising ways for children's health. There is a welcome move towards integration of general practitioner and health authority services because family health services authorities have been made accountable to regional health authorities, and the General Practitioner (GP) Contract also provides incentives for more preventive work to be carried out by the primary health care team. However, in linking payments to GPs to targets, for immunisation uptake for example, there is a danger that little effort will be put into improving uptake in situations such as inner city districts where targets are unlikely to be reached. Also, proposals that a greater proportion of GP salaries should come out of capitation fees means that extra financial pressure will be felt in deprived localities where small list sizes are essential for the provision of good quality care. The specification and agreement of contracts between purchasers and providers of health care must include measures of standards of quality of care but standards have not been set for the majority of conditions and situations. The requirement to audit health care in relation to standards as well as to health outcomes does provide real opportunities to make sure that children as a group and disadvantaged groups of children, are given priority and are appropriately targeted. Freeman (1990) has made the point that 'rights are meaningless without services'. There remains the serious concern that adequate and appropriate resources are not and will not be available to care for children in line with the agreed standards. For example, a greater availability of expert help is necessary to fulfil the requirements of the Children Act. In addition, if adequate and continuing training for professionals in the many new areas of work is not ensured, good intentions and practice may be severely compromised. Thought also needs to be given to the quality of environment required to promote satisfactory levels of health and development in children, and to incorporating these requirements into health policy and standards in health care (Graham, 1989). It is clear that there remain large differences in health and health care provision between groups of children reflecting other aspects of deprivation. Issues of equity must be addressed in the same spirit as recommended for Health for All (WHO, 1985). And the 'fundamental principle that the lives and normal development of children should have "first call" upon society's concerns and capacities and that children should be able to depend upon that commitment in good times and bad' (Convention on the Rights of the Child in UNICEF, 1991) will have to be incorporated unequivocally into health care policy and practice if our children and their health are to be given the value they deserve.

References

Aries, P. (1973) *Centuries of Childhood*, Penguin.

Anonymous (1990) 'Easing a childhood nightmare: personal view', *British Medical Journal*, **301**, p. 244.

Barker, W. and Anderson, R. (1988) *The Child Development Programme: An Evaluation of Process and Outcome*, Early Childhood Development Unit, University of Bristol.

Bone, M. and Meltzer, H. (1989) *The Prevalence of Disability Among Children*, OPCS Surveys of Disability in Great Britain, Report 3. London, HMSO.

Bradshaw, J. (1990) *Child Poverty and Deprivation in the UK*, London, National Children's Bureau for UNICEF.

Creighton, S.J. (1988) 'The incidence of child abuse and neglect', in Browne, K., Davies, C. and Stratton, P. (eds.) *Early Prediction and Prevention of Child Abuse*, London, Wiley.

Department of Education and Science and Welsh Office (1978) *Special Educational Needs. Report of the Committee of Enquiry into the Education of Handicapped Children and Young People* (Chair, HM Warnock), London, HMSO.

Department of Health and Social Security, Department of Education and Science, and Welsh Office (1976) *Fit for the Future: Report of the Committee on Child Health Services* (Chair: Professor Donald Court), London, HMSO.

Department of Health (1989) *An Introduction to The Children Act 1989*, London, HMSO.

Department of Health (1989) 'Health of the population: children', in *On the State of The Public Health for the Year 1988*, London, HMSO, pp. 61–2.

Dillner, L. (1991) 'Suffer the little children', *British Medical Journal*, **302**, p. 927.

Evans, P.M., Evans, S.J.W. and Alberman, E. (1990) 'Cerebral palsy—why we must plan for survival', *Archives of Disease in Childhood*, **65**(12), pp. 1329–33.

Freeman, M.D.A. (1987–88) 'Taking children's rights seriously', *Children & Society*, **4**, pp. 299–319.

Graham, P.J. (1986) 'Behavioural and intellectual development', in Alberman, E.D. and Peckham, C.S. (eds.) *Childhood Epidemiology: British Medical Bulletin*, **42**(2), pp. 155–62.

Graham, P. (1989) 'Social class, social disadvantage and child health', *Children & Society*, **2**, pp. 9–19.

Graham, P.J. (1990) 'Maternal employment', *Archives of Disease in Childhood*, **65**(6), pp. 565–6.

Griffin, J. (1986) *Well-Being—Its Meaning, Measurement and Moral Importance*, Clarendon Paperbacks.

Hogg, C. and Rodin, J. (1989) *NAWCH Quality Review—Setting Standards for Children in Health Care*, London, National Association for the Welfare of Children in Hospital.

Hogue, C.J.R., Strauss, L.T., Buehler, J.W. and Smith, J.C. (1989) Overview of the National Infant Mortality Surveillance (NIMS) Project, CDC Surveillance Summaries, *MMWR*, **38**, SS-3.

ILEA Research and Statistics Branch. 'School rolls from DES Form 7', in *Education Statistics 1988–89*. London, Inner London Education Authority.

Kosky, J. (1989) *Mutual Friends: Charles Dickens and Great Ormond Street Children's Hospital*, London, Weidenfeld and Nicholson.

Morris-Jones, P.H. and Craft, A.W. (1990) 'Childhood cancer: cure at what cost?', *Archives of Disease in Childhood*, **65**(6), pp. 638–40.

Moss, P. (1990) 'Work, family and the care of children: issues of equality and responsibility', *Children & Society*, **4**(2), pp. 145–66.

National Children's Bureau Policy and Practice Review Group (Chair: Professor Philip Graham) (1987) *Investing in the Future: Child Health Ten Years After the Court Report*, London, National Children's Bureau.

OPCS Social Survey Division (1989) *General Household Survey 1987*, London, HMSO.

Pearson, P. (1981) *Riverside Child Health Project*, Annual Report, Newcastle-upon-Tyne.

Pharoah, P.O.D. (1986) 'Perspectives and patterns in childhood epidemiology', in Alberman, E.D. and Peckham, C.S. (eds.) *British Medical Bulletin*, **42**(2), pp. 119–26.

Pharoah, P.O.D., Cooke, T., Cooke, R.W.I. and Rosenbloom, L. (1990) 'Birthweight-specific trends in cerebral palsy', *Archives of Disease in Childhood*, **65**, pp. 602–6.

Postman, N. (1983) *The Disappearance of Childhood*, W.H. Allen.

Scriven Report and Evidence and Children's Employment Commission's Report: Leichfield Report. Append, Part II, p 2, ss. 11,12; Franks Report Append, Part II, p K7, s 48; Tancred Evid. Append., p176 etc. quoted in Engels, F. 'Childhood in the Potteries' in Hoyles, M. (ed.) *Changing Childhood. A Publication to Mark the International Year of the Child* (1979) Writers and Readers Publishing Cooperative.

Sommerville, J. (1982) *The Rise and Fall of Childhood*, Sage.

Steedman, C. (1990) *Childhood, Culture and Class in Britain: Margaret Macmillan 1860–1931*, London, Virago.

Suranky, V.P. (1982) *The Erosion of Childhood*, Chicago University Press.

Troyna, B. and Hatcher, R. (1990) *Racial Harrassment in Schools*, Highlight no 92. London, National Children's Bureau with Barnardo's.

UNICEF (1991) *The State of the World's Children*, Oxford, Oxford University Press.

WHO (1946) *Constitution of the World Health Organisation*, WHO, New York.

WHO (1978) *Report of the International Conference on Primary Health Care*, Alma Ata, USSR, 6–12 September 1978. Geneva, World Health Organisation.

World Health Organisation Regional Office for Europe (1985) *Targets for Health for All*, Copenhagen, WHO.

Woodroffe, C. and Kurtz, Z. (1989) *Working for Children? Children's Services and the NHS Review*, London, National Children's Bureau.

SECTION 4

Protecting and Promoting Child Health

Introduction

In the previous section we referred to the rise, and the characteristics of, the New Public Health movement. The papers that comprise this section are underpinned by the philosophies espoused by this movement and also reflect the 'Health For All' values that run through this Reader.

Before reading through the papers in both this and the following section we want to alert readers to the concept of health promotion that we are using. 'Health promotion' is now a 'buzz' word in health care circles, particularly in nursing. Yet there is often ambiguity about both its meaning and how the concept is employed in day to day practice.

There is now, however, general consensus that health promotion has three complementary, interlinked components. Downie *et al.* have developed a model of health promotion which is the one to which most people now refer. This sees health promotion as three overlapping spheres of activity:

- preventive care;
- health education;
- health protection.

The first activity (preventive care) is one with which nurses (particularly community nurses) are very familiar. It includes such things as screening for and immunising against disease, and checking progress in such areas as normal growth and development, wound care or rehabilitation. The first paper (one of two in this section by Hall *et al.*) focuses on preventive care and advises on strategies for achieving high rates of childhood vaccination.

We then present a paper by Downie *et al.* In it they highlight the characteristics of health protection, necessary for the creation of health promoting environments (ones in which it is easier for people to make health-promoting life choices). The paper provides full and rich discussion of the role of government in creating regulations and policies which can either enhance or impede the health promotion of its citizens. They note that UK governments have never had consistent and strong fiscal policies for health protection and cite the case of legal drug (tobacco and alcohol) promotion as a particular example. We use the term (drug) promotion here because some government policies and relationships encourage use of these legalised drugs as they are a major source of revenue.

The paper by Pearson *et al.* is included because of its focus on illegal (as opposed to legal) drug use. It describes the ways in which people become heroin users, the stages and statuses of their involvement, and the concept of a drug use career. The notion of career is a very important one for therapists, who work with abusers to 'tap in' to their life-style, in order to seek to identify and influence their motivation to use and to change. It is a strategy very relevant to the practice of nursing and can be used, for example, in dietary, as well as drug abuse counselling.

Health protection is an activity which is particularly necessary for the healthy development of children. Responsibility for child health protection is shared between the state, parents or guardians, and health and welfare professionals. One difficult area of abuse in which health professionals may become involved is that of child abuse. In the second paper by Hall *et al.* strategies for managing a case of suspected child abuse are outlined.

We close the section by focusing on the newest challenge to public health: acquired immune deficiency syndrome (AIDS). As AIDS is a very high profile public health threat it is likely that nurses will be seen as a source of information about the disease. In the extract (taken from *The Nation's Health*) the current and potential size of the AIDS problem is identified and routes of transmission of the infection are discussed.

19

Immunization*

DAVID HALL, PETER HILL and DAVID ELLIMAN

How to achieve high rates of vaccination

- Give it a **high priority**. Devote time to organizing it within the practice. Give someone overall responsibility for vaccination within the primary care team.
- Be **enthusiastic** and convince parents that it is important. **Emphasize the benefits**.
- Be **well informed** and know the true contraindications.
- **Never say that a child should not receive a vaccination without being absolutely certain that this advice is correct**. There should be very strong grounds for denying a child the benefits of vaccination. If in doubt seek further advice from a community paediatrician, hospital paediatrician or community physician.
- **Know where to seek further advice locally**.
- Be **flexible** and vaccinate whenever the opportunity arises.
- **Liaise** closely with all others involved in vaccination in the District. This includes health visitors, DHA, Family Health Services Authority (FHSA), clinic doctors and the District Immunization Co-ordinator.
- **Obtain practice lists for patients under 5** from the FHSA and DHA at regular intervals.

Childhood vaccination

Vaccination of children has been shown not only to be a highly effective form of preventive care, but also to save money. Many vaccines have been in use for decades, but until recently the take-up rates were still, on average, below target figures set by the World Health Organization. The latest figures show that the average take-up of triple, polio and MMR immunization exceeds 90%.

*An extract from D. Hall *et al.* (1994) *Child Surveillance Handbook, Second Edition*, Oxford, Radcliffe Medical Press.

Introduction

In the GP Contract two target take-up levels have been set. To achieve the lower level of remuneration, an average of 70 per cent of children aged 2 years should have been immunized with the three groups of vaccines—diphtheria, tetanus and polio; pertussis; and MMR (mumps, measles and rubella). To achieve the higher level, 90 per cent will need to be immunized. It is obviously important that as many children as possible are immunized, irrespective of these targets.

Immunization schedules vary from District to District, but that currently recommended by the Department of Health is as follows:

Birth	BCG to those in high risk groups, i.e. likely to be in close contact with a case of tuberculosis. Hepatitis B to those babies whose mothers were Hepatitis B surface antigen-positive during pregnancy.
4 weeks	Hepatitis B (as above)—2nd dose.
8 weeks	Triple vaccine (diphtheria, tetanus and pertussis—DTP), oral polio (OPV).
12 weeks	DTP, polio and Hib.
16 weeks	DTP, polio and Hib.
26 weeks	Hepatitis B (as above)—3rd dose.
12–18 months	Mumps, measles and rubella (MMR).
Preschool (4–5 years)	Boosters of diphtheria, tetanus and OPV.
10–14 year-old girls	Rubella, if not already received MMR.
10–14 years	BCG, if tuberculin-negative.
School-leaving age (15–18 years)	Boosters of tetanus and OPV.

The change from the previous regimen, in which the primary course was given at approximately 3, 5 and 9 months, was introduced because:

- There is likely to be a higher uptake rate with only 4 weeks between injections and the course starting at 8 weeks old. This prediction seems to have been confirmed.
- There will be earlier protection against pertussis, which is most severe in children under 6 months.
- Concerns that this regimen would require a booster at 15–18 months are felt to be unfounded.

Haemophilus influenzae type b (Hib) vaccine was introduced into the UK on 1st October 1992. Hib is the most common cause of meningitis in children under four years old. Where the vaccine has been introduced, Hib meningitis has almost disappeared entirely. The vaccine is one of the safest in use. While it currently has to be given in a separate syringe from DTP, there is reason to believe that a combined preparation may be available soon. Parents must be reminded that the Hib vaccine prevents only one of several types of meningitis.

The intervals between the three doses of the primary course of DTP and polio should not be reduced below the new recommendation of 4 weeks. Any further reduction might impair efficacy. The timing of the preschool booster relates more to patterns of child care than to immunological factors. Now that many children start some form of day care from 3 years old, it seems logical to take this into account when giving the preschool booster. In Wandsworth we recommend that it is given at the same time as the preschool CHS visit, as long as two years have elapsed from the time of the third primary vaccination; however, at present this is not Department of Health policy.

Other vaccines

Other vaccines may need to be given in special circumstances. Hepatitis B vaccine should be given to those at risk by nature of disease-state or contacts. Those with some chronic disorders (severe asthma, cystic fibrosis, bronchopulmonary dysplasia, cyanotic congenital heart disease, etc.) should be given influenza vaccine. Tetanus boosters may be needed at the time of injury, depending on the circumstances. Rabies, yellow fever, hepatitis A, typhoid, Japanese encephalitis, tick-borne encephalitis, meningococcal and pneumococcal vaccines may be appropriate in some individuals.

Site of injection

Apart from BCG, and in some circumstances rabies, all injections should be given by intramuscular or deep subcutaneous injection. There is evidence that more superficial subcutaneous injections are likely to give rise to a greater number of significant local reactions. All intramuscular and subcutaneous injections should be given into either the deltoid region of the upper arm or the anterolateral aspect of the thigh. Vaccines should never be given into the buttocks as the efficacy may be reduced and there is a small risk of sciatic nerve damage. Intradermal injections should only be given by those who have had the requisite training and who use this route regularly.

The skin may be cleansed by swabbing, but vigorous attempts at sterilization are not needed. Do not use acetone; it is a serious fire hazard. Alcohol should be allowed to dry before the injection is given, otherwise it hurts, and may inactivate live vaccines.

Contraindications to vaccination

There are very few contraindications to vaccination, but myths abound. The true contraindications are set out below.

- Any vaccination should be postponed for any child who is **acutely unwell** with a fever or systemic upset. A mild illness without these features can be ignored. As soon as the child is well the vaccination should be given. Treatment with antibiotics is not, in itself, a contraindication.
- Children who are known to have had an **anaphylactic response to a constituent of a vaccine** should receive that vaccine only under hospital supervision, if at all. Minor allergic reactions to eggs or antibiotics are not relevant.
- Children who are **immunocompromised**, whether due to disease or treatment, or are **HIV-positive** should be referred to their consultant for advice. It should not be assumed that vaccination is to be postponed but it may often be overlooked.

- **Household contacts of individuals who are HIV-positive or otherwise immunosuppressed** should be given inactivated polio vaccine (IPV) rather than the oral vaccine (OPV) as the latter is transmissible.
- Pertussis vaccine should not be given to children who have had a **severe local or systemic reaction to a previous dose**. A severe local reaction is defined as 'an extensive area of redness and swelling which becomes indurated and involves most of the anterolateral surface of the thigh or a major part of the circumference of the upper arm.'

A severe general reaction includes any of the following:

- A fever equal to or greater than 39.5°C within 48 hours of injection.
- Anaphylaxis.
- Bronchospasm.
- Laryngeal oedema.
- Generalized collapse.
- Prolonged unresponsiveness.
- Prolonged inconsolable screaming.
- Convulsions occurring within 72 hours.

- Children with a **documented history of cerebral damage, a personal history of convulsions or a family history of febrile convulsions or idiopathic epilepsy** are at increased risk of a febrile fit following pertussis and MMR vaccinations. They are not at any greater risk of permanent adverse effects from the vaccines and should receive them. The Department of Health advice is that such children *should* receive pertussis vaccine. Parents of such children should give them paracetamol for 36–48 hours following vaccination against pertussis. Where a child has an 'evolving neurological disorder' the pertussis vaccine should be temporarily withheld until the picture becomes clear. As the pyrexia following measles/MMR vaccine occurs at an interval of 5–10 days after vaccination, prophylactic paracetamol is not appropriate. The parents should be told what to do in the event of a fever occurring. If such a child is under the care of a paediatrician, and there is any doubt as to whether either vaccine should be given, the paediatrician ought to be consulted first.

Mythical contraindications

Asthma; eczema; hayfever; snuffles; treatment with antibiotics or locally-acting steroids; being breast-fed; mother being pregnant; history of neonatal jaundice; previous clinically diagnosed infection with pertussis, measles, mumps, rubella, or polio; failure to thrive; stable neurological conditions such as cerebral palsy and spina bifida; and Down's syndrome have all been cited as reasons for withholding vaccinations. None of these are contraindications to any vaccination.

No allowance should be made for prematurity. The timing of the vaccination programme dates *from birth* not the expected time of delivery.

Table 19.1 The incidence of cases of diseases against which vaccination is available is shown for the years 1988–90. Deaths are shown in brackets

Disease	1988	1989	1990
Diphtheria	1 (0)	1 (0)	2 (0)
Measles	86,001 (16)	26,222 (3)	13,302 (0)
Mumps	–	20,713 (–)	4,277 (–)
Pertussis	5,117 (0)	11,646 (1)	15,286 (7)
Rubella	–	24,570 (–)	11,491 (–)
Tetanus	12 (5)	16 (2)	9 (1)
Tuberculosis	5,164 (478)	5,432 (443)	5,204 (390)

Why are high rates of vaccination not achieved more often?

Bearing in mind the very few contraindications that there are to the primary series of vaccinations, uptake rates of the order of 95 per cent are theoretically possible. Why is this level so rarely attained? There are a number of reasons:

- **Low priority**. Acute illnesses and child abuse attract publicity and hence resources at the expense of vaccination programmes.
- **Perceived low risk of diseases**. Many of the diseases against which vaccination is carried out are perceived as being rare. For diphtheria, polio and tetanus this is true, but for others, such as measles and whooping cough, the illnesses are still very common, frequently distressing and sometimes fatal. Table 19.1 shows how commonly these diseases occur in England and Wales. Encephalitis follows measles in between 0.1% and 0.2% of cases and can result in permanent disability. Mumps is the commonest cause of aseptic meningitis and is a significant cause of sensorineural hearing loss in children.

  While polio is rare in this country, it is still very common in developing countries. The disease may be acquired by infants travelling to such countries before they have been immunized.
- **Vaccination not seen as a positive activity**. Undue attention has been given to the very rare adverse effects of vaccination without pointing out the hazards of the diseases. Professionals seem to worry about being blamed for the adverse effects of a vaccination they have given, but are unconcerned by the far commoner situation of a vaccine being withheld for spurious reasons and the child suffering the ill effects of a preventable disease.

  Recent evidence suggests that pertussis vaccine rarely, if ever, causes any permanent harmful effects. In fact, recently published data from one of the British birth cohort studies showed that children who had not been immunized against pertussis were *more* likely to be intellectually retarded by the age of 5.
- **Lack of responsibility**. Vaccination is undertaken by GPs and the Community Child Health Services. Until recently, neither had overall responsibility. Thus low uptake rates could be, and often were, blamed on someone else. With the appointment of District Immunization Co-ordinators this should no longer be the case. The

Co-ordinator should be willing to offer any practice advice on setting up or improving an immunization programme and to help in individual 'problem' cases where there is doubt as to whether or not a child should be vaccinated.

- **Poor education**. The abundance of mythical contraindications and their propagation by professionals and public alike has caused understandable confusion for some parents. Better training of the professionals and adherence to official guidelines should help to dispel many of these myths. Ready access to a local expert who can offer speedy advice is often found to be helpful. Many Districts provide courses for doctors and nurses.

  Some Districts have Immunization Advice Clinics where children can be referred if there is doubt as to what vaccinations they should be given.
- **Poor information transfer**. Many parents will bring their children for vaccination with little prompting. However, a significant number forget or are reluctant and therefore need reminding. This cannot be done unless accurate records are kept and there is adequate transfer of data between all the professionals involved, i.e. DHAs, FHSAs, GPs, health visitors, etc. Only in this way can individual parents—and their doctors—be reminded of overdue vaccinations.

  Without efficient and speedy feedback, it is impossible to monitor the service being provided and attend to any inadequacies. Feedback to professionals at the grass roots allows them to monitor their own performance in comparison with others and to be alerted to any decline in uptake.

  DHAs will be offering such a service to GPs once DHAs and FHSAs have compiled accurate details of patients on GPs' lists.
- **Inflexibility**. Vaccinations should be performed not only by the doctor at set times during the day or week, but by any suitably trained person, doctor or nurse, whenever and for whatever reason a child is brought to see that professional, assuming the child is due for vaccination and no real contraindication exists. Practice nurses, clinic nurses and health visitors should all be trained to advise about and give vaccinations, without a doctor being present. If a child is a few days early for a vaccination it should not be put off. On any occasion that a child is seen the vaccination history should be ascertained and any gaps in the programme completed. MMR, DTP and polio vaccines can all be given together, as can Hib and MMR or Hib, DTP and polio.

  Opportunistic vaccination is one of the best ways of increasing uptake rates.

Commonly asked questions

Q. A child is adopted and the family history is not known—what immunizations should he receive?

A. He should receive all the vaccinations appropriate to his age. The only factor that may be of relevance is the HIV status of the mother. If there is any evidence to suggest that the mother may be HIV-positive, the adoption agency should be consulted.

Q. A child comes from abroad and the immunization status is unknown—what vaccinations should he receive?

A. Assume the child has only received those vaccinations for which there is documentary evidence and give full courses of the remainder.

Q. A course of vaccinations is interrupted by a longer interval than is recommended—should the course be restarted?

A. A course never needs restarting. The remaining dose(s) should be given at the same intervals as would have been appropriate had the course not been interrupted.

Q. Should a child receive one or more polio vaccinations before he is allowed to go swimming?

A. Polio has not been transmitted via swimming pools in the UK. The situation may be different in swimming baths or natural bodies of water in developing countries.

Q. A child has had a disease—should he receive the vaccination against that disease?

A. Only when there is microbiological proof that a child has had a disease should consideration be given to omitting the corresponding vaccine. It is unlikely that a child will have this level of proof of past infection with mumps, measles and rubella, and so MMR vaccination should rarely be omitted on these grounds. There are three antigenically distinct types of wild polio virus. It is therefore possible to have a second attack of polio. Even a serious attack of tetanus does not give lifelong immunity. Children may suffer invasive haemophilus disease on more than one occasion. Polio, tetanus and Hib vaccine should all be given even if a child has already had the respective disease. If a child has had a positive antigen test or culture for pertussis, the pertussis component of the triple vaccine can be omitted. **No harm will come by vaccinating a child against a disease he has already had.**

Q. Can more than one vaccine be given at the same time?

A. MMR, DTP, polio (IPV or OPV) and hepatitis can be given together, without any increase in adverse effects or reduction in efficacy. The same applies for DTP, polio and Hib, as well as for Hib and MMR. Each injection should be given at a separate site. Different vaccines should not be mixed in the same syringe.

Q. A child vomits soon after being given polio drops—should another dose be given?

A. The dose should be repeated if he vomits within 1 hour of the dose.

Q. The 'Statement of Fees and Allowances' (SFA) authorizes payment for tetanus vaccination given every five years, whereas the current Department of Health guidelines, 'Immunization against Infectious Disease', recommend that tetanus boosters should only be given every ten years. Which is correct?

A. There are a number of such anomalies. The SFA details what will attract remuneration, while the guidelines suggest the optimal course of action for the patient. The DoH guidelines should be followed.

Q. The Department of Health guidelines are different from the manufacturers' literature. Which is correct?

A. The manufacturer's literature is based on the original product licence and is often very conservative. The DoH guidelines are more likely to take account of experience since the vaccine was introduced and should be followed in preference to anything else.

Q. A child develops a nodule at the site of a DTP injection. Is this a contraindication to further doses?

A. Such nodules are quite common and may take months or, less frequently, years to resolve. They are not a contraindication to further doses. They may be more common with injections given too superficially and extra care should be taken with subsequent injections.

Q. A parent had a 'bad reaction' to a particular vaccine. Should her child receive the vaccine?

A. There is no convincing evidence that reactions to vaccines run in families and, in any case, it may be difficult to be sure that an event happening at the time of a vaccination is in any way related to the vaccination. A family history is therefore not relevant unless the suspected reaction was a fit, in which case it would be appropriate to recommend that the child should receive an antipyretic after DTP.

Q. Is recent immunization a contraindication to surgery such as tonsillectomy?

A. No.

Q. Is there a risk of MMR vaccine causing meningitis?

A. There have been some cases of mild transient meningitis with the Urabe strain of mumps vaccine virus which has now been withdrawn. The MMR II vaccine now in use contains the Jeryl Lynn strain and the rate of meningitis is much lower. Note that meningitis occurs in 80% of natural mumps and can be severe; vaccine cases have been mild and have left no sequelae.

Q. Should childhood immunizations be made compulsory, as in the USA?

A. In many states it is compulsory for a child to be immunized before school entry. Overall take-up rates are no better than those in Scandinavian countries where immunization is voluntary. More importantly, the take-up rate in 2-year-old children are significantly lower than in the UK. Professional knowledge and enthusiasm are much more effective than compulsion.

20

Health Protection*

R.S. DOWNIE, C. FYFE and A. TANNAHILL

This can be seen as the descendant of the great old regulatory public health measures which have had such an impact on the population's health over the last century. It may be defined as follows:

> Health protection comprises legal or fiscal controls, other regulations and policies, and voluntary codes of practice, aimed at the enhancement of positive health and the prevention of ill-health.

Health protection makes it less likely that people will encounter hazards in the environment, and that they will behave in an unhealthful manner, while increasing their chances of living in a positively healthful environment and having a lifestyle which promotes positive health. (It is the wider environment—political, legislative, social, etc., as well as physical—which is referred to here.) In other words, it is about making healthy choices easier choices.

The concept, and barriers to regulatory action, will now be illustrated through a series of examples, following which ethical considerations will be briefly explored.

Legal control

Examples include legislation concerning: the wearing of seat-belts in cars; the sale of alcohol and tobacco to minors; drinking and driving; the control of communicable diseases; and health and safety at work.

Fiscal control

A recent example of pro-health fiscal policy in the UK has been the imposition of differential taxation on petrol to make the unleaded variety cheaper, as an inducement to motorists to convert to this type of fuel in the interest of environmental protection.

---

*An extract from Downie, R.S., Fyfe, C. and Tannahill, A. (1989) *Health Promotion: Models and Values*, Oxford, Oxford University Press, pp. 51–55.

No Government has, however, had consistent and strong fiscal policies for health protection. Duties on tobacco and alcohol have been of particular concern to the pro-health lobby. It is widely accepted that the health problems associated with tobacco and alcohol in a society correlate with the levels of use of these drugs in that society, and that, over time, usage is inversely related to real price (ASH *et al.*, 1988; FCM, 1988). (The link between alcohol price and consumption has been demonstrated even for problem drinkers; Kendell *et al.*, 1983.) This is the rationale for widespread calls to increase alcohol and tobacco taxation (which forms a high proportion of the retail prices of these commodities) on health grounds. These calls generally fall on deaf (or un-listening) ears. Despite occasional health-motivated increases in duty, smoking and drinking remain cheaper practices (in real terms) than 40 years ago, when knowledge of ill-effects was less advanced.

Other regulations and policies

Regulatory action is not the exclusive province of Government. In recent years, for example, many employers (including health authorities/boards, who have a special exemplar role) have developed policies to promote non-smoking on their premises. Work-place policies on alcohol and problem drinking have also been becoming more common, as have canteen food policies.

So far we have concentrated on specific hazards, such as tobacco and alcohol. We should, however, remember that more fundamental aspects of public policy-making, such as those relating to housing, education, employment, and the prevention and alleviation of poverty, impinge on health. Health protection policies can address the full range of 'prerequisites for health' as identified by WHO.

Voluntary codes

These are in general poor substitutes for compulsion. The promotion and advertising of cigarettes, for instance, is regulated by a process of agreement between the tobacco industry and the Government, and breaches of the resulting voluntary code have been so frequent, and in many instances so crass, as to become legendary (Roberts, 1986; 1987).

Barriers to health protection

A major barrier to national regulatory action in favour of health appears to be a simple process of neglect—failure to look for, and give priority to, likely health consequences of public policy, such as fiscal policy. The 'Skoal Bandits' affair (DHSS, 1985) is perhaps a demonstration of what can happen when there is no proper mechanism for gearing action by the various Departments of the Government towards the protection of the nation's health.

Another problem is perceived clashes of the interest between Government Departments. Thus, it is often argued, deterrent increases in tobacco taxation are not overall in the national interest since tobacco revenue is the country's third largest source of income (after Value Added Tax and oil). In short, we cannot afford successfully to discourage smoking with any rapidity, especially as many more people might then live to collect their pensions.

This line of argument may be countered in three ways. Firstly, an economic analysis of a package of anti-smoking measures (including a rise in duty), based on a predicted 40 per cent resultant reduction in smoking, has suggested that, as well as saving many lives and much misery, the measures would result in an increase in Government revenue income from the higher prices paid by the remaining smokers (Atkinson and Townsend, 1977). Secondly, and more fundamentally, taxation is transferable: the same amount of revenue may be obtained by taxing something else (such as income), and so the case for the economic imperative of smoking is spurious. Thirdly, it is surely unacceptable for public policy (even if the economic reasoning were sounder) to preserve the status quo whereby one in seven deaths in England and Wales, for example, results from smoking. A national policy of compulsory euthanasia at retirement age would be a more honest, equitable, and effective means of achieving the desired economic objective!

The third barrier to health protection nationally stems from the enormous power of vested interests over public policy-making. Big business is in a strong position to oppose pro-health policies and perpetuate unhealthful ones, in the interests of profit. It is widely stated that progress towards a sensible, coherent food policy, for instance, is persistently hampered by the influence of the food and agricultural industries.

The impact of industry on policies which affect health is very clearly seen in relation to tobacco. The Zoos Bill episode of 1981 (Anonymous, 1981) is a case in point. More than 100 amendments to this hitherto uncontroversial Private Member's Bill suddenly materialized, with the result that another Bill, aimed at giving the Government power to control tobacco promotion, ran out of Parliamentary time. The latter had been expected to gain a majority. The amendments to the Zoos Bill were tabled by a handful of Members of Parliament (MPs), one of the principal participants being a parliamentary adviser to a major tobacco company, and others also having direct or indirect links with the industry. Not surprisingly this incident has been seen as a case of filibustering (an obstruction of legislation through delaying tactics) in which health lost out to darker motives. This raises the question of links between MPs and vested interests which damage health. These may be directly financial (through appointments with tobacco, alcohol, or related public-relations companies) or may involve constituency or trade union interests in industries. Contributions to political party funds might also be seen as potentially significant.

Political influence at the national level is reinforced by the power of vested interests over the public and the media. Power over the public is exerted by control over the availability and pricing of products for consumers (health education cannot succeed if advocated healthful goods cannot be found or afforded), by marketing strategies, and so on. Power over the media may take the form of lucrative advertising accounts 'with strings attached' (such as hints to magazines that business will be taken elsewhere if, say, anti-smoking features appear), or misinformation, and so forth.

These illustrations of constraints to health protection nationally are matched by interferences at more local levels. The raising of awareness of such local and national obstacles is an important component of type 3 health education as described by Draper *et al.* Given the enormity and power of the opposition it is easy to see why this type of work tends to be neglected.

It is, however, heartening to see professional bodies, such as the British Medical Association and the Royal College of Physicians of London, campaigning for health protection measures (BMA, 1986).

Ethical considerations

In many instances, attempts are made to justify antipathy to health protection on ethical grounds. Thus, it is often argued, it would be wrong to exert compulsory control on tobacco advertising or sponsorship because people's freedom of choice would be restricted. It is suggested here that the concept should be treated with scepticism. Failure to regulate powerful concerns which damage health serves to perpetuate the freedom of choice of those with a great deal of power (major business and others with vested interests in unhealthful products or activities) to exploit those with relatively little (the public).

In any case, society accepts a great deal of regulation for the common good: it is illogical that the manufacturers of cigarettes, the major preventable cause of serious illness and premature death, and alcohol, with its immense direct and indirect impact on social, mental, and physical health, should be treated so lightly. The contrast with the treatment of illicit drugs is striking; no-one, of course, makes a public case for the protection of heroin barons, for instance.

One specific ethical dilemma worth looking at here is the question of taxation of tobacco and alcohol products. The pro-health lobby often demands sharp and steep rises, outstripping inflation. In doing so they often meet the highly valid counter-argument that swingeing increases would hit the poorest most. It would be highly desirable if the question of large increases in duty were to be debated publicly. In the meantime, however, it would seem reasonable to take regular fiscal action such that the products do not become any cheaper in real terms.

References

Anonymous (1981) Commentary from Westminster. Blocking of Bill on tobacco advertising. *Lancet*, **i**, 1377–8.

ASH (Action on Smoking and Health), BMA (British Medical Association) and HEA (Health Education Authority) (1988) *Two good reasons for a tobacco pricing policy.* ASH/BMA/HEA, London.

Atkinson, A.B. and Townsend, J.L. (1977) Economic aspects of reduced smoking. *Lancet*, **2**, 492–4.

BMA (British Medical Association) (1986) *Smoking out the barons: the campaign against the tobacco industry*. Wiley, Chichester.

DHSS (Department of Health and Social Security) (1985) *Snuff-dipping—'skoal bandits'*. Letter from Chief Medical Officer, CMO(85)6.

Draper, P., Griffiths, J., Dennis, J. and Popay, J. (1980) Three types of health education. *British Medical Journal*, **281**, 493–5.

FCM (Faculty of Community Medicine) (1988) *Alcohol. The prevention of problems related to its use*. FCM, London.

Harrison, D.F.N. (1986) Editorial. Dangers of snuff, both 'wet' and 'dry'. *British Medical Journal*, **293**, 405–6.

Kendell, R.E., de Roumanie, M. and Ritson, E.B. (1983) Influence of an increase in excise duty on alcohol consumption and its adverse effects. *British Medical Journal*, **293**, 405–6.

King Edward's Hospital Fund for London (1989) *Blood cholesterol measurement in the prevention of coronary heart disease. Consensus statement*. King's Fund Centre, London.

Roberts, J.L. (1986) *Code busting by tobacco companies*. North Western Regional Health Authority, Manchester.

Roberts, J.L. (1987) *More honour'd in the breach . . . how the 1986 voluntary agreement on tobacco advertising is being broken*. Project Smoke Free, Manchester.

USNIH (United States National Institute for Health) (1986) *Health implications of smokeless tobacco*. Consensus development conference statement, Vol. 6, No. 1, NIH, Washington.

WHO (World Health Organization) (1984) *Health promotion. A discussion document on the concept and principles*. WHO, Copenhagen.

Winn, D.M. *et al*. (1981) Snuff dipping and oral cancer among women in the Southern United States. *New England Journal of Medicine*, **304**, 745–9.

21

Becoming a Heroin User and Heroin Using Careers*

GEOFFREY PEARSON, MARK GILMAN and SHIRLEY McIVER

This paper describes the ways in which people become heroin users, the stages and statuses of their involvement, and the concept of a 'career' in relation to their use of heroin. It is based on extensive fieldwork in the North of England during 1985.

Why do people use heroin, and how are they first introduced to it? Can people control heroin use, so that it remains merely an occasional recreational pastime, or is addiction an inevitable outcome of experimentation? Why do people take such risks with their health when the dangers of heroin are so widely known, or are many people still ignorant of its addictive properties? Is the drug in fact as enslaving as popular stereotypes insist, and are the horrors of withdrawal so engulfing as in the common notion of 'cold turkey'? Why is it that so many ex-addicts seem to say that 'coming off' is easy, but that 'staying off' is the most difficult part of abstinence?

Different statuses of involvement with heroin

There is no such thing as a 'typical' heroin user, nor a typical heroin user's career. Nevertheless, it is useful to think in terms of a simple four-phase model to describe levels of involvement with the drug through which a heroin user's career will pass.

1 The Non-User
2 The Initial Offer and Experimentation
3(a) Occasional Use on a Recreational Basis
3(b) The 'Grey Area' of Transitional Use
4 Addictive Use

*This is an abridged version of a chapter in G. Pearson (1986) *Young People and Heroin: An Examination of Heroin Use in the North of England*, London, Health Education Council. This paper is also available, in a longer version, in G. Pearson (1987) *The New Heroin Users*, Oxford, Basil Blackwell.

So, the non-user having been offered the drug will either accept it or reject the offer. If the offer is accepted and the person tries it on an 'experimental' basis, they might either discontinue their experimentation quite quickly because they do not enjoy the experience, or they might embark on a more prolonged period of experimentation. At this point they might begin a pattern of recreational use on a very occasional basis, and continue this pattern over a long period of time without becoming addicted. Or they might begin to use the drug more frequently and enter upon what we have called the 'grey area' of transitional use where it is not clear, either to themselves or others, whether or not they are becoming addicted—a phase of heroin use open to widespread misinterpretation in terms of the person's status of involvement with the drug, which is why we choose to call it the 'grey area'. And finally, if this pattern of transitional use continues for any length of time the heroin user will suffer an imperceptible drift into addiction.

Each of these phases can be thought of as different *statuses* of heroin involvement, and the passage between these different statuses as *transition points*. For health education purposes, these different statuses imply different *audiences*, with differing educational and informational needs. The transition points will also be crucial target areas for health education. Finally, each status will imply different possible *exit-routes* towards abstinence.

In moving from one status to another, conscious choices will sometimes make themselves apparent to the individual. But equally, a person can move imperceptibly from one status to another without any conscious decision-making. This is especially the case in the patterns of transitional use which take a person from the status of occasional user to compulsive user and addiction. At this fateful transitional point it is not uncommon for a heroin addict to say that they were taken by surprise when they first experienced withdrawal symptoms, sometimes to the extent that they did not identify what these symptoms were.

There is nothing inevitable about the passage from one status to another in the career of a heroin user. Some people do slide rapidly into habitual use and addiction, following the pattern of progressive decline and escalating drug consumption which characterises the dominant stereotypical image of the heroin addict. But other people can, and do, arrest their involvement at different points in this hierarchy of statuses. So that some people discontinue their heroin use after a brief flirtation with the drug, whereas others maintain stable patterns of occasional use over long periods of time (cf. Zimberg, 1984). But because the hidden figure of experimental or recreational use is unknown, it is not possible to say what proportion of heroin users follow the pattern of progressive decline into addiction which is commonly (but wrongly) assumed to be the inevitable consequence of heroin use.

Exit-routes also vary considerably. Different motivations trigger them, different methods are used in order to come off heroin, and different timescales are involved. Some people try to make a clean break with heroin, while others try to withdraw themselves slowly by gradually reducing their intake. Some try to do it with professional assistance, whereas others do it on their own. And a crucial distinction must be made between 'coming off', which for many heroin users is relatively effortless, as against 'staying off' which has been repeatedly described to us as much more difficult.

This simple model could undoubtedly be refined, and it will be overlaid with important considerations such as whether a person smokes heroin or injects it. For example, an exit-route for someone who injects might first involve moving onto smoking heroin for a time and overcoming 'needle fixation' before attempting to come off the drug completely. Nevertheless, this simple model will serve usefully as a framework for our subsequent discussion which will focus on crucial points of transition: the circumstances of the initial offer; experimentation and the perceived benefits of heroin use at this stage; the 'grey area' of transitional use into addiction; and finally exit-routes and the process of 'coming off' and 'staying off' heroin.

However, first it is important to recognise that even habitual heroin use is compatible with a wide range of lifestyles and patterns of use (cf. Stimson, 1973; Stimson & Oppenheimer, 1982). Before moving onto a consideration of different statuses of involvement, it will be useful to exemplify what some of these different patterns of habitual use amount to, on the basis of experiences that we have gathered together in our research.

Kevin started smoking heroin four years ago in a circle of friends and at its peak his habit amounted to 1 gramme of heroin daily. He supported his habit by shoplifting, for which he was caught more than once. It was when he was facing a further Court appearance, which seemed likely to result in a custodial sentence, that he discovered the motivation to enter a treatment programme.

Joe had a pattern of heroin use, stretching back for nearly ten years, which involved episodic binges during which he would consume the drug hungrily. When he felt that his habit was spiralling out of control, he would register for a methadone-reduction programme whereupon he would remain abstinent for as long as 18 months before starting his next binge.

Julie maintained her heroin habit, and that of her boyfriend, for nearly two years by prostitution. At one time they were consuming 1½ grammes daily, costing something like £600 per week, which she said she could earn easily by a couple of hours work per night.

When Harry first tried heroin he had several thousand pounds in the bank, consisting largely of redundancy money from when he had been made unemployed. He quickly developed a heavy habit of more than a gramme smoked daily and was always generous with his friends who also smoked heroin, so that he blew all his money in a matter of months. When his debts began to increase he stopped using heroin and he now receives methadone.

Carol first tried heroin with a girlfriend, and says that she did not know what it was at the time. She became heavily involved with a circle of heroin users for 12 months, but she now receives methadone while still buying a £5 bag of heroin every other week and enjoying 'a little toot'.

The initial offer and experimentation

Very little is known in any detailed way about early patterns of heroin use. The beginning user is elusive, and not only because the practice is illegal and therefore kept well hidden. A person who tries heroin will sometimes quickly discontinue use, either because they find that they are unable to maintain a supply of the drug, or because it makes them feel ill and they have no desire to continue, and there is no reason why people such as this should come to the notice of public authorities or researchers. Only those who sustain their heroin use over time are likely to come to public notice, and then because of their involvement in crime, ill health, or domestic difficulties. There is no reason to suppose that the early experiences of those people who do come to public notice should correspond to the experiences of those who do not. So that what follows might only be a partial reconstruction of early experiences with heroin.

Nevertheless, a number of certain features of the circumstances of the initial offer can be briefly summarised.

1 The initial offer will always be made in the context of a friendship network.
2 The stereotype of the 'pusher' and the 'free sample', so beloved of the news media, is false and unhelpful for health education purposes.
3 There is no guarantee whatsoever that the known dangers of heroin will deter people from accepting the initial offer. Indeed, an emphasis on the dangers of heroin might sometimes even enhance the sense of risk and excitement to be enjoyed from the drug and increase the likelihood that the initial offer will be accepted.
4 Nor is there any guarantee that because a person has refused an offer of heroin in the past, they will not accept in the future.

The first time that a person is introduced to heroin it will be by a friend, and not by a so-called 'pusher'. This point is so important that it cannot be emphasised too strongly. Indeed, this makes it more likely that the offer will be accepted, because the context of friendship (or kinship) will make the drug seem that much safer than if it had been offered by a stranger. It is indeed a sobering fact that if the stereotype of the 'pusher' and the 'free sample' to lure people into addiction were true, then its possibilities for epidemic growth within a friendship network would be considerably reduced.

When asked how they first got into heroin, our informants offered different versions of the same story:

> 'I was just gave some, for nothing like, by a mate. And the feeling is different, I liked the feeling . . . and after that I started buying my own bags, £5 bags and that. I just got into it that way' (Colin, 23 years, Manchester)

> 'It's like everything else, the heroin came round and . . . I was curious so I tried it and I liked it. . . . There was a few of us, we were all good mates and that like, we all tried it and eventually everyone just got hooked' (Eddie, 21 years, Merseyside)

The early experience

What does it feel like when a person first tries heroin? Often enough it makes them feel sick, and sometimes this is the end of their heroin using career. But other people persist with heroin, in spite of the nausea, which is hardly surprising in view of the fact that initial encounters with other drugs (including those that are socially sanctioned, alcohol and tobacco) often make people feel ill until they learn how to take the drug properly and how to handle its effects and interpret them as enjoyable. The first surreptitious 'drag' or 'swallow' on a cigarette, with its attendant effects of dizziness or nausea; the 'never again' feeling which accompanies the first hang-over, or the sickness from excessive drinking: these experiences lay a sound foundation upon which people will persist with drugs which are not immediately experienced as pleasurable, having learned that these are inhibitions which must be overcome if an intoxicant is to be enjoyed. And in this respect there is no reason why heroin should be different from other drugs.

If the likelihood that heroin will make someone feel ill cannot be relied upon to deter them from continuing use, then what are the pleasurable effects? Often in the accounts of ex-addicts we hear only of the painful and enslaving absorption into the drug: 'the monkey on your back'. But a major reason why people use, and continue to use heroin, is that they enjoy it. This is sometimes a difficult thing for health education to admit to, but it is true nevertheless.

Precisely what is the nature of this enjoyment? Here we enter into an area of difficulty, because drug users do not employ a very complex vocabulary by which to describe and label the internal states experienced when under the influence of a drug. So that words such as 'stoned', 'buzz', 'high' and 'wrecked' not only sum up the limits of this restricted vocabulary, but are also employed to describe the effects of a variety of substances (cannabis, amphetamines, opiates) which are otherwise totally dissimilar.

A typical description of the initial effects of heroin, then, will often be set in a characteristic vagueness:

> 'First, when I was on it, like, I donnow . . . it made me feel dead pleasant, I donnow . . . as if I never had a care in the world, d'you know what I mean? It wasn't like a "high" . . . . It was just like . . . you haven't got a care, y'know, it was just different' (Paul, 24 years, Merseyside)

Sometimes heroin's effects were described, in straightforward and immediate terms, as simply pleasurable:

> 'It was just the *nicest* drug going. You feel just *great*! Just . . . phoo . . . blows your mind, like, you start nodding and . . .' (Eddie, 21 years, Merseyside)

Some people described heroin's effects as peaceful and relaxing:

> 'With smoking, it comes on you gradually and you just feel dead relaxed and dead tired, and what have you . . .' (Mick, 23 years, Manchester)

Whereas other people described the initial effects as a feeling of great personal power with an immediate impact:

> 'As soon as you chase it, it just hits you straight away and you just feel like the boss, like . . .' (Jack, 22 years, Merseyside)

And there were those who liked the helpless feeling of being 'wrecked' and 'gouching', which is a common British expression for the North American term 'nodding off', and which comes through in this Liverpudlian's version of drug argot as 'grouching':

> 'So what's so special about heroin?'
> 'The way you take it, I loved it, like . . . And the hit's brilliant. . . . You just sit there and just . . . like helpless. You must look bad and all that, because I've seen me mates and thought they did, like. And, I'm just sitting there grouching, it's brilliant' (John, 19 years, Merseyside)

If the active elements of heroin's effects were open to a wide variety of forms of description and interpretation, these people were nevertheless in agreement that they liked the drug's effects. Another common feature in many of the accounts that we were given was the drug's capacity to take away a person's worries:

> 'I'd just finished with my girl . . . and I suppose I was on a bit of a downer myself like, a bit depressed and all that. And as I say I took some heroin, and all my worries that I had just seemed to float away . . . . When I had heroin, I didn't have a problem. I didn't have any worries' (Paul, 24 years, Merseyside)

In many of the accounts that we were given an ambivalence surrounded descriptions of the drug's pleasures, which is hardly surprising since many of the people whom we talked to were trying to stay off heroin. Indeed, sometimes it was not easy to get people to talk about the enjoyable aspects of heroin use at all, in that they preferred to dwell upon the damage which heroin had caused in their lives. At one extreme, in an interview with a self-help group of ex-users the group-leader vetoed any discussion of the pleasures of heroin at all. The group's philosophy involved a total renunciation of drug experiences, which is common to organisations such as Alcoholics Anonymous, and even to think about the pleasures of heroin was defined as a sign that a group member might relapse.

The early experiences of heroin use, from the accounts that we have been given, suffer from a wide variation. For some people the drug is an instant 'buzz' or 'hit'. For others it is a matter of relaxation. For some it brings an enhanced sense of personal power. For others it means being 'wiped out' and 'wrecked'. But with different shades of emphasis, one common feature was the ambivalence felt towards the drug, while another was that heroin 'took your worries away' and made people feel 'at ease' with themselves and in their minds. Indeed, if anything it was this cushioning effect from external pressures which caused people to form an initial attachment to the drug and which then led them onto a regular pattern of consumption which eventually resulted in addiction.

On occasion, this feeling of release from external pressures and worries was so all-consuming in a person's recollections of their early heroin use that the positive drug-effects (in the sense of a 'buzz' or a 'hit') were almost entirely absent from their account. And this seemed to be particularly so where someone's construction of the subjective meaning of their drug-use was closely tied to their experiences of social deprivation. In other words, where heroin appeared to 'solve' a person's difficulties with housing, unemployment or low income.

The question of occasional non-addictive use

If there is very little research on early patterns of heroin use, except as reconstructed from the experiences of addicts and ex-addicts, then the occasional user who only takes heroin on a recreational basis is even more elusive. Indeed, there are authoritative traditions within the addictions field which question whether heroin use is even possible without eventually becoming addicted. Nevertheless, a substantial body of research evidence on non-compulsive opiate use has been collected by Zinberg and his colleagues in the USA, where occasional heroin use on a recreational basis is known within the drug culture as 'chipping'. This has established beyond doubt that stable patterns of non-addictive heroin use can be sustained if certain rules are adhered to (cf. Zinberg, 1984). Zinberg's work, which contains a useful summary of research in this little explored area, has also attempted to identify what these rules, rituals and routines amount to. Briefly, the necessary underlying supports which can sustain a non-compulsive pattern of opiate use include the following: access to a knowledgeable network of controlled drug users who can offer advice to the novice; strict adherence to rules on the frequency of use, so that the drug is only used on certain occasions such as at weekends and at no other time, and never on consecutive days; the existence of other valued commitments in a person's life such as employment, family life and recreational pursuits which conflict with opiate use; and a circle of friendship which includes non-users as well as users.

In Britain a smaller study by Blackwell (1983) identified similar features within the lifestyles of controlled opiate users, while also pointing to the way in which people sometimes move between different statuses of involvement with heroin.

Transitional use: mistaken identities in the 'grey area'

Addiction does not follow on instantly from experimentation with heroin, and although the rate at which a person becomes addicted probably varies between individuals it will have been necessary to use the drug regularly on a daily basis for some time before the actual development of a 'habit'.

The transition into compulsive, addicted use is clearly an important change of status in the career of a heroin user, and it will often be characterised by an imperceptible drift—a 'grey area' where a person's growing involvement with heroin is unclear and open to misinterpretation. We can identify two kinds of such misinterpretation within this transition, each of them with its own attendant dangers. The first is where a person believes themselves to be addicted when in fact they are not. The second is when a person does not believe that they are addicted, when in fact they are.

The first case of mistaken identity is probably more common than is usually recognised. In one locality a drug squad officer reported to us that he had often noticed that people who had been arrested on drug charges did not exhibit any withdrawal symptoms when they were held in custody on remand, even though they believed themselves to be heroin addicts. His explanation of this phenomenon was that people who claimed to be heroin addicts when they were not were 'showing off' in front of their friends, and one thing which certainly has to be reckoned with is that in some localities being a 'smack-head' is assuming something of a heroic status. However, this is not necessarily a conscious choice, and we can identify a number of subtle, interacting influences which play a part in these misrepresentations of self within the 'grey area' of transitional heroin use.

Perhaps the most important is that in the absence of a well informed drug culture a person might be a victim of the mythology of heroin's 'instantly' addictive powers, and therefore pursue and consume the drug in fear of withdrawal before an actual physical dependence has been established. In a situation such as this a person's mistaken belief that they are addicted will quickly become a 'self-fulfilling prophecy', and a number of ex-users whom we talked to described in their own terms how these mistaken identities might arise and then lead eventually to addiction.

> 'I think people get the wrong ideas, you know, people who've got started on it . . . and they've smoked it for a month or two months, and then they haven't got it one day. Well, alright, you know, they might feel a bit rough. But they start, y'know, they've got it in their heads that they're going through withdrawal symptoms. So they're out to get more to make them feel that bit better because they were feeling rough . . . and before you know it, they *are* hooked on it' (Paul, 24 years, Merseyside)
>
> 'When you get hooked on it you get, sort of, psychologically hooked at first. Do you know what I mean? You're saying, "I *need* this . . . I need it", like . . . and you don't. But you buy it again, and then one day you just wake up and you're fucked' (Eddie, 21 years, Merseyside)

An alternative set of reasons why a person might embark upon a regular pattern of heroin use even before they become addicted, is that it gives them some meaning in life, either in the shape of an identity (I'm an addict) or a status within the peer group.

Auid *et al.* (1985) have also described how an assumed addict-identity can give people not only local status, but also other forms of social-psychological reward in the shape of sympathy from one's family and friends. Declaring oneself to be a 'junkie', and thereby assuming a helpless victim status, might then be understood under the right circumstances as a form of 'attention-seeking'. It has been pointed out to us on more than one occasion that it is not unknown for a young offender to claim addict-status when appearing before a Court, thereby hoping to secure a sentence which involves 'help' rather than 'punishment'.

As a person becomes more deeply involved with a heroin using network, they also become increasingly identified with group activities which centre around drug use. In order to gain acceptance within this group of acquaintances, it might then be necessary to magnify one's familiarity with heroin. Tall stories abound in drug-using circles about so-and-so who took twenty 'dikeys' at one go and really 'gouched out'; about how awful it was the other day when you were 'turkeying' and couldn't get a 'bag' anywhere; or how someone had escaped from the clutches of the law by 'legging it' when the drug squad appeared around the corner.

Equally important in this respect is that the life of a heroin user is an extremely active one, in which a person needs to be constantly on their toes—knowing who is who in the drugs scene; who sells the best 'bag' and where you buy it; how to avoid getting 'burned' by a dealer, and how to know the difference between brick-dust and the real thing; constantly hustling for the money for the next bag. A study of street addicts in New York showed how this hectic cycle of activity could assume more importance in a person's life than the effects of the drug itself (cf. Auid *et al.*, 1985). This corresponds with the argument advanced by Peele (1985) that people become addicted to activities just as much as they become addicted to substances. And it also squares with the commonly reported experience by ex-users that 'staying off' heroin was much more difficult than 'coming off' the drug, because the day seems so empty without the drug and its associated flurry of activity.

One can see, then, that within this 'grey area' of transitional use there is ample scope for a person to adopt harmful self-identifications with the addict lifestyle prior to the actual onset of dependence, in such a way that these generate a 'self-fulfilling prophecy'. But it is equally true that a different kind of mistaken identity can be assumed, whereby addiction overtakes someone without them realising how deeply involved they had become with the drug. In some people's accounts of their transition into habitual use, their experience of how this came about was simply passed over in a sentence:

> 'I just got into it, buying a bag every day because I had money then, from the redundancy money and that, and before I knew it like, I was dependent on it . . . I needed it' (Malcolm, 23 years, Manchester)

The impression that is so often given in accounts of a heroin user's early experimentation and transition through the 'grey area' into addiction is one of inevitability. In retrospect, the transition no doubt feels that it was inevitable. But the 'grey area' of transitional use does not necessarily take this form, and people can and do arrest their involvement and so avoid what would otherwise be the inevitable consequences of daily heroin use.

It is reasonable to suppose that over a period of weeks and months certain conscious choices and decisions are made. And also that these decisions would sometimes involve various kinds of subterfuge, by which people hide from themselves the obvious consequences of their actions. Perhaps the most common form which these subterfuges take is revealed in the often repeated expression, 'One little toot won't do me any harm', a self-deception whereby someone says to themselves that they will do it again today, but not tomorrow. And then when tomorrow comes, the same act of bad faith: 'One more little toot. . . . Just one more little chase'.

One of the characteristics of accounts given by heroin users and ex-users is that they rarely embrace any recognition of their own motivation and agency. So that the drift into addiction is remembered only as something in which one played a passive role—as if the user were powerless in the face of a relentless pharmacological process, and then later driven by the overriding concern to avoid symptoms of withdrawal.

References

Auid, J., N. Dorn & N. South (1985) 'Irregular Work, Irregular Pleasures', in R. Matthews & J. Young (eds), *Confronting Crime*, (Sage).

Blackwell, J.S. (1983) 'Drifting, controlling and overcoming: opiate users who avoid becoming chronically dependent', *Journal of Drug Issues*, vol. **13**, no. 2.

Peele, S. (1985) *The Meaning of Addiction: Compulsive Experience and its Interpretation*, (Lexington).

Stimson, G.V. (1973) *Heroin and Behaviour*, (Irish UP).

Stimson, G.V. & E. Oppenheimer (1982) *Heroin Addiction*, (Tavistock).

Zinberg, N.E. (1984) *Drug, Set and Setting: The Basis for Controlled Intoxicant Use*, (Yale UP).

22

Growing Threats to Public Health*

B. JACOBSON, A. SMITH and M. WHITEHEAD

HIV and AIDS: the newest challenge to public health

AIDS, or acquired immunodeficiency syndrome, is the most serious worldwide threat to public health to emerge in the last ten years. In the UK alone, where the problem is still much smaller than in the USA, Africa and many other EC countries (see Figure 22.1), there were more than 3,100 reported cases by March 1990. Of these, 56 per cent had already died. Although the number of AIDS cases has now plateaued, this has not been the case for those who are HIV positive. In 1988 it was estimated that the costs of hospital treatment (assuming no major advances in therapy) for HIV/AIDS patients ranged between £20–30 million,[1] but this does not include costs incurred in the community or the potentially large costs of prophylactic treatment if it is decided to use the drug Zidovudine (AZT) or other drugs on a large scale in asymptomatic HIV positive people.

Anxiety about AIDS stems not only from its incurable nature or from uncertainties about the growth of what is a new, and still little-understood epidemic, but from the realisation that its prevention requires changes in lifestyle that raise profound ethical issues. While our understanding of AIDS has grown enormously since the first case was diagnosed in 1981, there are few things that can be said with absolute certainty at such an early stage in the development of the epidemic. We are aware that many of the statements made today, may need revision in years to come.

AIDS is the end point in a wide spectrum of incompletely documented diseases caused by infection with the human immunodeficiency virus (HIV) which was first isolated in 1983. Approximately 50 per cent of those infected with HIV will have developed AIDS after ten years of infection, but this may be higher in certain sub-groups—especially those with co-existing sexually transmitted disease.[2]

---

*B. Jacobson, A. Smith and M. Whitehead (1991) Growing threats to public health, in *The Nation's Health*, King Edward's Fund for London, London, pp. 64–68.

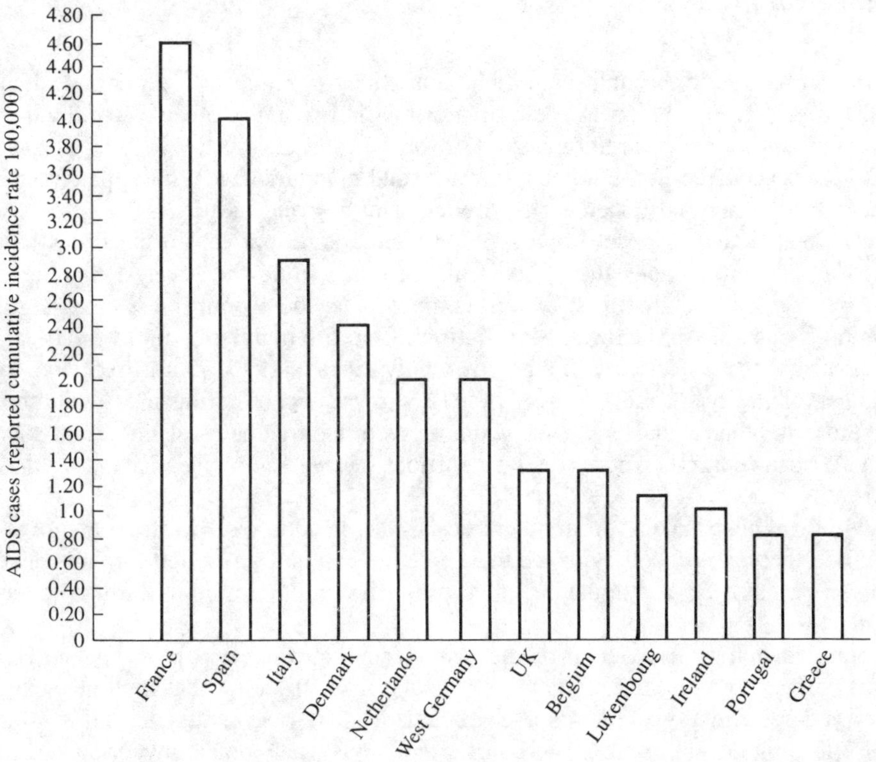

Source: World Health Organization. Global statistics to March 1990. *AIDS*, 1990, **4**: 375–376.

Figure 22.1 Cumulative incidence of AIDS in the EC to March 1990

Ways of transmitting HIV infection

All the evidence so far confirms that HIV cannot be transmitted by ordinary social or occupational contact.[1,3–5] Follow-up for periods of up to two years shows that household and non-sexual, close contacts of AIDS patients have not become HIV positive.[6] Proven cases of health care workers becoming HIV positive through casual exposure associated with caring for a patient are hard to document.[5] Even health care workers who have accidentally exposed themselves to HIV-infected blood run a very low risk of becoming HIV positive themselves[7]—a much lower risk than exposure to hepatitis B virus where 6–30 per cent of staff accidentally exposed become infected.[4] In a UK study of 150 laboratory workers exposed to blood or body fluids from patients infected with HIV, none had become HIV positive themselves in the first nine months of follow up.[8]

Sexual transmission

HIV can be transmitted through semen, blood and blood products[1,9,10] and cervical and vaginal fluids.[10] The commonest route of transmission so far identified worldwide is sexual, with considerable variation across Europe. In the UK up to 1990, 80 per cent of AIDS cases occurred in the homosexual/bisexual population. A similar pattern was evident in the Netherlands, Denmark, Sweden, Norway and the Federal Republic of Germany. In Italy and Spain, however, 66 per cent and 63 per cent respectively have occurred among intravenous drug users. In Scotland, while the greatest number of AIDS cases has been, and still is, among homosexuals, the proportion is changing as more intravenous drug users develop AIDS. In the Scottish population intravenous drug users comprised the majority of HIV positive individuals in 1990, so it is expected that the number of newly diagnosed cases of AIDS in intravenous drug users will soon exceed those in homosexuals.[11] Heterosexual transmission is the most important route in many African countries where equal proportions of men and women have developed AIDS.[12]

HIV virus has been isolated from other body fluids, including saliva, tears and breast milk. While there is no good evidence that infection can be transmitted through saliva or tears,[9] evidence is accumulating that transmission is possible through breast milk.[13,14]

Most information we have so far on the relationship between sexual activity and HIV infection comes from research among homosexual men. It shows that multiple sexual partners and receptive anal intercourse are independent risk factors for HIV infection.[15,16] Bleeding during or after intercourse, and any sexual contact involving semen, blood or excretions of infected partners were associated with a high risk of becoming HIV positive.[17]

More recent evidence shows that the HIV virus can also be transmitted heterosexually both from men to women and women to men,[18] and that multiple partners[19] and sex with prostitutes is associated with a high risk of becoming HIV positive in some African countries[20,21] and parts of the USA and Europe.[22] The presence of genital ulcers and sexually transmitted disease increases the risk of transmission. Research on the sexual partners of AIDS sufferers, and of haemophiliacs who are HIV positive, suggests that the virus may be more readily transmitted from men to women than from women to men.[23]

Transmission through transfusion of blood and blood products

Transfusions of blood and blood products were the second most important source of HIV infection in the UK until screening of all blood donors and heat treatment of blood products were introduced in 1985. Those most affected were haemophiliacs who formed the second largest group (6 per cent) of AIDS cases in March 1990. Research in British haemophilia centres shows that in 1986, 44 per cent of people with haemophilia A and up to 60 per cent of severe haemophiliacs (who needed multiple transfusions) were HIV positive by 1986.[24]

Transmission through injecting intravenous drugs

Those who inject intravenous drugs are at high risk of developing AIDS even though they still form only a small proportion (about three per cent in 1990) of the total number of AIDS cases throughout the UK. Evidence from the USA, where intravenous drug users accounted for nearly one in five AIDS cases in 1986, suggests that the potential of this route of viral transmission has been hitherto underestimated.[25] The explosion of infection among intravenous drug users in Spain, Italy, Scotland and Thailand, further reinforces this concern. The virus is easily, and most rapidly, spread among intravenous drug users, and those most at risk of becoming HIV positive are those who share injecting equipment[26] and those who inject frequently or who go to 'shooting galleries'.[27] Although evidence is scanty, the injection of intravenous drugs may be a more efficient way of transmitting the virus[28] than sexual intercourse, and this is evidenced in the very short period over which groups of drug users who are known for sharing 'works' have become HIV positive.[29–31]

European intravenous drug users with AIDS are much younger than other AIDS sufferers: three-quarters are under 30,[31] and by September 1986 over 50 per cent of intravenous drug users in one Edinburgh general practice were HIV positive.[26]

HIV infection can also be transmitted from a pregnant woman to her infant child during pregnancy, birth and shortly after. There have been 39 cases of AIDS in children in the UK up to 1990, 24 born to mothers who were infected. Four of these mothers were intravenous drug users, five acquired the infection through transfusion, and ten through heterosexual transmission.[11] The risk of an HIV positive woman transmitting the virus is high, probably about 20–40 per cent in most studies, but the recent European Collaborative Study underway in ten countries, including Scotland, suggests that transmission rates may be lower at 13 per cent.[32]

Predicting the future size of the HIV/AIDS epidemic

Attempts to make predictions have resulted in widely differing estimates for the number of people likely to become HIV positive and to develop AIDS. For such predictions to be useful we need to know more about the sexual behaviour of the population at risk; about changes in sexual behaviour over time; about the relationship between HIV infection and eventual disease outcome; and how long it takes from infection with HIV to the development of AIDS. Extrapolations from past UK and American data, or even from models which make assumptions about these largely unknown aspects of HIV infection, can lead to an unhelpfully alarmist view of possible future trends.

Predictions for England and Wales have been made by two major working groups in recent years, and illustrate how difficult a task it is in this field. The first was set up by the Chief Medical Officers of England and Wales, and the report of the working group (the Cox report)[33] was published in November 1988. At that time the number of reports of AIDS cases had been increasing exponentially in the homosexual category, with only a slight indication that the pattern of growth might be changing. Based on the information available at the time, the Cox report estimated that there were between 20,000 and 50,000 people infected with HIV in England and Wales at the end of 1987, of whom 13,000–30,000 were homosexuals. This gave a projection of 2,000 to 10,000 *new* AIDS cases by the year 1992, with a cumulative total of between 10,000 and 30,000 cases by that date.[33]

However, these predictions have been proved too pessimistic, mainly because there has been a marked decline in transmission of HIV among homosexual and bisexual men, resulting from an apparently major change in behaviour in the homosexual population in the mid-1980s. The second working group reporting in January 1990 (the Day report),[34] more than halved the predictions for new AIDS cases given in the Cox report. The Day report estimated that the number of infected homosexuals at the end of 1988 was in the range 8,750 to 17,500, much lower than the Cox estimates. The projections for new AIDS cases among homosexuals in 1993 were in the range 875 to 1,500.

By contrast, the report pointed out that the increase in AIDS cases in injecting drug users and heterosexual contacts was still in an exponential growth phase (similar to the early phase of growth in homosexual and bisexual men). If this exponential spread continued, then by 1993, the Day report predicted that two-thirds or more of new AIDS cases would arise from the injecting drug users and heterosexual contact categories, compared with just seven per cent at the end of 1989. On the other hand, there was also some evidence that the exponential growth phase might be easing up in these two categories, in which case there may be little new transmission taking place in either group and only minor increases in cases will be seen in the next few years.

With this range of uncertainty in mind the working group projected that in 1993 the overall number of new cases of AIDS would be between 1,175 and 4,825. The projected number of AIDS deaths was 750 for 1990 and 1,540 for 1993, with a total by the end of 1993 of 6,380 AIDS deaths since the start of the epidemic. Unlinked, anonymous HIV testing programmes, as recommended in the Day report, will reduce some of the uncertainty in the predictions of future cases.[34]

Notes

1. Wells N. *The AIDS virus. Forecasting its impact.* London, Office of Health Economic, 1986.

2. Anderson, R. The AIDS epidemic in the UK: past trends and future projections. In: UK Health Departments and HEA (eds). *HIV and AIDS: an assessment of current and future spread in the UK.* London, HEA and UK Health Departments, 1990.

3. Anon. Latest UK figures on AIDS. *British Medical Journal*, 1987, **295**: 1004.

4. Anon. *AIDS—a public health crisis.* Population Reports, Series L, no 6. Baltimore, Johns Hopkins University, July–August 1986.

5. Geddes, A.M. Risk of AIDS to health care workers. *British Medical Journal*, 1986, **292**: 711–712.

6. Friedland, G.H., Brian, M.D. *et al.* Lack of transmission of HTLV-III/LAV infection to household contacts of patients with AIDS or AIDS-related complex with oral candidiasis. *New England Journal of Medicine*, 1986, **314**, 6: 344–349.

7. Gazzard, B.G., Wastell, C. HIV and surgeons (ed). *British Medical Journal*, 1990, **301**: 1003–1004.

8. McEvoy, M. Porter, K. *et al.* Prospective study of clinical laboratory and ancillary staff with accidental exposure to blood or body fluids from patients infected with human immunovirus. *British Medical Journal*, 20 June 1987: 1595–1597.

9. Acheson, E.D. AIDS: a challenge for the public health. *The Lancet*, 22 March 1986: 662–665.

10. Adler, M. ABC of AIDS: development of the epidemic. *British Medical Journal*, 1987, **294**: 1083–1085.

11.World Health Organization Collaborating Centre on AIDS. *AIDS surveillance in Europe*. Quarterly Report No. 25. Update at 31st March 1990.

12. Melbye, M. The natural history of human T lymphotropic virus-III infection: the cause of AIDS. *British Medical Journal*, 4 January 1986, **292**: 5–11.

13. Lepage P. Postnatal transmission of HIV from mother to child. *Lancet*, 1987, **ii**: 400.

14. Clebunders, R. *et al.* Breastfeeding and transmission of HIV. *Lancet*, 1988, **ii**: 147.

15. Kingsley, L.A., Detels, R. *et al.* Risk factors for seroconversion to human immunodeficiency virus among male homosexuals. *The Lancet*, 14 February 1987: 345–348.

16. Evans, B.A., Dawson, S.G. *et al.* Sexual lifestyle and clinical findings related to HTLV-III/LAV status in homosexual men. *Genito-urinary Medicine*, 1986, **62**, 6: 384–389.

17. Darrow, W.W., Echenburg, D.F. *et al.* Risk factors for HIV infection in homosexual men. *American Journal of Public Health*, 1987, **77**, 4: 479–483.

18. Anon. Who will get AIDS? *The Lancet*, 25 October 1986: 953–954.

19. Winkelstein, W., Samuel, M. *et al.* Selected sex practices of heterosexual men and risk of infection by the HIV. *Journal of the American Medical Association*, 1987, **257**: 1470–1471.

20. Melbye, M., Bayley, A. *et al.* Evidence for heterosexual transmission and clinical manifestations of human immunodeficiency virus infection and related conditions in Lusaka, Zambia. *The Lancet*, 15 November 1986: 1113–1116.

21. Van de Perre, P., Carael M. *et al.* Female prostitutes: a risk group for infection with human T-cell lymphotropic virus type III. *The Lancet*, 7 September 1985: 524–526.

22. Skidmore, C. AIDS and intravenous drug users. *Health Education Journal*, 1987, **46**, 2: 56–57.

23. May, R. HIV infection in heterosexuals. *Nature*, 1988, **331**: 655–656.

24. UK Haemophilia Centre Directors. Prevalence of antibody to HTLV-III in haemophiliacs in the UK. *British Medical Journal*, 19 July 1986, **293**: 175–176.

25. Moss, A.R. AIDS and intravenous drug use: the real heterosexual epidemic. *British Medical Journal*, 1987, **294**: 389–390.

26. Robertson, J.R., Bucknall, A.B. *et al.* Epidemic of AIDS related virus (HTLV/LAV) infection among intravenous drug abusers. *British Medical Journal*, 22 February 1986, **292**: 527–529.

27. Marmor, M. Des Jarlais, D.C. *et al.* Risk factors for infection with human immunovirus among intravenous drug abusers in New York City. *AIDS*, 1987, **1**: 39–44.

28. Fuchs, D., Dierich, M.P. *et al.* Are homosexuals less at risk of AIDS than intravenous drug abusers and haemophiliacs? *The Lancet*, 16 November 1985: 1130.

29. Brettle, R.P., Bisset, K. *et al.* Human immunodeficiency and drug misuse: the Edinburgh experience. *British Medical Journal*, 15 August 1987, **295**: 421–424.

30. Robertson, J.R., Bucknall, A.B.V. Regional variations in HIV antibody seropositivity in British intravenous drug users. *The Lancet*, 1986, **i**: 1435–14.

31. Ancelle-Park, R., Brunet, J.B. *et al.* AIDS and drug addicts in Europe. *The Lancet*, 12 September 1987: 626–627.

32. European Collaborative Study. Children born to women with HIV infection: natural history and risk of transmission. *The Lancet*, 1991, **337**: 253–260.

33. Department of Health and Welsh Office. *Short-term prediction of HIV infection and AIDS in England and Wales: report of a working group* (Chairman Sir D. Cox). London, HMSO, 1988.

34. *Acquired immune deficiency syndrome in England and Wales to end of 1993: communicable disease report (Day report)*. London, Public Health Laboratory Service, 1990.

23

Child Protection*

DAVID HALL, PETER HILL and DAVID ELLIMAN

Management of a case of suspected child abuse

The prime concern is the welfare of the child and if this conflicts with the needs of the parents, then the parents have to take second place.

Members of the primary care team such as the GP and health visitor are likely to know the preschool child and his family much better than any other professional, whereas the school child is probably best known by his teachers. They will often be the first to suspect abuse and will be intimately involved in the management of the child and his family.

In every Borough there should be agreed guidelines on the management of child abuse and these should be kept to hand and consulted in every case. The following plan of action should be considered in the light of such local advice.

How urgent?

If the possibility of abuse arises during a consultation, the urgency of subsequent action will depend on a number of factors.

- **The severity of any injury** and the need for immediate medical treatment. This must take priority.
- **The nature of the abuse**. Emotional abuse and non-organic failure to thrive do not require urgent action whereas non-accidental injury (NAI) may do. Sexual abuse, if an acute episode, may require relatively urgent examination to obtain forensic material.
- **The age of the child**. A young child may be in more imminent danger than a school child.
- **The abuser**. If this is a member of the household, consideration should be given as to whether or not the child can safely return home.

*An extract from D. Hall *et al*. (1992) *Child Surveillance Handbook*, Oxford, Radcliffe Medical Press, pp. 65–67.

- **The informant**, if any. If a child makes an allegation of abuse it should be taken very seriously and it should be made obvious to the child that this is the case. If it appears, in the child's eyes, that nothing is happening the allegation may be retracted and an opportunity lost. This is especially important in suspected sexual abuse.

Unless the well-being of a child is in immediate danger it is rarely necessary to examine him without the consent of a parent or guardian. If a parent refuses to give consent, the child may still be examined if he is himself willing and mature enough to give consent. Alternatively, a Court Order may be sought. A child of sufficient understanding may refuse to be examined. Bearing in mind the likely antagonism that such a course of action could produce, it should never be undertaken lightly.

Whenever there is a significant suspicion of abuse the Social Services Department should be contacted after the treatment of any acute injuries has been carried out. The parents should be told of the immediate plans. Depending on the circumstances of the individual case and the strength of concern, the doctor should share his concerns with the parent. In some cases it may be appropriate to be absolutely frank, in others it may be better to say something such as 'I cannot explain these injuries/findings and I wish to seek further advice.' Doctors who suspect child sexual abuse (CSA) but have little experience of dealing with it may find it difficult to raise the subject, yet the parent may be relieved to find that the doctor is prepared to discuss it.

Detailed notes of the examination and any discussions with the parent(s) and other professionals should be made immediately and in your own records. Remember that such notes may be called in evidence before a court and that the parents may have access to them.

After discussion with the social worker, a number of courses of action are possible:

- **Examination by another doctor**. In the case of suspected sexual abuse, a detailed examination should be carried out only after a detailed history ('disclosure interview') has been taken. Young children should be interviewed by someone specially trained to do so. The examination should then be carried out by an approved doctor who may be a paediatrician, a specially trained forensic medical examiner or occasionally a gynaecologist. Repeated examinations often produce conflicting opinions (the signs may change over time) and are traumatic to the child. If emotional deprivation or non-organic failure to thrive are under consideration, a further expert opinion will be necessary.

  When non-accidental injury (NAI) is suspected, it may be helpful to have a further opinion when there is doubt as to the aetiology of the injuries.
- **Removal of the child to a safe place**. Rarely is it necessary to take a child away from its home. (Remember that social workers do not have a right of entry to a child's home—only police officers have this right.) If it is necessary to remove a child from its home, this should be arranged by a social worker. The Children Act, 1989 makes provision for a child to be assessed medically, against his parents' wishes, but without being removed from them.
- **Calling of a case conference**. The purpose of a case conference is for professionals to share information and to decide the most appropriate course of action in the child's best interests. Parents will almost always be invited for part of the conference, but professionals should always be given an opportunity to share information and concerns before the parents are brought in.

If abuse is confirmed, and the child is felt to be at continuing risk, the child's name will usually be put on the **Child Protection Register**. This confers no rights to any agency and has no legal standing. It does, however, signify the level of concern and usually results in continuous monitoring of the family.

As a result of the case conference, a plan for future management ('child protection plan') will be drawn up. If there are continuing worries about the family, the primary health care team will have an important role in supporting and monitoring the family. Minutes of the case conference should always be sent to the GP. These are confidential and should be filed in a secure place. Social Services Departments are currently considering whether minutes should be circulated to parents. If in doubt about what decision has been made in a particular case, the chairperson of the conference should be consulted.

Points to remember in the management of child abuse

- Do not panic.
- Keep local guidelines to hand along with details of how to contact the local Social Services Department.
- Take any allegation, especially by a child, seriously.
- Record full and accurate details of the history and examination. Make sure you date and time your notes. The parents will have access to your notes and they may be used in legal proceedings.
- Consult with the Social Work Department at an early stage.
- Try to attend any case conferences, especially the first. The primary health care team often has unique information to offer. If unable to attend, send a written report or speak directly to the conference chairperson.
- Keep the key worker informed about any subsequent worries you may have about the family. If there is no key worker, inform the Area Social Services Department. Record all such contacts.
- If in doubt at any stage consult the Social Services Department, the Community Child Health Services or the Hospital Paediatric Department.

Further reading

An introduction to the Children Act 1989. (1990) HMSO, London.

Child abuse trends in England and Wales 1983–1987. (1989) NSPCC, London.

DHSS (1988) *Child protection: guidance for senior nurses, health visitors and midwives*. HMSO, London.

DHSS (1988) *Diagnosis of child sexual abuse: guidance for doctors*. HMSO, London.

Home Office, DoH, DES, Welsh Office (1991) *Working together under the Children Act 1989: a guide to arrangements for inter-agency co-operation for the protection of children with abuse*. HMSO, London.

Meadow, R., ed. (1989) *ABC of child sexual abuse*. British Medical Journal, London.

The medical aspects of child abuse. (1989) A report of the International Committee for Child Health of the Children's Research Fund. The Children's Research Fund, London.

White, R., Carr, P. and Lowe, N. (1990) *A guide to the Children Act 1989*. Butterworths, London.

SECTION 5

New Directions for Child Health

Introduction

Rethinking 'health' has been a major activity during the last two decades and has been occurring in all developed countries, including the UK. With regard to thinking about health it can be said that a paradigm shift has occurred, one which places the recipients of health care at centre stage, instead of health professionals. This paradigm shift is characterized by (among other things):

- empowering people to become involved in decisions about their own health;
- greater sensitivity to differences in population groups;
- health professionals working in partnership with people to promote health and reduce the trauma caused by illness experiences.

The papers collected in this section represent these themes. They are wide ranging in terms of their focus, and the geographical settings from which they were drawn, but all have direct applicability to UK health settings.

The first three papers focus on empowerment as a central theme. Kalnins *et al.* use the goal of health promotion to look at how a previously disenfranchised group (children) might influence their health. In their paper they advocate a shift in thinking about children as recipients of health promotion efforts, to children as partners in health promotion efforts. Central to this shift is the need to accept children's competence to make and implement decisions. New directions in research and practice are identified and discussed.

In the second paper, Gott describes an innovative health promotion project that is currently occurring in Canada. It is characterized (like the previous paper) by a belief in young people's ability to make and enact their own health related decisions. A particularly noteworthy feature of the project described in this paper is the use of new technology (computer bulletin boards) to promote health. Contrary to popular belief it was found that use of new technology by adolescents did not impede their social contacts and development, in fact it promoted them.

Molloy, in her paper on Community Mothers, also describes an innovative project, the central feature of which is handing control of childbearing advice and supervision over to mothers themselves, rather than maintaining exclusive control of supervision of parenting by public health nurses. In the Community Mothers model, collaboration between health professionals (family development nurses) and 'lay' mothers is described. Particularly noteworthy here is the fact that the mothers who the family development nurses work with are socially and economically disadvantaged, and, in the past, would have experienced greater, rather than less professional control.

Other (health service) disadvantaged groups are frequently those from minority populations. In a report of her work on babies from different ethnic groups Bundy explores patterns of disease and handicap caused by consanguinity (parental kinship by blood relationship). She has found that the perinatal mortality rate and the malformation rate for Pakistani babies is greater than that for other ethnic groups. Some reasons for this are advanced, and some strategies for intervention are identified.

The section concludes with a paper by Vehviläinen-Julkunen which explores client–public health nurse relationships in child health care. Suggestions for nursing practice and further research are made.

24

Children, Empowerment and Health Promotion: Some New Directions in Research and Practice*

ILZE KALNINS, DAVID V. McQUEEN, KATHRYN C. BACKETT, LISA CURTICE and CANDACE E. CURRIE

Introduction

The notion that health is related to the ability of an individual or group to realize aspirations and satisfy needs as well as to cope with the environment is broadly accepted in contemporary health promotion. This idea has roots in the WHO conceptualization of health promotion. In this view health promotion is seen as a process of enabling people to increase control over, and to improve their health (WHO, 1986). It follows that one task of health promotion is to empower individuals and groups to do so. This view of health promotion arose, in part, from a belief that when constrained by factors such as poor health, inadequate housing, low self-esteem, etc., people may not have command of the necessary power to alter the conditions that affect their health, nor believe themselves able to take control.

Three principles may be seen as central to the notion of empowerment. The first, that health promotion must address problems that people themselves define as important. The second, that health promotion involves effective participation of the public, alongside experts, in problem solving and decision making. The third, that health promotion works effectively when it is in harmony with a healthy public policy. In this paper we focus on the first two of these principles and their implications for pre-adolescent children in the primary school grades who are still 'children' in the sense that they are economically and legally dependent on their families, and, many would assert, cognitively limited to what is concrete and observable.

We argue that acceptance of health promotion as a process of empowerment has major implications for how we perceive children's health and design health promotion programmes for them. We believe that a shift will be necessary from thinking about children as recipients of health promotion efforts on their behalf to accepting children

*This is an abridged version of an article first published in *Health Promotion International*, Vol. 7, No. 1, pp. 53–58, 1992.

as active participants in the whole process. In turn, this will entail the acknowledgement of children's concerns about health as valid in their own right; and a recognition of their competence to make and implement decisions. Our intention in presenting this conceptual analysis of the meaning of empowerment for children's health promotion is to stimulate critical discussion of the place and role of children in health promotion, and to suggest some new directions in research and practice.

Accepting children's views and opinions as valid in their own right

Acceptance of the principle that health promotion must address problems perceived by the public as important in the context of their everyday lives requires understanding health as children themselves see it and within their own relevant social contexts.

Within health promotion research and practice, little attention has been paid to how children perceive health, to what they see as major health problems or to what they would like to learn about health. Instead children's health problems have been identified by adults from the perspective that children must be protected from conditions that lead to unnecessary morbidity or mortality, either during childhood or later in life. Thus injuries, a leading cause of death in children, have been a major focus of concern. Dental health has been selected as a target for preventive action and among attitudes and behaviours, eating, exercise, smoking and alcohol use are given priority because of their relationship to cardiovascular disease and cancer, the major causes of ill health and death among adults (Smith and Jacobson, 1988).

There are examples of studies in which children have been asked to talk about health from their own perspective. In the analysis of children's accounts of health however, the children's views have been compared, implicitly or explicitly with those of adults. The development of the child's concept of health has been analysed within a framework of age-related development stages derived from Piaget (Natapoff 1978; Bibace and Walsh 1980). Other studies have approached children's accounts of health through the Health Belief Model, seeking to verify its generalizability to children (Dielman *et al.*, 1982). These approaches rest on a cognitive model of the child's world of health. They assume that a better understanding of how children think about health will lead to more effective health promotion approaches with children by identifying appopriate methods of changing health knowledge, attitudes and behaviours.

Undoubtedly, an epidemiologic approach with its focus on risk factors and healthy behaviours is an important one because children must be protected from conditions that can affect their health regardless of whether they feel the need for such protection. Given the embeddedness of children in their families, schools and peer groups, and their cognitive capacities, it would be irresponsible of adults not to guide children into what is considered good for their health based on a broad adult overview of the factors which determine health. At the same time, within an empowerment model of health promotion, it is equally important to acknowledge children's own views and concerns about health and accept these as valid. Children's perceptions of health may involve priorities, evaluative processes, ideas of what is possible, and social spheres of relevance different from those of adults. It is, therefore, essential to understand what is special about children rather than to expect them simply to absorb and accept adult definitions. To fully understand children's perceptions we must search out the principles according to which they interpret their world rather than measure the extent to which they have incorporated adult standards. A vivid demonstration of this point in a health context is to be found in the experiences of the Pioneer Health Centre in Peckham, South London which served the community from 1935–39 and from 1946–50. This centre was set up to provide a holistic health promoting social environment based on the family. In its early stages the centre included a variety of organized activities for children. Surprisingly, these were poorly attended. Yet, it was evident that the children enjoyed the centre because they continued to attend although, for safety reasons, they were barred from using on their own the two greatest attractions of the centre, the swimming pool and the gymnasium. Adults felt that the children were wild and disruptive. For some months the social organizer tolerated chaos but meantime observed the children's individual needs. She then introduced a ticket system which allowed children individual access to all of the facilities and allowed them to use these in the way they chose. Once the children were able to manipulate the environment to their own learning and playing purposes, order ensued. In an analysis of the Peckham experience, Stallibrass (1989) noted that the ability to exercise choice and to learn by doing are crucial elements in the environment and that adult 'experts' may be obstacles to children's realization of what is important and satisfying.

Few studies have attempted to study children's views about health in the context of their everyday lives. Findings from such studies indicate that children see health in the context of interactions and negotiations with events and people in their environment. They do not think about health or health behaviour in the abstract. For example, they perceive health in terms of conflict situations in which courses of action they know are good for their health are pitted against pressures from family and friends. Decisions about how best to behave in these situations are based on a recognition that certain matters are decided by adults; others are resolved by routines; and yet others require deliberations before a decision can be reached (Kalnins *et al.*, 1991). Studies have also shown that to resolve health dilemmas, children engage in various forms of negotiation or exchange. They seek out alternative behaviours that are slightly less unhealthy or they deliberately ignore what is healthy by deciding that they will make up for it the next day. To children, health is very much a matter of having to make pragmatic decisions about situations and actions which may appear mundane and trivial to adults (Backett 1989; Kalnins *et al.*, 1991).

Children also demonstrate a keen awareness and concern about health at a community level. Surveys which ask them to indicate places and things in their communities that correspond to adjectives such as dangerous, dirty, happy, peaceful etc. have been carried out on a city-wide basis (e.g. Seattle, USA; Kidsplace Executive Board, 1986) or on a neighbourhood scale (e.g. Edmonton, Canada; Edmonton Board of Health, 1988). The results again show that, for children, health is defined in pragmatic terms. Health has to do with fear of people such as drunks and drug-dealers, the dangers of crossing busy streets, lack of recreational facilities, being home alone, and coping with stray dogs.

Research which maps children's health behaviour from the point of view of their social contexts is not extensive. But, already it is becoming clear that they perceive health behaviour as the outcome of complex processes in which what is good for health must be balanced against the pressures and realities of their daily lives. The findings suggest that an important component of health promotion for children should be lifeskills training which provide children with an understanding of and with opportunities to practice the skills they require to resolve the health problems they encounter (cf. Anderson, 1986; Hopson and Scally, 1981; Tones, 1990 for discussions of health lifeskills). Among adolescents, lifeskills approaches have already been used extensively and successfully in Social Influences programmes to prevent smoking. These programmes generally include several of the following components: the health consequences and social consequences of smoking; critical awareness of the social influences from peers and the media to smoke; and the development of skills to resist pressures to smoke (see Botvin and McAlister, 1991; Botvin and Wills, 1985). The available research on children's concepts of health and the promise of lifeskills approaches as an effective health promotion strategy both suggest that serious study of children's views and health behaviours from their own perspective must continue in order to uncover the salient features of health in the contexts of their everyday lives.

Accepting children's competence to make and implement decisions

So far, little attention has been paid to the possibility of children's participation in any health promotion efforts other than those which involve their personal health habits. A review of policy documents and health education programmes reveals an underlying assumption that children must be protected from immediate and long-term health problems. They are perceived to be cognitively and socially immature, and therefore, as having to be taught and guided into proper health behaviours, or cared for through the provision of health services. A few examples will suffice to illustrate this prevailing view.

While the health needs of children are acknowledged in health policy and health service planning documents, the role relegated to them is that of passive recipients of the efforts of adults on their behalf. Children along with other special groups such as women, native peoples and minority groups are specifically classified as disadvantaged and vulnerable to a variety of problems which can undermine their health. These range from open abuse to more indirect, yet powerful, social pressures to adopt lifestyle practices detrimental to health. For example, the Canadian health promotion planning document, *Achieving Health for All*, notes that children have already been the beneficiaries of improved prenatal and neonatal care and that preventive measures are helping them to overcome inequalities arising from health problems associated with dyslexia, hyperactivity and speech and hearing problems. The report also notes that children need to have clean and supportive environments at home and school that nurture their development and protect them from physical and psychological abuse (Epp, 1986). There are, however, no suggestions that children should be given the power or the resources to participate in making any health decisions other than those which affect their personal health. Similar sentiments are found in British documents (Department of Health 1991). Health strategies for children are defined in terms of equalizing mortality and morbidity rates among different socio-economic groups, encouraging parental involvement in childrearing through the provision of knowledge and skills, and joint initiatives such as improved surveillance systems among health and social service agencies.

Acceptance of the principle that public participation is a fundamental feature of health promotion that is based on empowerment means that, children have to be seen as partners in health promotion rather than as a special group needing protection. This conception implies an acceptance that children are competent to represent themselves, to make health decisions and to participate in their health care. As yet, health promotion programmes explicitly based on a belief in children's competence are rare. Perhaps this is because there is a danger that if children are empowered to select and address problems they perceive as important they may later be blamed for ineffective solutions, thus again producing health promotion strategies that blame the victim. Despite this danger, a few programmes, explicitly based on a belief in children's competence have been adopted in a variety of settings and we present an overview of a few of them by way of illustration.

With respect to personal health care, for example, Lewis and his colleagues allowed children in grade five to decide for themselves when to visit the school nurse, and to do so without asking the teacher's permission (Lewis *et al.*, 1977). During the consultation with the nurse, they were asked to suggest ways of coping with their problem and allowed to choose the treatment they wished. Their choice was respected as long as it did not pose a threat to their health and welfare. When the nurse felt the choice was less than optimal, other treatment options were reviewed and alternatives discussed for 'the next time'. Analysis of utilization patterns indicated that only a few children abused the system. Perhaps the most intriguing finding was that the children's patterns of visitations closely approximated those of adults. This suggests that children, when given the opportunity to make decisions for themselves, will closely mimic established societal patterns. A similar acceptance of prevailing norms has been observed in experimental schools in which children participate in a full course of study although there are no requirements for classroom attendance and no examinations (Neill, 1962). Thus when children are given more decision making power the scenarios of anarchy depicted by Golding in his novel '*Lord of the Flies*' do not materialize (Golding, 1960).

In school, where children spend a large part of their lives, health education is a low priority in the curriculum or may not have an assured place at all. Teachers may consider themselves ill-prepared to teach about health issues because they perceive these as being concerned with medical matters or with sensitive issues. To young people, health education comes across as moralizing or being concerned with matters of ill health remote from their own lives (e.g. Scottish Health Education Group/Scottish Consultative Council on the Curriculum, 1990). To enable children to take an active part in enhancing their health the WHO has proposed the Healthy School concept. A Healthy School is defined as a community to which all children can relate and one that they have the right to change. Health is fostered through '. . . the whole ethos established by the atmosphere of the school, its code of discipline, the prevailing standards of behaviour, the attitudes adopted by staff towards pupils, and the very values implicitly asserted in its mode of operation (Scottish Health Education Group/ Scottish Consultative Council on the Curriculum, 1990)'. In Britain, this view of school health education has been articulated in a comprehensive health education curriculum '*Health for Life*' which spans primary and secondary education (Williams *et al.*, 1989). Healthy School objectives can also be achieved through assemblies in which children and teachers are given an equal voice to comment on what is happening in the school (e.g. Brookes, 1991; Ministry of Health, Province of British Columbia, 1990). Some of the changes that children have instituted include changing the food offered in the school cafeteria, organizing a paper recycling program, organizing an alcohol and drug-free graduation party, instituting a student-based system for conflict resolution, and implementing a clean-air, smoke-free policy for school buildings and property. It is hoped that the Healthy Schools concept will be endorsed by Ministries of Education in different countries. If so, it will be the first setting in which the participation of children in determining conditions which affect their health is institutionalized.

At a community level, children's participation in health promotion has been demonstrated in both underdeveloped and developed countries. In developing countries the acceptance of children's competence is the underlying basis of the Child-to-Child program (Aarons *et al.*, 1979; Hawes, 1988). This programme developed from the observation that older children play a major role in looking after younger children. They not only dress, feed, and play with their younger siblings but are also responsible for safeguarding them from injury and caring for them when they are ill. Child-to-Child teaches them to do so in the healthiest manner possible. Guidelines have been developed to teach children to prepare and administer oral rehydration therapy, to observe simple safety precautions at home, to stimulate cognitive and social development through play, and to seek out community health resources. The children are taught to see themselves as 'health scouts' who can actively and directly influence the health of their community. Although critics have expressed fears that children may be exploited as cheap labour, supporters of the programme argue that they are helping children to do what they are already doing but to do it better. Whatever the case, there is little doubt that the design of this programme is based on an acceptance of children's competence to make and implement decisions.

In developed countries, the idea that children should have a say about conditions in their communities has resulted in broad-based and politically visible programmes to create cities that are more responsive to and supportive of children and youth. These programmes, variously labelled as Kids Place (Seattle, USA), Kids City (Santa Monica, USA), or Kids Beat (Edmonton, Canada) have several features in common. Children are involved in the definition of community problems from their perspective. This is accomplished by asking them, through schools and youth groups to participate in questionnaires, interviews, public forums and focus groups to express their concerns and to suggest solutions. They are also invited to participate in committee meetings and boards to implement changes. The end result of these programmes has been the formation of broad coalitions of city government, business and youth groups. For example, in Seattle USA, the city which pioneered the concept of Kids Place, children's concerns are now on the agenda of many organizations which have expanded their programmes to include special events of interest to children and families. The sheer number of organizations involved has ensured a visible effect and created the image of Seattle as a desirable city in which to live. It has also led to the acceptance of children as a constituency equal to other constituencies whose needs and wants must be considered in policy and planning.

In summary, the examples cited above illustrate that meaningful ways to assure that children have a voice in matters that affect their health can be devised. It is worth noting in the Healthy Schools example that when children are given opportunities to make decisions, they strive to address health issues they appear to ignore when the initiative comes from adults. It may be that approaches such as Healthy Schools are enabling a 'silent majority' of children who care about their health, to express their concerns and to do something about them. Perhaps in our efforts to protect children, we have fallen into the trap of focusing almost exclusively on correcting the negative aspects of children's health behaviours rather than encouraging what is positive. Accepting children's competence as the starting point for health promotion endeavours may redress this imbalance.

Conclusion

In our discussion of health promotion as a process of empowerment, we have presented the view that this conception has major implications for children. We have argued that its realization will require an acceptance of children's views and perceived needs as valid, and an acceptance of their competence to make health decisions about the conditions that affect their health. These implications place an onus on researchers to develop new methods to investigate children's health from perspectives different to those currently in vogue and to develop concepts and models which place children's health in broader social contexts. On practitioners and policy makers, they place an onus to examine seriously the assumptions about children which underlie health promotion programs and policy.

References

Aarous, A., Hawes, H. and Grayson, J. (1979) *Child-to-Child*, McMillan, London.

Anderson, J. (1986) 'Health Skills: The power to choose', *Health Education Journal*, **45**, 19–25.

Backett, K.C. (1989) 'Health-related beliefs and behaviours of young children', end of Award Report to ESRC XG10250001. Swindon, U.K. (Unpublished).

Botvin, G. and McAlister, A. (1981) 'Cigarette smoking among children and adolescents: Causes and prevention', in C.B. Arnold (Ed.), *Annual Review of Disease Prevention*, Springer, New York.

Botvin, G. and Wills, T.A. (1985) 'Personal and social skills training. Cognitive-behavioural approaches to substance abuse prevention', in U.S. Department of Health and Human Services (Ed.), *Deterring Drug Abuse Research Monograph Series*, Monograph, **63**, 8–49.

Brookes, O. (1991) 'Where do I fit in?' *Scottish Child*, April/May, 10–11.

Department of Health (1991) *The Health of the Nation: A consultative document for health in England*, HMSO, Cm. 1523, London, p. 81.

Dielman, T.E., Leech, S., Becker, M.H., Rosenstock, I.M., Horvath, W.J. and Radius, S.M. 'Parental and child health beliefs and behaviour', *Health Education Quarterly*, **9**, 2 & 3: 60/56–77/73.

Downie, R.S., Fyfe, C., Tannahill, A. (1990) *Health Promotion*, Oxford University Press, Oxford.

Edmonton Board of Health (1988) *Kidsplace Project: A Report of Survey Results.*

Epp, J. (1986) *Achieving Health for All: A Framework for Health Promotion*, Department of National Health and Welfare, Ottawa.

Golding, W. (1960) *Lord of the Flies: a novel*, Faber & Faber, London.

Hawes, H. (1988) *Child-to-Child: Another path to learning*, Unesco for Education, Hamburg.

Hopson, B. and Scally, M. (1981) *Lifeskills Teaching*, McGraw-Hill, London.

Kalnins, I.V., Yoshida, M. and Kellmer, M.J.K. (1991) 'Decision making strategies of 9–12 year old children in everyday situations involving their health', (Unpublished).

Kalnins, I.V. and Love, R. (1982) 'Children's concepts of health and illness—and implications for health education: An overview', *Health Education Quarterly*, **9**, 8–19.

Kidsplace Executive Board, *Kidsplace Report: The State of Seattle's Children*, 1986.

Lewis, C.E., Lewis, M.A., Lorimer, A. and Palmer, B.B. (1977) 'Child-initiated care: The use of school nursing services by children in an adult-free system', *Paediatrics*, **60**, 449–456.

Ministry of Health, Province of British Columbia, Office of Health Promotion. (1990) *Healthy Schools.*

Natapoff, J.N. (1978) 'Children's views of health: A developmental study', *American Journal of Public Health*, **68**, 995–1000.

Neill, A. (1962) *Summerhill: A Radical Approach to Education*, Gollancz, London.

Scottish Health Education Group/Scottish Consultative Council on the Curriculum, Joint Working Party on Health Education in Schools. (1990) *Promoting Good Health*, Scottish Health Education Group, Edinburgh.

Smith, A. and Jacobson, B. (eds.) (1988) *The Nation's Health: A Strategy for the 1990's*, King Edward's Hospital Fund for London, London.

Stallibrass, A. (1989) *Being Me and Also Us: Lessons From the Peckham Experiment*, Scottish Academic Press, Edinbugh.

Tones, K., Tilford, S. and Robinson, Y. (1990) *Health Education: Effectiveness and Efficiency*, Chapman & Hall, London.

WHO (Europe) (1986) 'A discussion document on the concept and principles of health promotion', *Health Promotion*, pp. 73–76.

Williams, T., Wetton, N. and Moon, A. (1989) *Health for Life 1: Health Education Authority Primary School Project*, Nelson House, Surrey.

Williams, T., Wetton, N. and Moon, A. (1989a) *Health for Life 2: Health Education Authority Primary School Project*, Nelson House, Surrey.

25

E ZOOT: Health Promotion by Use of an Electronic Bulletin Board System (BBS)*

MARJORIE GOTT

Introduction

This paper describes one of a number of case studies analysed for an international European Community project: Telehealth and Telemedicine at the Electronic Home (Gott, 1993). In it, a qualitative research approach has been used.

The decision to study health promotion with adolescents was prompted by the health potential they represent. They present our greatest opportunity for achieving a healthier future. These young people are the parents, the citizens, the leaders of tomorrow. Investing in them means investing in the future.

In choosing to look at an initiative operating in Canada there was recognition of 'the moral and intellectual leadership that Canada has provided in the field of health promotion' (Cunningham, 1992).

The electronic bulletin board system (BBS) is called E ZOOT. It is one prong of a co-ordinated community education, inter-agency approach to the development of freedom skills in adolescents. It is complemented by initiatives such as 'Two Way Street: Parents, Kids and Drugs'. This is a publication in co-operation with the Royal Canadian Mounted Police, based on the recognition that most young people do not use drugs, but they are being called on to make their first decisions about them at an increasingly early age. One teenager wrote, in an Alberta essay contest:

> Teenagers want to be told that they are somebody and can be somebody without using drugs or alcohol. We want to be reassured of our place in life and know that we are accepted and deserve our parents' love.

The objective of the personal development style of primary prevention is to empower people to do their own prevention. In this model, agencies do not do prevention to people; prevention does not happen until individuals do it. To be most effective,

---

primary prevention needs to be global, rather than disease specific. This is recognised in the statement of E ZOOT design objectives (1987):

> Prevention of intoxicant problems is not, and should not become, a major focus or priority . . . it is only one of the many hazards to be alert for.

The level set for prevention work can also be problematic. If fixed too high, the preventee in a low risk situation will wonder what all the fuss is about, and so fail to identify with the programme; if set too low, giving central life issue more weight, observers will wonder why a (publicly funded) addictions agency is doing all this 'human stuff'. This latter perspective will be a central concern of funding bodies, particularly during a time of both generalised economic recession, and public spending cuts.

The position adopted by the Alberta Alcohol and Drug Abuse Commission (AADAC) was to develop a framework that allows people to:

> . . . move from big picture to specific focus, as the situation demands . . . (this way) individuals will be in a much better position to conduct their own prevention, priorities will be according to circumstances, and everyone will have a better idea of what the addictions agency is up to. (E ZOOT Co-ordinator)

The System

E ZOOT is a multiline electronic BBS using telephones, linked by modems, to personal computers (PCs). It is aimed at teenagers and young adults and allows users to:

- leave public and private messages in over twenty areas;
- review or download files containing information about alcohol, drugs, and healthy lifestyles;
- upload or download public domain computer software.

E ZOOT began as a one line computer BBS using a PC and a modem (handling 2400 bps), connected to a PC. A used PC was donated by the local telephone company. The software was obtained free from a source in Toronto. It is a 'Shareware' program and is easy to use. The (24-hour) E ZOOT service is offered free within the Edmonton toll area. Most people in Alberta have access to a telephone, and local calls are free.

User demand was high, and in 1992 E ZOOT was upgraded to four incoming telephone lines/modems.

Health promotion information is collected by the systems operator, transcribed, then is available (free) to read, or download. Health related queries raised by users are either answered by moderators direct or networked to specific helping agencies, with information routed back through E ZOOT.

Moderators

Moderator volunteers from AADAC staff moderate discussions and keep them on track. All new users are subject to call-back verification, to prevent obscenities being entered on the bulletin board (this was instituted after a problem in the summer of 1992). A Moderator describes the system:

> If we see an issue on the BB of potential exploitation or a lurking adult with a negative motive . . . on one occasion we were very uncomfortable with what was going on and we called the police in. Another occasion we had a young person who appeared to us to be suicidal, we worked that through and made sure that that young person got to the service required in order to remain safe.

Service description

E ZOOT is offered by Community Education Services (CES) Edmonton, a prevention education unit of the AADAC. The goal is to serve programs aimed at increasing understanding, building personal competence, enhancing public awareness, and encouraging community action in the prevention of substance abuse.

A member of the team describes its origins:

> In 1981 AADAC undertook a very large adolescent prevention campaign. This had many facets, including the evolution of peer support as an initiative, the development of a youth magazine called Zoot Capri that youth would receive in their homes; it was an adjunct to school curriculum rather than distributed in school. Also, AADAC had been sitting on curriculum development committees with Alberta Education for all levels, elementary, junior high and high school, and there were particular aspects of alcohol and drug prevention initiatives in the curriculum, so there was development of curricula materials: posters, handout materials, and a parent education component, and an allied professional education component, so that teachers, nurses, counsellors, those involved with youth, would be involved as well.
>
> The context of Zoot Capri was to provide a health promotion vehicle that would, in a very subtle way, influence the behaviour of youth towards positive self esteem, the development of skills and competencies, the choice of health alternatives for behaviour that would increase the strength of the young person to withstand the pressures that would lead to dependence on alcohol and other drugs. So then that came from a very positive perspective of empowering youth and the networks supporting youth.

It was recognised at the outset that the system would be used if it was adequately advertised, and 'user friendly'. 'User friendliness' poses a particular problem with regard to systems design. Generally, in computer generated activities, form rules function. When form rules, function can be both obscure and inaccessible, thus being demotivating for users.

Process was a particularly relevant topic for E ZOOT designers as the goal of E ZOOT is to enhance the 'freedom skills' of users. This means handing over control in both the process (encouraging 'browsing'), and content (encouraging personal autonomy).

In North America access to a telephone is less problematic than it is in Europe, also, local calls are free. Access to PCs however may be more difficult, and, recognising this, AADAC staff and the Telephone Pioneers of North America assisted with the set-up of three (donated) PCs in youth clubs in two deprived city areas, and in the Adolescent Treatment Centre in Edmonton.

There is evidence of thorough and collaborative evaluation:

> Mental Health Services did a survey a couple of years back and asked kids where they would go for help for suicide, unplanned pregnancy, for mental health, for family problems, and they put AADAC for practically everything.

The format is also seen as accessible:

> It was a real motivator for kids . . . they're already interested in computer technology, they're the ones who play Nintendo, get into computer games, and for them its a motivating way to reach them . . . I mean, kids in grade 2 class in South Edmonton are talking to friends all over the world via computer. Unlike ourselves who have had to become acquainted with it in our middle years (which is easier for some than it is for others!) these kids are growing up seeing this as a naturally available tool and if we just continue to provide posters and print material and so forth we are eventually going to get behind the times. (Service Manager)

Users

Due to E ZOOT's promise of anonymity, very little demographic information relating to users is held; however it is known that most users are between the ages of 14 and 18 years, and most (85%) are male. It is interesting to note however that this is less than the average sex split for use of bulletin boards. E ZOOT Annual Report notes that figures for other BBs are all over 90% male.

A **message thread** is defined as reciprocal message exchanges of three or more messages between two or more BBS users in which a common theme or topic is developed and discussed. A message thread begins when a new topic for discussion is introduced. It is fully underway once there are two or more related replies to the initial message. It has concluded once there can no longer be found any messages which relate to the initial topic. A message thread can also be considered complete if its topic has evolved to a point where it is no longer related to the initial topic. When this occurs a starting point for a new thread should easily be identifiable.

Three hundred and two messages from the message area 'relationships', were collected over a five-week period (5 February–10 March, 1992). Twenty-two separate message threads were identified from the 302 messages. These included conversations related to sex, sexuality, help with meeting girls/women, the perfect relationship, rape and alcohol.

Of the 22 identifiable message threads, 17 began as a request by a user for advice or information, while seven began through the introduction of a new topic by a participant. Continuation of the message thread is dependent on the reaction by the advice seeker to the comments of the advice giver(s).

Message threads can be simple or complex. A complex message thread shows a greater willingness to engage in open conflict. Complex threads are shaped by topics which allow for, and encourage, open uninhibited debate.

Mary's query

A message thread began rather innocuously in the 'relationships' area when a user named Mary asked: 'How does alcohol affect someone's life?'

This simple question generated a heated debate totalling 37 responses and reactions over a 13-day period. Including the moderator, 12 users took part in the discussion. Three replies were sent to Mary, and her six-word question was her single contribution to the entire message thread. On the screen, the thread looks like this:

> By Aquaman
> To Deadhead
> Re Alcohol
>
> Are you saying that if (your friend) drank his life would be full of excitement and fervour? Like hell. You are so often mentioning 'dependency' in terms of relationships and how it is so crippling, but yet you present yourself as being dependant on alcohol for all your social needs.
>
> (Reply)
> By Deadhead
> To Aquaman
> Re Alcohol
>
> Hee hee, alcohol is a positive part of my life, just like 90% or so of the rest of the population. I present myself as dependant? I'd like some proof of that. Since you will have a real hard time finding proof, let me give you some: . . . OH I NEED BOOZE, I NEED BOOZE BAD, I CAN'T LIVE WITHOUT IT . . . . There you go . . . :-) (**note smile**) . . . For ALL my social needs? Whadya mean? So socially, all I need is a bottle? Please prove it noble sir. My social life is unbounded, unlike some people I know . . . .

Users are extremely inventive in their use of noting and using what are normally regarded as 'non verbal' elements of communication in their verbal messages, (see the smile :-) above).

A typical message might be: 'I didn't mean to SHOUT (grin).'

Social interaction

It is often alleged that use of the new technologies reduces social interaction. Whilst this could well be true for personal 'game' systems, it is certainly not true for all technologies: 'Until recently, the notion that social and or cultural data could exist in the computer mediated communications (CMC) context has been overlooked or discounted' (Jackson 1993). Jackson goes on to quote a study by Myers (1987) in which it was found that the CMC environment of an electronic BBS could be seething with an abundance of social activity. Myers' findings reveal that a unique form of interaction exists and that BBS messages provide an ideal forum for uninhibited, anonymous communication (particularly valuable for teenagers). 'Anonymity is part of the magic' (Myers 1987).

The team were asked whether they thought use of a BBS limited social interaction:

> Kids at dances are a lot more involved with one another because of knowing one another via the BB. Many set up meetings to get together; once they get to know each other on the BB they want to meet each other and get together. For those who don't want that they can still reach out, this is a faceless person you are meeting on the BB, but not a cold medium; actually a very warm medium in the sense that people needing to, can reach out. (Team Member)

> The way it's offered is another form of empowerment . . . boys' and girls' clubs having problems keeping teen (age) members; wherever an E ZOOT has been located they are pulling those teens back and the kids can't always get onto the BB straight away . . . so other dialogue is going on while they are waiting to get on to the (one) computer in the club . . . discussions are going on re staying in school, family problems, . . . so the BB is like a carrot that tempts the teens back into the clubs. (Service Manager)

As indicated earlier, a common practice by BB users is the creation of 'smilies' through the combination of keyboard characters to punctuate/illustrate points that they are trying to make. These need to be viewed by turning this page sideways:

:-)	=	smiling face
;-)	=	wink and smiling face
:-(	=	sad face
d:-)	=	smiling face with baseball cap
B-)	=	smiling face with glasses

The future

There is now a solid core of regular system users and many calls for extension of the service have been made. For these to be met, more resources are needed, plus a new computer with a greater capacity and handling speed.

> Our success has been one of our blocks in the way it's grown so fast, and it's got so much potential that it could consume this entire unit. (Service Manager)
>
> (J agrees): We're in a time in our government in Alberta when our government are trying to manage a debt, and as a government agency we feel accountable to that situation; also as tax paying citizens we do, but here you have a really incredible potential and to keep it reined in has been quite a challenge.

Another desired change is that the needs of community partners (as opposed to individual users) should be made a priority. It is recommended that two additional (dedicated) phone lines be added in youth clubs in two other downtown areas.

The heavy use of E ZOOT by males and its under use by females is a source of concern, but the team have seen the user gap narrow (slowly) over the last two years. It is believed that provision of computers in youth centres, with support for female use encouraged by staff, will help to shift the use. Teachers are also aware of the problem and are working on it with AADAC. The Zoot Capri magazine also promotes the use of the bulletin board, and positive messages to build the self-esteem of young females.

Evaluation

E ZOOT is an outstanding example of good practice in adolescent health promotion. A social model of health is used, and exploited to its full potential. All of the Health for All principles enshrined in the Ottawa Charter are evident. Service provision has been reorientated towards community responsive health promotion; the creation of supportive environments for the making of healthy lifestyle choices is evident, as is collaboration with other providers and networks to develop healthy public policy.

Costs are very low. Donated and reconditioned PCs have been used; donated software was traded, and the network expanded. Four Modems cost less than 800 CD (£400.00). Staff costs have increased only slightly (the employment of a systems operator), but existing staff have shifted priorities to run E ZOOT.

The service began modestly; planned growth is also modest, in line with the quality of service staff know they can deliver within budget limitations. It is gratifying to note that, although AADAC has suffered a budget cut, E ZOOT work has been protected.

Service access is not a major problem for the population served. Many young people have home computers, and, in areas of deprivation, computers have been available in schools and youth centres. The fact that local telephone calls are free must help enormously (note: rental charges for lines are made).

Ethical issues were quite problematic to the team who gave a lot of thought to how they could moderate use, yet have the BB belong to the users. The system they have evolved (roving moderators, together with a call-back verification facility) seems to be working well.

Major risks for young people are substance abuse (alcohol, tobacco, 'soft' and 'hard' drugs), sexually transmitted diseases and AIDS. Young people with low self-esteem are more likely to take health risks than those with high self-esteem; additionally, youngsters who take one health risk are more likely to take others (i.e. they are susceptible to a cluster of threats). The behaviour change approach that offers most chance of success with these young people is a broadly based lifeskills approach which builds esteem, and thus equips youngsters to cope with a range of threatening situations, rather than just one.

At E ZOOT a lifeskills approach is employed to promote the building of mature, reflective behaviour. The indications are that this socially responsive health promotion approach is more likely to include sustained behavioural change than the narrow medically based, negative risk reduction approaches that are the norm in so many European health education campaigns.

Hansen and Graham (1991) report findings from a project that had a similar goal to that of the E ZOOT team (reduction of drug use):

> The findings of this study suggest that the key to changing substance abuse patterns (legal and illegal drugs) requires changing sociological factors that account for the onset of use . . . particularly, establishing conservative norms within adolescent friendship groups may effectively reduce demands that otherwise may serve to promote substance use.

Nutbeam *et al.* (1991) have commented that traditional health education campaigns appear very naive in their approach to influencing health behaviour among young people. They are seen as naive in terms of both the message and the form of provision (mass media, 'top down', individualistic, education programmes).

According to Castanheira (1991):

> Most of the programmes to promote adolescent health are neither on the right track nor in the right direction. The right track for health promotion is the community.

At E ZOOT a social model of health is used, and exploited to its full potential. Additionally, service provision has been reorientated towards community responsive health promotion. The creation of supportive environments for the making of healthy lifestyle choices is also evident, as is collaboration with other providers and networks to develop healthy public policy.

References

Castanheira, J.L. (1991) 'Promoting the health of adolescents: are we on the right track?' *International Journal of Adolescent Medicine and Health*, Vol. **5**, No. 2, pp. 113–125.

Cunningham, R. (1990) *Promoting Better Health In Canada and the USA*, Department of Politics, University of Glasgow, Scotland.

Gott, M. (1993) *Telehealth and Telemedicine in the Electronic Home: Final Report*, European Foundation for the Improvement in Living and Working Conditions, Dublin, Irish Republic.

Hansen, W.B., Graham, J.W. (1991) 'Preventing alcohol, marijuana, and cigarette use among adolescents: peer pressure resistance training versus establishing conservative norms', *Preventative Medicine*, Vol. **20**, pp. 414–430.

Jackson, J. (1993) *Exploring computer-mediated communication structures on a electronic bulletin board: a unique context for anonymous interaction*. Department of Sociology, University of Alberta, Edmonton.

Myers, A. (1987) *In* Jackson, J. (1993) *Exploring computer-mediated communication structures on a electronic bulletin board: a unique context for anonymous interaction*. Department of Sociology, University of Alberta, Edmonton.

Nutbeam, D., Aaro, L. and Wold, B. (1991) 'The lifestyle concept and health education with young people: Results from a WHO international survey', *Journal of the Institute of Health Education*, Vol. **29**, No. 3, pp. 98–103.

26

Community Mothers Programme*

BRENDA MOLLOY

The Community Mothers Programme is situated in the Eastern Health Board, Republic of Ireland. The Eastern Health Board is a statutory organisation and serves a population of 1.2 million people, this being one third of the total population of the Republic of Ireland. The Programme extends throughout the whole of the Eastern Health Board area which incorporates the counties of Dublin, Wicklow and Kildare.

This Programme is a support Programme for first and second-time parents with infants in the 0–1 age span, with plans to extend it to children up to two years. It operates in areas of social and economic disadvantage and aims to give power to parents developing their latent skills and restoring confidence and self-esteem, so that they tackle their own problems in their own way. The model is one of parent empowerment.

The disadvantaged areas consist of both traditional working class communities with extended family networks and a strong mother/daughter tie and also large urban housing estates to which families from close-knit inner city communities have been relocated in recent years. In the latter, the fabric of community that the people were used to is no longer there, and basic facilities are lacking in many instances. A lot of people feel alienated and there is no sense of community. There are problems of unemployment, poverty, poor housing, low educational attainment, apathy and powerlessness. In the urban housing estates young mothers are isolated from their extended families. This is particularly acute for the young single parents. Nationally, over 10% of all births are to single parents and a disproportionately high percentage come from the lower socio-economic groups where as many as 70% of births are to single mothers.

Method of delivery

Experienced mothers with common demographic and life histories are recruited as Community Mothers in these areas to give support and encouragement to parents in the rearing of their children. They emphasise health care, nutritional improvement and overall development. The Community Mothers are trained, monitored and guided by

*This is an abridged version of a report first published by Community Care Service, Eastern Health Board, Dublin (1992).

Family Development Nurses. Each unit consists of one Family Development Nurse working in equal partnership with fifteen to twenty Community Mothers and deals with approximately one hundred and fifty referrals of first and second time parents per year.

At present there are ten Family Development Nurses, one hundred and fifty Community Mothers visiting a thousand parents in the home each year. The Programme is co-ordinated with administrative back up. The parents are visited in their own homes by a Community Mother once a month for the first twelve to eighteen months of the infant's life. The parents are acknowledged as the experts and the key agents for change and are supported while they achieve their own goals for their children. A behavioural approach is used in which parents are encouraged to undertake agreed tasks. Illustrated cartoon sequences that show the alternatives available to parents in coping with various child-rearing problems are used.

Parent and child groups have evolved in a number of areas. These groups are facilitated by the Community Mothers and parents and cater for approximately four hundred and fifty parents per year. The expectation would be that the parents who attend would become more connected to the community in which they live. Other significant outcomes are ante-natal visiting, support for breast-feeding mothers in the form of groups and home visits and also developmental initiatives with the Travelling community. Approximately fifty Traveller parents are receiving monthly home visits from the Community Mothers and Family Development Nurses. Many of the Community Mothers have benefited from their involvement in the Programme through self-development and increased self-esteem. While a number have found paid employment others have become involved in other community endeavours and adult education eg. personal development courses. The Family Development Nurses and Community Mothers are also involved in building up active relationships in their areas as a basis for mutual support and for exchange of ideas, with other agencies and community groups.

The training process for the Family Development Nurses and Community Mothers is demand led and encourages initiative and innovation. There is an initial orientation which is not based on theory but, instead, the Family Development Nurses and Community Mothers are familiarised with strategies and resources. This allows them to attempt Programme visits from an early stage. Following this initial orientation, the Family Development Nurses and Community Mothers are supported individually and in groups on a monthly basis in order to build confidence, build on knowledge and exchange ideas. The Programme has been evaluated and it is achieving its goals of parent capacitation and empowerment. On-going evaluation of Programme development and initiatives remains an integral part of the Programme.

In this paper we focus on one part of the Community Mothers Programme—their work with Travelling families. Participants describe the Programme.

The Family Development Nurse's perspective

This is my third year working with the Community Mothers. My respect for their skills and values has grown and we are working more in partnership. My professional expertise is valued by the Community Mothers who appear to see me as a facilitator and friend. The last year has been difficult with obstacles of all kinds impeding our ideas and progress. With the help and encouragement of the Community Mothers, the Programme and I have survived.

My colleague and I visit six Traveller families each month. This is a big achievement. We are accepted and welcomed into the caravans and my colleague is overcoming her fear of dogs. A more holistic approach is needed when working with marginalised people and we need to spend more time and thought with the Travellers if their needs are to be met.

During the last months, we visited two camp-sites. One is an official serviced site, the other a large field with no amenities. We visited six families. The women are avid for information to improve the lot of their many children. The cartoons are helpful as illiteracy is a big problem. Literacy classes are greatly needed and perhaps classes could be organised on the field. Alcohol abuse, lack of employment and play areas, all compound the hardships of the women. Perhaps bringing a service to the people rather than people to the services would be more beneficial.

Keeping appointments is not a problem. The women enjoy the visits from settled people. We hope to continue visiting and perhaps modify some of the cartoons.

My perception is that now the settled community needs to be educated in the Travellers' way of life and perhaps then their lot could be improved but without loss of identity. Closer liaison with the police, teachers, local residents and the Travellers themselves might be helpful in overcoming a lot of prejudices.

Primary Health Care is the Community Mothers Programme in action.

The Community Mother's perspective

I had been a Community Mother for three years and had enjoyed it immensely but I thought I needed a break. However, my Family Development Nurse asked if I would try working with the Travellers and so, I decided to give it a try.

There is a halting site not too far from me with about fifty families staying in it. So, with two babies to locate, I went up to the site. The first thing I noticed were the dogs which put me off a bit. I tried hard to find the two people I wanted, only to be told they were 'Gone off.' I headed for home, disappointed that I didn't get to see even one of the babies but extremely grateful that I hadn't been eaten by the dogs. The next day I decided to try again and did in fact make contact with one of the mothers. She was a young girl with a beautiful baby boy and she was delighted that I had called and invited me in. We had a great chat and I found that she had great values for herself and her baby.

Unfortunately, after only three visits, she moved on. This is the most disappointing thing about working with the Travellers.

I am visiting another lovely girl at the moment. She is a single girl, rearing the baby on her own but with fantastic help from her family who live in trailers all around her. I have become very good friends with her father who is about seventy and is able to tell me about everyone on the site which will help when I am looking for the new mothers. Of course, he nearly got my life story out of me before he volunteered any information. He has been living on the site for nine years but will take off to Kerry now for a couple of months and return in September.

I have gone in the mobile clinic with the Public Health Nurse who works with them and she has introduced me to a good few mothers so I suppose they will get used to me being around.

I have learned to ignore the goats, horses and greyhounds but it's the little dogs you have to watch, as I discovered when one of them ran after me on a recent visit.

I hope to have six mothers in the Programme by September which is the time they will all settle down here before the Winter.

I hope to continue working with them for a good while and help them in any way I can. I also hope that some settled people's attitudes will change towards the Travellers and that they won't treat them as second class citizens as there are good and bad people in every society.

The parents' perspective

A boost to my confidence

My name is Sandra and I am sixteen. I have a six month old baby boy named Christopher. I was first told about the Programme by a friend of mine who is also visited by the Public Health Nurse. To me the Programme sounded very interesting but I didn't think that I would be approached because I was so young.

When the nurse asked me did I want to participate, I jumped at the chance because I know just how hard it is starting from scratch on your own and I hoped that I could help girls like me. I was trained by someone who has now become a good friend to me. I found the training very exciting and always looked forward to her visits. I learned things about babies that I probably would never have learned otherwise. It has boosted my confidence and enthusiasm about meeting people and also in looking after Christopher.

At first I was very nervous about offering the Programme but both girls accepted and so far all has gone very well.

I think that it is a great idea and would have loved to have availed of the Programme myself. As it is, I'm learning it all anyway!

Mother, Area 10

Somebody cares

My name is Susan and I am the mother of a ten month old bouncing bundle of joy named Emma.

Even though Emma is the apple of our eye, the last ten months have been filled with some anxiety such as whether or not the baby is feeding well, or whether she is getting the proper nutritious food she needs to develop or whether she is stimulated enough in areas of mental and physical development. In general were were anxious to know if we were doing the right things for our new baby.

You will always find people, mostly women, unfortunately, who are ready and waiting to lead you and give their advice on how to raise your child. These people do not mean to seem as if they know everything about child-rearing although some do! I found some of their advice confusing and complicated and most people would say to me, 'Pay no attention, do your own thing'. But, when you look at these people who have two, three or four children, a young inexperienced mother like me is bound to get somewhat confused.

This is where the Community Mothers come in. My Community Mother is experienced and friendly, she does not push any 'tips' onto you and expect to see them carried out. What she actually does is to sit down and listen to you. To have another mother sitting down in a friendly, warm atmosphere, in the security of our own home, discussing and explaining ideas about our baby and ourselves is what I found most comforting. I say, 'our baby', because my husband, Thomas, likes to sit in on these discussions, which saves the bother of passing on information and getting it confused in the process.

I have found that the Community Mothers are not only interested in the baby, but in the mother too. They guide you on what is nutritious for yourself as well as the baby. And it makes it a little bit more comforting to know that somebody cares as much for your welfare as well as your baby's.

At the end of every visit my Community Mother would always hand me an information sheet which often referred to the talk we'd just had. These sheets were done in a simple cartoon form with tips, for example on feeding, dangers in the kitchen, nutrition and diet for both mother and baby. I found these sheets a simple and effective way of getting the message across.

Mother, Area 4

27

A Prospective Study on the Health of Birmingham Babies in Different Ethnic Groups: Interim Findings*

SARAH BUNDEY

Introduction

Health patterns of immigrants are likely to be different from those of indigenous English people for several reasons. The immigrants may be newly exposed to viruses or antigenic stimuli that are rare in their own countries. They often belong initially to lower social classes and so suffer deprivation and poverty. They may be puzzled by our patterns of health care and not make full use of them. They may have different genetic susceptibilities to polygenic diseases and they may show different frequencies of single gene conditions. They may be unused to our diet and our social habits such as drinking and smoking. They may have different customs such as marriages between blood relations.

Many of these features particularly affect the frequency, severity and natural history of diseases of adult life, and have been the subject of various useful studies (Beevers, 1983; Cruickshank and Beevers, 1989). One observation made by paediatricians in Birmingham has been that there is a high frequency of chronic handicapping diseases amongst Pakistani children, and it has been suggested that this may be due to the high frequency of parental consanguinity. However, another explanation could be that handicapped children are preferentially brought to England or to Birmingham by their parents in order to search for treatment. We therefore planned a study on the health of Birmingham children by prospectively following babies born here. The findings of the study relating to the basic data and the first four weeks of life have already been published (Bundey *et al.*, 1990, 1991).

*This is an abridged version of Chapter 8 in Bittles, A.H. and Roberts, D.F. (eds) (1992), *Minority Populations: Genetics, Demography and Health*, Proceedings of the twenty-seventh annual symposium of the Galton Institute, London, 1990, London, Macmillan in association with the Galton Institute, pp. 143–155.

Table 27.1 Distribution of minority ethnic groups in the West Midlands conurbation

		Percentage of children aged 0–4 in four ethnic groups†			
	*Number of children 0–4 yrs**	*Caribbean*	*East African and Indian*	*Pakistani*	*Bangladeshi*
Birmingham	63 588	4.9, 10.0	9.7, 11.4	12.5, 13.2	1.6, 1.6
Sandwell	18 149	2.6, 5.3	15.4, 18.1	4.0, 4.2	1.4, 1.4
Dudley	17 733	1.0, 2.0	2.5, 3.0	3.4, 3.6	0.2, 0.2
Wolverhampton	15 625	3.6, 7.6	21.5, 25.4	1.4, 1.5	0.2, 0.2
Walsall	16 058	0.8, 1.7	9.1, 10.7	5.2, 5.5	0.8, 0.8
Solihull	11 256	1.3, 2.7	0.7, 0.8	0.2, 0.2	–
Coventry	19 124	1.1, 2.1	12.5, 14.7	2.7, 2.8	0.6, 0.6

*1981 census.
†The first number gives ethnic group as defined by birthplace of head of household (1981 census); the second number is adjusted upwards to account for those heads of households of ethnic minority groups who were born in the UK (Bundey *et al.*, 1990).

Previous work

Population

Birmingham and indeed most of the West Midlands conurbation is multiracial (Table 27.1) with the highest percentage of Pakistani families being found in Birmingham. Within Birmingham itself, the distribution of ethnic minority groups is uneven, with very few being found in the North and South Health Districts. Indians, Afro-Caribbeans and Bangladeshis are found predominantly in the West Health District, and Pakistanis predominantly in the Central and East Health Districts (WMRHA, 1984). The Afro-Caribbeans come mainly from the West Indies, in particular from Jamaica, but about 5 per cent are from the continent of Africa. Of the West Indian adults, 50–60 per cent were born in the UK. Of the Indian adults, about 70 per cent were born in India, the remainder being born in East Africa or the United Kingdom. Few Pakistani or Bangladeshi adults were born in the UK. The Pakistani families mainly come from the rural areas of Mirpur in the Kashmiri region of North Pakistan and the Bangladeshi families mainly come from Sylhet.

Collection of data

At the outset of the study, births occurring on weekdays at three maternity hospitals in Birmingham which serve the West, Central and East Health Districts were documented. The study was carried out between January 1986 and the end of April 1987 and only births to city residents were included. Briefly, mothers were interviewed in the postnatal wards by a Research Associate who could speak Asian languages as well as English. Information was collected on health, ages, race of both parents, whether they were consanguineous, history of previous pregnancies, amount of antenatal care, diet and drug or alcohol consumption during pregnancy. The interview was supplemented by data from hospital records relating to the mother and baby. Altogether, 4934 babies were enrolled in the study.

Perinatal and neonatal mortality

The first analysis of these births concerned early mortality rates and these have been reported (Bundey *et al.*, 1991). In brief, the perinatal mortality rate for the Pakistani babies was significantly greater than that for European babies. Some but not all of the excess mortality could be explained by the occurrence of autosomal recessive diseases in the offspring of consanguineous parents. Another explanatory factor was the high frequency of severe congenital heart disease in Pakistani babies. Other races did not appear to be particularly predisposed to serious problems although the higher rate of twinning in Afro-Caribbeans led to a greater risk of prematurity.

Further follow-up

Following the documentation of deaths occurring in the first four weeks of life, any subsequent illnesses, disabilities or deaths occurring in the children were ascertained by searching through the child health register, the regional hospital statistics on inpatient admissions, the death notifications to the District Medical Officers, and the computerised lists of hospital record numbers accorded against names and date of birth. Permission for these searches was obtained from the mothers (at the time of the initial interview), from the District Medical Officers of the five Birmingham Health Districts and from the five District Ethical Committees. Hospital records relating to children in the study were scrutinised to determine if an illness was genetic or had some other cause.

Follow-up of 4934 children enrolled in the study will continue until they enter school at the age of five, and indeed the type of school entered will be one objective observation. So far the follow-up has continued for three years and the interim results are presented here. They are necessarily incomplete, and one source of error arises from the fact that we have not yet ascertained how many of the original cohort of babies are still living in the city of Birmingham.

We have documented serious malformations, but have excluded the following: talipes that did not require surgery, syndactyly or polydactyly, Poland syndrome, umbilical hernia, cardiac septal defects that did not require operation, and pyloric stenosis. Under serious chronic diseases, we have included chronic epilepsy but have excluded febrile convulsions, asthma and eczema.

We were also interested in documenting diseases caused by single genes and have categorised them as follows. Autosomal dominant and X-linked disorders are self-explanatory. Autosomal recessive disorders are subdivided into: (a) certain or undoubted autosomal recessive diseases, because of distinctive clinical features and listing in McKusick (1988); (b) probable autosomal recessive diseases, because the clinical features are usually but not always caused by recessive genes, such as unexplained microcephaly, or severe congenital deafness in the offspring of healthy parents; and (c)

Table 27.2 Serious malformations in 4934 index babies

Type of malformation	*Ethnic origin and numbers* of babies*					
	European	*Afro-Caribbean*	*Indian*	*Pakistani*	*Bangladeshi*	*Other*
Multiple malformation	1	0	0	4 (4)	0	0
Congenital heart	7	1	1	10 (7)	1	0
Gut malformations	4	2	0	0	0	1
Joint	7	0	1	6 (6)	1 (1)	0
Kidney (including hypospadias)	5	0	1	2 (2)	1	0
Eye	1	1	0	1	0	0
Skull, CNS and NTD	1	0	0	2 (2)	0	0
Cleft lip† palate‡	5	0	0	0	0	0
Chromosomal abnormality	6 (1)	1	2	2 (1)	0	1
All malformations†	37 (1)	5	5	27 (22)	3 (1)	2
Total babies	2432 (10)	509 (3)	625 (32)	956 (657)	216 (29)	196 (20)
Malformation rate per 1000 (and 2 s.e. range)	15.2 (10.2–20.2)	9.8 (1.0–18.6)	8.0 (0.8–15.2)	28.2‡ (17.4–39.0)	13.8 (0–29.6)	10.2 (0–24.2)

*The number in parentheses refers to those babies with consanguineous parents.
†20 of the 79 malformed babies had died.
‡Equals 16.7 for non-consanguineous parents and 33.5 (19.5–47.5) for the offspring of consanguineous parents.
s.e. = standard error of the mean.

doubtful autosomal recessive conditions, those where the clinical features represent a recessive condition in a minority of instances, for example, Potter's syndrome or non-specific mental retardation.

Results

Malformations

Malformations are listed in Table 27.2. However, malformations at birth give a somewhat misleading impression since, during the period of the study, neural tube defects would have been recognised in the first half of pregnancy, which would then probably have been terminated. This means that their rate of about 2/1000 (Carstairs and Cole, 1984) should be added to the malformation rate for Europeans, Indians and Pakistanis.

The malformation rate for Pakistanis given in Table 27.2 is considerably greater than that for other ethnic groups, particularly so amongst the babies of consanguineous parents, of whom 22 out of 657 (33.5/1000) had a serious malformation. This rate is significantly higher than that for Afro-Caribbeans and Indians.

Chronic diseases and disabilities

The most common of these was mental retardation with or without other problems. Some of these babies were premature, had evidence of an intrauterine infection or were asphyxiated at birth. For others however the delay in development is unexplained. At present it is not certain which children will be graded as severely retarded; however they all presented with developmental delay before three years of age, and some very much earlier. The rate of mental retardation was 0.6 per cent for Europeans, 0.8 per cent for Afro-Caribbeans and Indians, and 2.4 per cent for Pakistani babies. All the Pakistani babies who have been listed here as having mental retardation or some other chronic disability had consanguineous parents. The rate of chronic disabilities in Pakistani children is significantly greater than the rates in other ethnic groups.

Discussion

Our main interest lay in determining to what extent the practice of close consanguinity in Pakistani parents resulted in an increased incidence of autosomal recessive diseases or of polygenic malformations in their children. The health of babies in other ethnic groups did not reveal any significant problems; the finding of two Afro-Caribbean babies with sickle cell disease was predictable.

Analysis of the high perinatal mortality of Pakistani babies (Bundey *et al.*, 1991) did not show an obvious effect of parental consanguinity, presumably because of the small numbers inevitable in a prospective study, and because many other factors can cause stillbirths or neonatal deaths. However a large study from Pakistan (Shami and Zahida, 1982) had documented significantly increased mortality in the children of consanguineous parents, even though the overall perinatal mortality rate in Pakistan is about 50/1000, and the overall death rate in months one to twelve is about 39/1000. Such high background rates might have obscured any effects of parental consanguinity but did not do so.

In considering problems occurring after the perinatal period, we first had to assess whether our ascertainment of problems occurring in the first three years of life of the 4934 babies was complete. Eight babies had Down's syndrome, which fits the expected incidence of one in 600, and two babies had cystic fibrosis which also fits the expected incidence. Five children have X-linked recessive disorders (2/1000 males) which approaches the estimate of 2.3 to 3.0/1000 males predicted by Polani (1990). Six children have autosomal dominant disorders (1.2/1000) which is less than the 7/1000 predicted by Carter (1977), but one would expect only a small proportion of dominant disorders to be detected at such young ages. The incidence of confirmed or probable autosomal recessive diseases in European babies is 1.2/1000, less than the 2.0–3.0/1000 expected (Carter, 1977; Polani, 1990). In contrast, the rate of known autosomal recessive diseases in Pakistanis is 14.6/1000, and increases to 25.1/1000 if probable autosomal recessive diseases are included. These incidences which are ten to twenty times those in Europeans must be due to the parental consanguinity which is often closer than first-cousin relationships.

The increased risk of perinatal mortality is gradually becoming known to the Pakistani community. It is not surprising that such awareness has been slow; after all, Pakistani couples in Pakistan have a 5 per cent chance of losing a child in the perinatal period and about a further 4 per cent chance of losing a child during the next eleven months, so they can only be pleased at the dramatic fall in mortality on moving to the UK.

The striking feature in the present study is the excess of malformations and chronic handicapping conditions in the offspring of consanguineous Muslims. The prevalence of such conditions in European children is 2.5 per cent, in Pakistani children it is 6.5 per cent and in the Pakistani children who are the offspring of consanguineous parents it is 9 per cent. It was expected that all autosomal recessive diseases of Pakistani children would be found among those with related parents because of the high background level of consanguinity (Roberts, 1988). The level of consanguinity is much less in Bangladeshi families than in Pakistani families and there is correspondingly less morbidity although the figures are small. We have insufficient data in other ethnic groups to study the effects of parental consanguinity.

Implications of these findings for health care

Since one in 11 of the offspring of consanguineous Pakistani couples has a serious malformation or chronic handicapping disease, it is important that Pakistani mothers should be offered careful ultrasound examination in each pregnancy and that their babies should be carefully screened for developmental problems. In these ways diagnoses of serious problems can be made earlier, an offer can be made to terminate a pregnancy if the fetus has a severe inoperable malformation, or prompt medical or surgical treatment can be instigated for others. In addition, warning may be given about any recurrence risks.

It will be valuable to have Pakistani health education offers to explain to Pakistani mothers about tests during pregnancy, and about the importance of looking out for any problems in a child, such as congenital deafness. Such a health education programme is planned in Birmingham, with support from the Central Birmingham Health Authority and the Save the Children Fund. One way in which these health workers could help is by explaining to mothers that it is useful for doctors to know about other ill children in the family, since the presence of other consanguineous unions sometimes means that the same disease occurs in cousins and other relatives. This is particularly important if prompt treatment of a metabolic disease is crucial. One mother in our study never mentioned that her sister had a child who died with non-ketotic hyperglycinemia and so the diagnosis in her similarly affected baby was unnecessarily delayed; although in this instance, earlier treatment would not have saved the baby.

Once an autosomal recessive disease has occurred in a child, genetic counselling is useful not only for the parents but also for other members of the family, since the presence of one consanguineous union in a Pakistani family is usually accompanied by others. For example, if the brother or sister of an affected child marries a first cousin, the risk for the same disorder occurring in a child of this union is at least one in 24. If the affected child in due course marries a first cousin, the risk for his or her offspring is at least one in eight. Genetic counselling therefore should be made available to other members of the family, preferably with the help of Pakistani health education workers.

Should any efforts be made to discourage the practice of marrying cousins? Darr and Modell (1988), who studied the pedigrees of 100 Pakistani women in Bradford, concluded that their level of consanguinity was greater than that of 900 Pakistanis from Lahore, and also that the practice of marrying one's cousin was beneficial in providing extended support and friendship in an alien country. They felt that any attempt to discourage consanguineous marriages would do more harm than good.

In Birmingham there seems to be a tendency for Pakistani women who marry relations to be younger than those who do not (Bundey *et al.*, 1990) but this is not significant statistically and there is no other evidence that the practice of consanguinity is actually increasing. Indeed, the impression gathered from genetic clinic interviews is that young Pakistanis who have been educated in the UK do not wish to marry their cousins (Syeda, 1988). It therefore can be predicted that the current high consanguinity rate of Pakistanis in the UK, and its associated untoward effects, is a temporary phenomenon. In the meantime, doctors should take the opportunity to document and investigate the autosomal recessive diseases that occur in Pakistani children. Experience in Birmingham suggests that about half of these diseases are new.

References

Beevers, D.G. (ed.) (1983) 'Ethnic differences in common diseases', *Postgraduate Medical Journal*, vol. 59, pp. 615–71.

Bundey, S., H. Alam, A. Kaur, S. Mir and R.J. Lancashire (1990) 'Race, consanguinity and social features in Birmingham babies: a basis for prospective study', *Journal of Epidemiology and Community Health*, vol. 44, pp. 130–5.

Bundey, S., H. Alam, A. Kaur, S. Mir and R.J. Lancashire (1991) 'Why do UK-born Pakistani babies have high perinatal and neonatal mortality rates?', *Paediatric and Perinatal Epidemiology*, vol. 5, pp. 101–14.

Carstairs, V. and S. Cole (1984) 'Spina bifida and anencephaly in Scotland', *British Medical Journal*, vol. 289, pp. 1182–4.

Carter, C.O. (1977) 'Monogenic disorders', *Journal of Medical Genetics*, vol. 14, pp. 316–20.

Cruickshank, J.K. and D.G. Beevers (eds) (1989) *Ethnic Factors in Health and Disease* (London: Wright).

Darr, A. and B. Modell (1988) 'The frequency of consanguineous marriage among British Pakistanis', *Journal of Medical Genetics*, vol. 25, pp. 186–90.

McKusick, V.A. (1988) *Mendelian Inheritance in Man*, 8th edn (Baltimore, Md: Johns Hopkins Press).

Polani, P.E. (1990) *The impact of genetics on medicine*, Harveian Oration 1988 (London: The Royal College of Physcians).

Roberts, D.F. (1988) 'Conclusion', in S. Bundey and D.F. Roberts (eds), *Health and Consanguinity in Immigrant Populations in Britain, Biology and Society*, vol. 5, pp. 32–7.

Shami, S.A. and Zahida (1982) 'Study of consanguineous marriages in the population of Lahore (Punjab), Pakistan', *Biologia*, vol. 28, pp. 1–15.

Syeda, W. (1988) 'Muslim couples and genetic counselling', in S. Bundey and D.F. Roberts (eds), *Health and Consanguinity in Immigrant Populations in Britain, Biology and Society*, vol. 5, pp. 22–4.

West Midlands Regional Health Authority (1984) *Ethnic minorities in the West Midlands Health Region* (Birmingham: WMRHA).

28

Client–Public Health Nurse Relationships in Child Health Care: A Grounded Theory Study*

KATRI VEHVILÄINEN-JULKUNEN

Introduction

Field services in public health nursing have existed in Finland for 50 years, with child health concerns being a major focus from the early years to the present. Public health nurses have played a key role in running the child health care system. During the first year of a child's life he or she is examined about 12 times, of which about eight to nine examinations are by a public health nurse and the rest by a physician. In practice, the participation of mothers with their children in the health centre activity is 100%, especially in the group with children under 1 year of age (Health Care 1987; Lauri 1989).

This historically important work of public health nurses has challenges. Critical comments about the services usually deal with the content of the public health nursing and especially the manner in which services are given, i.e. the relationship between the client and the provider of services, in this case usually a public health nurse. According to Finnish research studies clients often want to get more information and guidance from public health nurses. Clients wanted to receive support as parents.

Little systematic examination

It can be argued that, although there has been much discussion and debate about the public health nurse–client relationship in Finland and abroad, there has been little systematic examination of what constitutes this relationship and the factors that influence its development (see Chao 1989; Luker & Chalmers 1989; Pearson 1991). Theoretical models (e.g. Lauri 1981, 1989; Clark 1986) developed in this field approach these interactions mainly from the perspective of the public health nurse, somewhat neglecting the role of the client. For example, the meaning of the child's presence in the situation is systematically neglected; usually it has been taken for

*This is an abridged version of an article that was first published in *Journal of Advanced Nursing*, Vol. 17, No. 8, pp. 896–904, 1992.

granted. This leads to examination of the concept of client in this system: who is the client—the parent, the child or both?

Also, the studies of interaction in nursing have focused primarily on hospital patients, and especially on certain aspects of verbal communication (e.g. Macleod Clark 1983; Faulkner 1984; Athlin 1988; Leino-Kilpi 1990). One could ask to what extent studies of hospital patients are comparable to what happens in health care. The methodological orientation has been mostly positivistic; in order to support pre-existing theories or models the analyses have been quantitative (May 1990). Thus interesting questions arise as to how public health nurses interact with their clients.

Aims of the study

The purpose of this paper is to describe the relationships between clients and public health nurses in child health care. This paper is a part of a large qualitative, grounded theory study about the content and patterns of interaction in child health care in Finland. In this study empirical data were used to build up a descriptive theory or, as in grounded theory, a substantive theory about the interaction between the client and the public health nurse. The aim of the study was to produce a theoretical construct that would be understandable and accessible to people working in child health care.

Data collection and analysis

The data were analysed using the grounded theory approach, especially qualitative comparative analysis. The grounded method is a systematic research approach to the collection and analysis of qualitative data for the purpose of generating a theory that will further understanding of social and psychological processes. Descriptions of how grounded theory study is done are illustrated in various sources (Glaser & Strauss 1967; Glaser 1978; Chenitz & Swanson 1986; Strauss 1987; Strauss & Corbin 1990; Janhonen & Vehviläinen-Julkunen 1991).

Observations

The data about the content and patterns of interaction were collected by non-participant observation (Wilson 1985) and formal and informal interviews in addition to written essays. Data collection started in January 1988 and ended in January 1990. The basic data were collected so that the researcher observed public health nurse–client interactions during visits to child health clinics in seven health centres out of 23 in the North Savo region of Finland; three of them were in towns and four in rural areas.

For public health nurses (PHN) to be observed, the criteria were different working experience and age. The average age of the public health nurses was 37 years, range 26 to 60 years. Thirty per cent of them had worked 15 years or more as a public health nurse, 40% from 3 to 15 years and 30% under 3 years. Eighty per cent of public health nurses had children of their own.

As for the clients, all of these visits were with children under 1 year of age. Usually, children were 8–10 months old. The mothers' (M) average age was 27 years, range

20 to 44 years, 70% were married, only one was unmarried and five were living with the child's father.

Observations were made in the daytime during normal working hours for public health nurses. According to field notes taken during this time, 1554 interactions (from 20 visits) with public health nurses were analysed in terms of conditions, strategies and consequences. Non-participant observation was used (see Benoliel 1975; Wilson 1985; Chenitz & Swanson 1986). The researcher usually sat in the corner of the room and used a tape-recorder, which was placed in a good location with respect to the public health nurse.

The verbal content of the interaction was tape-recorded so that the researcher could concentrate on nonverbal aspects of the interaction. The researcher made notes about the room, the interaction and its patterns. In addition, a total of 40 interviews were conducted, which dealt with the observed interactions. These interviews were used to complement and interpret the observations.

Analysis of data

Analysis of the data was based on what had been written about grounded theory, especially qualitative comparative analysis. Data collection and analysis are not two discrete processes. They are related circularly; as data are collected they are analysed and this initial analysis guides and focuses further collection of data (Glaser 1978; Wilson 1985; Strauss 1987). Analysis of the data started with line-by-line analysis of written observational and interview data, so-called open coding. Codes were given for the contents and patterns of each interaction. These substantive codes were written on the margins of the written documents from the observations. Then all the codes were compared, and subcategories were formed from these coded properties.

The data about interaction were first classified according to eight categories of the contents of consultations using line-by-line analysis. Then categories of relationships were formulated from these properties and substantive codes. The categories of relationships describing the interaction were formulated from verbal and nonverbal patterns (Janhonen & Vehviläinen-Julkunen 1991).

Findings

A description of the patterns of interaction or relationships between client and public health nurse used is presented in the following sections:

1 relationship between mother and child during the visit;
2 relationship between public health nurse and child during the visit;
3 relationship between mother and public health nurse during the visit.

The aim was to look at the interactions from the child's point of view and relationships between child, mother and public health nurses were described by using the patterns of interaction.

Table 28.1 Relationship between mother and child during the visit

Category	Properties
Persuasive relationship	Trying to get the child to do something Explaining to the child what is to be done
Tender relationship	Expressing affection for the child Touching the child when comforting him/her Holding the child in her arms Kissing the child Chatting with the child Calling him/her by name
Protective relationship	Warning the child not to touch things

Relationship between mother and child during the visit

The relationships between mother and child during the situation were called tender, protective and persuasive. The formulations of these relationships are presented in Table 28.1. The category tender relationship consisted mainly of nonverbal patterns, usually the mother touching the child. This showed whose child the child really was—he was the mother's (love relationship). The touching was called 'comforting touching', because it was associated with the child's fears or crying. The mother held the child in her arms, comforting him or kissing the child when he started to cry. The child might also be afraid of public health equipment or actions.

The persuasive relationship was described as including the explanations to the child about what was going to happen next, what the public health nurse was doing. The aim of this activity was to make the child co-operative and to help the public health nurse with measurements.

> [PHN to child] Look I have a bead here. You can take it. [The child did not take it.]
> [M to child] Take it when she gives it to you. Show her how beautifully you can take things and move them from one hand to another.

The protective relationship was illustrated by the mother warning the child not to touch the public health equipment or liquids. The aim was to protect the child from accidents.

> [The child crawls to the public health cupboard and the mother forbids it] Be careful, you just may not touch it; it is dangerous for you . . . go there.

Relationship between child and public health nurse during the visit

The relationship between child and public health nurse was described as one of persuasion and entertainment. The persuasive relationship was described as containing

Table 28.2 Formulation of persuasive and entertainment relationship categories describing the relationship between child and public health nurse

Category	Properties
Persuasive relationship	Trying to get the child to do something Praising the child for doing something Explaining to the child what she is going to do
Entertainment relationship	Whistling Chatting Touching when doing rituals Telling the child he/she is the most important Mimicking

[the] public health nurse's attempts to get the child to do something, to complete the rituals or explain to the child what the nurse was going to do to her (Table 28.2).

> [PHN to child] Look what kind of beads I have here; you can take them. Yes, just like that. There it is, take it also in your other hand, please take it.

Entertainment relationship meant whistling to the child or praising the child, saying that he was climbing beautifully. Usually entertainment was connected with the child's crying; nurses tried to prevent crying by entertaining the child (Table 28.2). The aim of this entertainment relationship was to prevent crying and keep the child co-operative. With his co-operation, the public health nurse was able to assess the child's development.

> [Child starts to cry while being measured. PHN to the child] Look, Mike, what I have here. [PHN makes strange voices and whispers, showing toys to the child] This nice, Mike? Now, well, you are already smiling; better.

Public health nurses touched the children when measuring them. This pattern was called 'informative touching', because the nurses used touching only when they wanted to know something about the child's development. Some of them used mimicking when communicating with the child or played hide-and-seek without saying a word.

Relationship between mother and public health nurse during the visit

The relationship between mother and public health nurse could be described as a relationship supporting self-confidence. This main relationship was formulated for later analysis, making it easier to handle the data later on (Table 28.3). It was formed from the patterns: good to see you again, information sharing and advising, encouraging, calming, joking, negotiating, listening and silence. It was described as supporting self-confidence, because the individual needs information and advice, encouragement, calming and joking to get support for her self-confidence. Joking was used as a form

Table 28.3 Relationship between mother and public health nurse as described by the patterns of interaction

Category	Pattern
Relationship supporting self-confidence	Good to see you again Information sharing and advising Negotiating Encouraging Calming Confirming Joking Listening Silence Nonverbal communication

of encouragement. All of the concepts fit under the category called relationship supporting self-confidence. For example, in an interview, one young mother described it this way:

> When I talk with the public health nurse, I get information about my child's growth and care . . . . I can tell her about my uncertainty, there I get self-confidence in taking care of my child.

The mutual relationship between mother and public health nurse could be said to be the main relationship in the situation, because they were both talking about the child. First, the patterns of mutual interaction, subcategories, properties and substantive codes were described and after that relationships describing the patterns were formulated (categories). The nonverbal communication was taken from the observations. In the following section, the patterns are described in more detail.

Nonverbal communication

Nonverbal communication included data about proximity, orientation in the room, speaking level, physical appearance, direction of gaze and eye contact. In these data by the mother and public health nurse, touching was not used when greeting. As for proximity, there was a desk for the public health nurse, and the mother and public health nurse were sitting at the desk. In most cases the mother was not behind the desk, but they sat quite close to each other.

Both mother and public health nurse moved around the room when measuring the child and at the same time talked to each other. This was called orientation or how people position themselves in situations. Both parties could be said to be at the same speaking level in such situations. The physical appearance of the public health nurses was not very formal; they did not wear uniforms. The gaze and eye contact were direct, expressing an interest in each other.

Verbal communication

Good to see you again

The interaction started with the pattern called 'good to see you again'. This was described as containing a greeting, and it started with the public health nurse fetching the mother from the waiting room. It could be described as an invitation to talk. In the waiting room, they usually greeted each other but did not shake hands, and started to talk about the child or mother. In the interviews, the public health nurses explained why they went to the waiting room. They wanted to see how the mother handled the child when she undressed it.

> [PHN] How are you? It has been 2 months since we met last time; are you already working?
> [M] Yes, started 1 week ago.

Information sharing and advising

At this stage, information sharing and advising were combined into one category, because they contained the same elements. In the relationship between public health nurses and mothers, information sharing was described as containing information gathering, information giving and advising as a basis for working in the situation. Usually either one of the participants was asking questions or inquiring and the other was explaining. This might be direct questions such as 'Does the child sit?' Answer: 'Yes'. Then they asked questions by using examples. The public health nurses inquired about the situation at home or ascertained whether the mother was going to work. This was described as containing, on the public health nurses' part, answers to the questions, giving information or advice, advising by using written material, giving orders to mothers and explaining alternatives.

> [PHN] What does he eat when he wakes up in the morning, porridge?
> [M] Yes, porridge and milk, then he sleeps a few hours . . .
> or
> [PHN] Did you see the dentist? Was everything all right?
> [M] Yes, we did.

Another example concerns advice:

> [PHN] Where do you keep the flowers?
> [M] He reached them, they are not so low.
>
> [PHN] When he gets the doors open, you must pay special attention to accidents, they may really occur. Washing liquids and things of that sort are dangerous. And what about the electrical outlets? Have you already covered them as was said last time?
> [M] Yes we have, like it said in the papers.

Information sharing was used on the part of the public health nurses when they talked about the child's development (physical, psychological, social, behaviour), about events during development and influences on development (life situation, education, incidents), talking about formalities (rituals), the relationship between parties, about being a mother and situational matters during the visit.

On the part of the mother, information sharing and advising included answering questions, telling about and explaining situations, telling why she did something, explaining why and how the child did something and talking about situations, fears or feelings.

> [M] How much does he weigh?
> [PHN] He has gained 500 g; that is enough and is good; it is just fine.

An example of explanations follows:

> [PHN] What about the spots on his shoulders? I remember them from last time.
> [M] I put some cream on and they disappeared but I noticed one thing. When Matthew had a sweater on with buttons on the shoulders, they . . .

Mothers used this pattern when the interaction was about events during development that influence development, formalities, relationships between parents, being a mother and relatives. They did not use this pattern when discussing situational matters during the visit.

Confirming

The confirming pattern, on the other hand, included the public health nurses' inquiries about whether the mother had carried out the decisions made during the last visit. Mothers usually wanted confirmation about situations where they disagreed with relatives about caring for their child. Confirming was described as ensuring that the family or mother had done a certain thing for the child before coming to see the public health nurse. For instance:

> [PHN] Did you try the milk for Laura as I told you to last time?
> [M] I gave it like you told me to do. If I remember right, you said that I can give . . .
> [M] Must I be careful with food, including milk, because we have allergies in our family?
> [PHN] Yes, if there are allergies in the family, during the first year you must be careful what you give the child.

On the other hand, the mother might be uncertain about her child's illness or other advice received from professionals and relatives. Often she seemed to be asking for confirmation of the decisions of others.

[M] We had to take Mark to see doctor. Well, they said it was babypox [mother describes symptoms]
[PHN] As you described the symptoms, it is really clear. First the child gets fever—no other symptoms—and after that eczema. That really confirms it.

Encouraging

The encouraging pattern was described, in terms of the public health nurse, as containing assurance, convincing the mother, encouraging the mother to do things or persuading her to do something. On her part, this meant hesitation and wondering if she did the right thing for the child. The aim was to get encouragement. Generally, the public health nurse was giving encouragement and the mother was waiting for encouragement.

[M] Some skin problems have been coming up. It was my fault, I did put some cream with scent on her, that might have done it . . . . I stopped this; I have not done it much after.
[PHN] Yes, you did the right thing when stopping, however, during the wintertime the child's skin usually gets dry . . .

Mothers could be interpreted as asking for encouragement in the situation. Encouragement was also given by praising the child or expressing positive feelings about the way the mother–child dyad worked.

[PHN] This Mike is such a nice boy, he always charms us here. He is not shy with us here at all.
[M] Yes, yes.

Public health nurses used encouragement during the interaction when the child's physical and social development was concerned and when talking about relatives. Mothers used it when talking about the child's physical development, life situation, rituals and situational matters during the visit.

Calming

The pattern of calming was described as calming the mother when she was worried about the child's reactions. Calming was differentiated from the encouragement pattern, because this was connected firmly to some special occasions such as accidents. These occasions had worried the mother and made her really anxious; she had real fears.

The interviews afterwards with clients supported this description. The mother might say, 'I was terribly worried about Laura when she got the fit of anger, whether I did the right thing . . .'. The public health nurse said, 'You did the right thing: these things are not rare with children . . . it is usually a normal situation . . .'. In the calming pattern explanations were usually used—the worries of the mothers were explained as normal situations.

Negotiating

For the public health nurse, the negotiating category consisted of admitting and suggesting something to the mother. On her part, this meant admitting, accepting, agreeing and explaining or obeying suggestions. It also meant that the mother might be sure about the child's care and the public health nurse was admitting that the mother was right. The category was called negotiation because the mother and public health nurse had the same aim. The situations might also start out with the mother not agreeing with the public health nurse at first, but they ended up with a mutual aim.

> [M] Have you got shoes for the child to use in the house?
> [M] No, she wears socks.
> [PHN] Because she is standing, it is worth getting shoes for her. The age matters but when she is standing . . .
> [M] Well, are you sure she will wear them?
> [PHN] Yes, quite, when she [the situation continues by the nurse explaining shoe sizes, models, etc.].

Public health nurses used this negotiating stance only when talking about the child's physical development, referring to professionals or talking about matters concerned with being a mother. Mothers used it several times when talking about physical development, psychological development, incidents, rituals, reference to professionals and situational matters during the visit.

Joking

In general, joking was rarely used in the interaction. When used, the basic aim of joking was to encourage the mother to make some decisions concerning the child. Joking included humour which was described by laughing, and teaching the mother, e.g. about keeping the child in bed beside her. Mothers made jokes about themselves. One mother explained laughingly how the child had independently searched for her breast during the night. The public health nurse also laughed.

Listening

Listening included the mother listening to the public health nurses' explanations or vice versa. It could be described as paying attention to each other in the situation.

Silence

Silence was very rare, and when it occurred it usually lasted only a few seconds—when the public health nurse was filling in forms or the child's hearing was being tested. This was strictly related to the time frame of the visit.

Discussion

This study started from the argument that while there has been much discussion about nursing relationships in health care, there has been little systematic research about this area abroad or in Finland. In this paper, some information about client–public health nurse relationships in child health care has been produced. The patterns of interaction were classified in this study from the perspective of relationships starting from the child's perspective; an approach for which no similar information exists.

Implications for nursing

For nursing practice the results indicate the importance of the public health nurse–client interaction, especially the use of mutual negotiation. The interaction skills of the public health nurses during the visits should be emphasized. It should be obvious that the knowledge obtained in this study about the child's presence and meaning in the situation can sensitize nurses to use their skills more consciously to work with the whole family. This may demand different skills from those needed in working mainly with adults.

Various aspects of nursing research arise in this study. First, we must carefully study the meaning of continuity and confidence in the nurse–client relationship. In particular, the question of continuity which relates to the situation-based relationships between clients and public health nurses demands more research. This body of knowledge should be enlarged to look at the phenomena involved on a larger scale so that the cautiously built substantive theory outlined here can later be formulated as a formal theory.

In the present study home visits were not included in the data collection. Observations of fathers attending the child health care clinics would also enlarge the overall picture of the services and thus enlarge the body of knowledge about client–public health nurse relationships or interaction in nursing.

Further research is also needed on how the relationships change, when the clients are children of different age groups and their mothers or fathers. More information about these relationships would give a new perspective to nursing activities in child health care.

References

Athlin, E. (1988) *Nursing Based on an Interaction Model Applied to Patients With Eating Problems and Suffering from Parkinson's Disease and Dementia*, Umeå University Publications, Umeå.

Benoliel, J.Q. (1975) 'Research related to death and dying patient', in *Nursing Research* vol. 1, (Verhonick, P.J. ed.), Little, Brown, Boston, pp. 189–227.

Chao, Y. (1989) 'Theoretical thinking in nursing: implications for primary health care strategies', in *Theories and Models of Nursing, Recent Advances in Nursing 24*, (Akinsanya, J.A. ed.), Churchill Livingstone, Edinburgh.

Chenitz, W.C. & Swanson, J.M. (1986) *From Practice to Grounded Theory: Qualitative Research in Nursing*, Addison-Wesley, Menlo Park, California.

Clark, J. (1986) 'A model for health visiting', in *Models for Nursing*, (Kershaw, B. & Salvage, J. eds), John Wiley & Sons, Chichester.

Faulkner, A. (1984) *Communication*, Churchill Livingstone, Edinburgh.

Glaser, B.G. (1978) *Theoretical Sensitivity. Advances in Methodology of Grounded Theory*, The Sociology Press, Mill Valley, California.

Glaser, B.G. & Strauss, A.L. (1967) *The Discovery of Grounded Theory: Strategies for Qualitative Research*, Aldine, Chicago.

Health Care (1987) Finland's Official Statistics, National Board of Health, Health 3. Valtion painatuskeskus, Helsinki.

Janhonen, S. & Vehviläinen-Julkunen, K. (1991) 'Grounded theory in nursing education and nursing practice research', Vård i Norden 3. (in press).

Lauri, S. (1981) 'The public health nurse as a guide in infant child care and education', *Journal of Advanced Nursing*, **6**, 297–303.

Lauri, S. (1989) 'Changes in national child health care policies and their effects on the public health nurses' work in child health care in Finland', *Journal of Advanced Nursing*, **14**, 1034–1037.

Leino-Kilpi, H. (1990) *Good nursing care, on what basis?* Academic dissertation, University of Turku. Annales Universitatis Turkensis, ser D, medica-odontologica 49, Kirjapaino Pika Oy, Turku.

Luker, K.A. & Chalmers, K.I. (1989) 'The referral process in health visiting', *International Journal of Nursing Studies*, **26**(2), 173–185.

Macleod Clark, J. (1983) 'Nurse–patient communication—an analysis of conversation from cancer wards', in *Nursing Research. Ten Studies in Patient Care*, (Wilson-Barnett, J. ed.), John Wiley, Chichester.

May, C. (1990) 'Research on nurse–patient relationships: problems of theory, problems of practice', *Journal of Advanced Nursing*, **15**(3), 307–315.

Pearson, P. (1991) 'Clients' perceptions: the use of case studies in developing theory', *Journal of Advanced Nursing*, **16**, 521–528.

Strauss, A. (1987) *Qualitative Analysis for Social Scientist*, Cambridge University Press, New York.

Strauss, A. & Corbin, J. (1990) *Basics of Qualitative Research. Grounded Theory Procedures and Techniques*, Sage Publications, London.

Wilson, H.S. (1985) *Research in Nursing*, Addison-Wesley, Menlo Park, California.

SECTION 6

A Partnership with Families

Introduction

Family centred care is now universally accepted as the main element in the philosophy of child health nursing. It is now an expectation of parents that they will be involved to a considerable degree in the care of their children when they are admitted to hospital. This requires that the parents, and indeed other family members, be regarded as equal partners in the delivery of care to the child. However, even where this is fully accepted by staff in principle, it does not necessarily mean that it will happen in practice. The details of what is required to establish successfully a genuine partnership will vary accordingly to the setting, the nature of the child's condition, and particular features of each child and family. It has been argued that, if a real sharing of care is to occur, then negotiation must take place to establish who is to be responsible for each aspect of care.

In the first paper in this section, Callery and Smith look at the issue of role negotiation between nurses and parents of hospitalised children. Their study showed that senior staff describe themselves as negotiating with parents, whereas more junior staff describe their role as encouraging and advising. The balance of power in the nurse–parent relationship is in the nurse's favour, and therefore it is clearly the nurse's choice whether to adopt a negotiating strategy or not. The implication for nurse education is that negotiating skills may need to be taught to allow the nurse to fulfil this new role effectively.

In the second paper Anne Casey outlines the partnership model of care which she has pioneered at Great Ormond Street. The nurse, the child and the family are three elements which interact in a variety of ways depending on the type of clinical setting. There is a great deal of flexibility in the model, so that it can be used in radically different care settings.

Dearmun, in the third paper, examines how the partnership philosophy can be practised in dealing with the specific problem of pain management. In addition to improving the quality of pain control, Dearmun argues that the involvement of parents also has the effect of reducing parental anxiety and stress, and in this way contributes to the overall well-being of the family. The paper concludes by noting that a successful partnership depends on both the acceptance by nurses that parents can contribute to this area of care, and the adoption of nursing approaches to empower parents to fulfil their role as partners.

The issue of partnership is also implicit in the paper by Whyte, which details a research project she undertook looking at the way four families coped over a 5-year period with the burden of cystic fibrosis. The report uses the families' own account of their experiences to describe the complex effects that chronic, life threatening illness have on the health of the family as a whole. The involvement of community specialist nurses in helping the families to cope and maintain their integrity as a unit is detailed. Whyte argues that the 'partnership with parents' philosophy needs to extend to a relationship with families and that the use of a term such as 'family nursing' would reinforce this concept.

The coping needs of parents of critically ill children are examined in the paper by Carnevale. Using a self reporting method, the main stressors and coping strategies of five sets of parents are analysed. One of the principal stressors identified was parental role conflict with professional staff. The paper concludes by suggesting strategies which could help to resolve this conflict.

The final paper in this section looks at the difficulty of delivering family centred care in the critical care setting. Rushton identifies eight elements of family centred care, which she believes can overcome the many problems of developing a close partnership with families of children in the critical care unit.

29

A Study of Role Negotiation Between Nurses and the Parents of Hospitalized Children*

PETER CALLERY and LORRAINE SMITH

The role of the parent of a hospitalized child has changed considerably over the past 30 years. Where parents were previously expected to hand responsibility for care over to their child's nurses, there is now an expectation that parents will be extensively involved in the care of their hospitalized children. The negotiation of roles between nurses and parents has been advocated by workers concerned about conflicts between nurses and parents. However, it is not known whether such negotiation takes place between nurses and parents. It is clear that power is not evenly distributed between nurses and parents: issues of territory, stress, anxiety, uncertainty, control and conflicts arising from parental competence all place the parent in a weaker position. It is argued that the nurse holds the initiative in the decision about whether negotiation takes place. A small study is described in which nurses were invited to describe their response to their perception that a parent wanted to increase or decrease her or his involvement in her or his child's care. The critical incident technique (Flanagan 1954) was used to collect data. Nurses' responses were categorized into categories of 'encouragement', 'explanation/advice' and 'negotiation'. Responses were then placed in more specific subcategories. The inter-rater reliability of the categorization was measured. Owing to the limitations of the study, the results can only be regarded as suggestive. Nevertheless, significant association was found between the category of response and the grade of staff, with a stratified pattern of category of response demonstrated. The implications of the study for future research are discussed.

The role of patient

The definition of the patient role as summarized by Anderson (1973) might at one time have described the role of the parent of a sick child as much as that of the child herself:

> When a person assumes the role of patient he exchanges freedom,

---

*This is an abridged version of an article first published in *Journal of Advanced Nursing*, Vol. 16, No. 7, pp. 772–781, 1991.

> autonomy and self-direction for controls. At the same time he gains protection, care and freedom from responsibility.

However, major changes in the expectations of the parents of hospitalized children have occurred over the last 30 years and the modern-day parent of the hospitalized child is often expected to play a major part in the care of her or his child. This role can even include procedures which nurses would see as an extension to their own role. What is not clear is the extent to which parents and nurses negotiate mutually satisfactory roles in hospital. What is evident in the popular literature is that the expectations of the parent's role have changed: there is now an assumption that parental participation in care is desirable and should be a feature of children's nursing (Bishop 1988, Goodwin 1988).

Nurses' expectations of parental participation

There is no consensus amongst children's nurses about what form parental participation should take and how far that participation should extend. Stull & Deatrick (1986) reported a study undertaken in order to produce a form for the assessment of parental participation in care. They found disagreements amongst nurses about what was appropriate parental participation:

> Direct care activities are the types of activities the parents most frequently planned and in which they actually did participate. Since the participation was highest in these activities, there was the most confusion from nursing staff as to the appropriateness of the parent's interactions. For example, parents reported that a first shift nurse said it was okay to bathe their child post-operatively whereas an evening shift nurse said it was not possible.

It could be that such inconsistencies have their roots in the nurses' individual understandings of the nature of nursing.

Stull & Deatrick's (1986) assessment form appears to rest on the assumption that parental participation, and by implication nursing, consists of observable behaviour. Of course, there are many other ways of conceptualizing nursing and, by implication, the nature of parental participation.

Parents' expectations of parental participation

Knafl & Dixon (1984) used semi-structured interviews and field observation in order to analyse fathers' participation in their children's hospitalization. They suggested that fathers fell into two categories: those who performed their usual role in an unusual setting (76% of the 62 fathers in the study) and those who took on increased responsibilities. The former and larger group is described in terms of passivity:

> These fathers did not ask nurses for assistance even when they identified a problem with their child. Rather they waited for the nurse independently to recognise the problem. Their participation in the actual care of the child was limited to the caretaking activities they usually did at home.

This description is puzzling, for it appears extraordinary that the fathers were prepared to ignore a problem which they had identified with their child. However, Knafl & Dixon (1984) indicated that this group of men saw their role in child care as limited:

> These men did not participate in preparing the children for hospitalization, a task they assumed either their wives or professionals would perform.

Knafl & Dixon (1984) report that all but one of their sample of fathers were employed, and describe them as 'ethnically a diverse group [although] most families were white and from the middle class'. Thus it is not possible to determine whether the type of occupation of the fathers was related to their behaviour group.

In contrast to the majority, the smaller group of fathers was more active: they

> adopted an expanded role [and] participated actively in their child's care. They initiated care when they believed it was necessary and emphasised the importance of interacting directly with their child's physician. They usually had only minimal expectations of nursing staff.

The picture painted by Knafl & Dixon (1984) is not one of partnership but of control by one or other group: either the nurses remained firmly in control and the fathers were passive or the father took the initiative and expected little of the nurses. Both possibilities offer a recipe for frustration and conflict.

Power and control

In the absence of a similar analysis of mother–nurse relationships, it is difficult to disentangle the effect of gender and/or family roles on the father–nurse relationships. However, it is clear that Knafl & Dixon's (1984) analysis suggests relationships where power and control are central issues. They argued for negotiation of roles between nurses and parents:

> it is crucial that nurses explicitly discuss with parents how they would like to participate in their child's care and how the nurse and the parents might work together in determining what their respective roles and levels of participation will be.

There is only limited evidence of what parents feel about these issues. A magazine survey (*Your Family Under Five* 1987) provides some anecdotal evidence, although the data must be treated with caution. Fifty-four per cent ($n=?$) of the self-selected sample of parents felt the nursing care their child received was good: this percentage might be seen as a cause for concern. It is only possible to speculate on how to interpret this comment from a mother:

> The only time we saw a nurse was in the morning to make the beds and take the temperatures. If the children who hadn't their mothers there wanted anything, one of the mothers had to get it for them.

This might be 'simple' bad practice. Alternatively, it might reflect a clash of expectations held by the mother and the nurse: the mother expecting the nurse to care for the children, the nurse expecting the mother to care and to ask for help when needed. It could suggest a lack of negotiation between nurse and mother.

Negotiation of roles

The expectations of the parent of a hospitalized child have changed enormously over the past 30 years. Where previously parents were expected to remain separated from the children, now they are expected to stay with them in hospital and be involved in the child's care. Such a realignment of roles does not take place without major adjustments by both nurse and parent. It has been argued that the roles of nurse and parent should be negotiated. It is not known whether this actually occurs in practice: it is only by understanding the interaction of nurses and parents better that improvements can be made in the negotiation of relationships.

Definitions of negotiation

One definition of 'to negotiate' given by the *Oxford English Dictionary* (OUP 1971) is: 'to hold communication or conference (with another) for the purpose of arranging some matter by mutual agreement; to discuss a matter with a view to some settlement or compromise'. However, Strauss (1978) complains that dictionary definitions

> give no clear guidance for making distinctions between negotiation and agreements arrived at without negotiation, nor between negotiation and other modes of attaining desired ends—such as persuasion, education, appeal to authority, or the use of coercion or coercive threat.

Strauss (1978) went on to state:

> negotiation generally will stand for one of the possible means of getting things accomplished when parties need to deal with each other to get these things done. The choice of negotiation as a means is neither fortuitous nor divorced from the social conditions under which it is made.

Strauss (1978) thus provides useful limits to the dictionary definition. The result is a mixture of a negative and a positive definition. When examining a behaviour, three criteria can be applied:

1 Was a non-negotiation mode of attaining an end used?
2 Was negotiation chosen as a mode?
3 Was there communication for the purpose of arranging some matter by mutual agreement? (*Oxford English Dictionary*)

The balance of power between nurses and parents

There is wide agreement that negotiations must be considered within their context; that negotiation does not take place within a vacuum (Druckman 1977, Rubin & Brown 1975, Strauss 1978). It is, therefore, necessary to consider the relative positions of the nurse and the parent of the hospitalized child, as this provides part of the context within which negotiation may or may not take place. Of particular importance is the balance of power and control within the relationship of nurse and parent.

Territory

Rubin & Brown (1975) consider the physical context of negotiation (they use the term 'bargaining' synonymously with 'negotiation'):

> The four physical components of bargaining structure. . .—site location and neutrality, physical arrangements at the site, communication availability and use, and time limits—both reflect and exert a powerful influence on the nature and quality of the bargaining exchange.

The hospital ward provides a context in which the nurse has a more powerful position than the parent: 'the site location' is one that is as familiar and controlled to the nurse as it is unfamiliar and confusing to the parent. The nurse attends the site in an occupational role, usually in uniform, whilst the resident parent is camping out in the hospital —however convenient the facilities that might be provided—removed from his or her home where control and privacy can be exercised.

Stress

In addition to the disadvantage of being a guest in someone else's work-place, the parent has the additional disorientation and tasks provided by stress. Stress in the parents of children hospitalized with chronic disabilities was examined by Hayes & Knox (1984). Their qualitative analysis of interviews with 40 parents suggested that 'the key to the parents' stress experience' lay in the changes in their usual parenting role that hospitalization required:

> In describing the nature of the changes required, parents identified the need to understand the illness experience; become familiar with the

> hospital environment; adapt to their changing relationship with the child and other family members; and negotiate with health professionals about their child's care.

In addition to these extra demands on parents, Hayes & Knox (1984) suggested that:

> Parents perceive their role in their hospitalized child's care differently than health professionals do, and it would appear that much parental stress is attributable to the 'space' between health care workers' understanding of parents' experience, and parents' own comprehension.

Anxiety

A further contributor to the stress of parenting a hospitalized child is anxiety. Teichman *et al.* (1986) investigated the anxiety reactions of hospitalized children and their mothers. Mothers were more anxious in the day hospital than in the traditional hospital used in the Teichman *et al.* study. They speculate that the increased anxiety was associated with mothers taking greater responsibility for care in the day hospital.

Uncertainty

It has been suggested by Mishel (1983) that perceived uncertainty has a major influence on the experience of parenting a sick child. She suggests that uncertainty 'hampers clear appraisal of events and limits coping'. A consideration of the causes of uncertainty in the parents of hospitalized children illustrates the dependence of parents on nurses and others for information. The parent may have many different sources of information in the hospital—his or her own observation, previous life experiences, different nurses, doctors, physiotherapists, other parents, and so on—which may provide ambiguous or even contradictory information.

Competence

Parents who are used to coping with the needs of chronically ill children face additional stresses when their child is hospitalized. Ferraro & Longo (1985) suggested that power conflicts between nurses and families who are used to caring for their child at home result when they confront the 'usual' model of care for acutely ill children, described as 'crisis intervention'. Ferraro & Longo (1985) suggested that it is the very competency and confidence which families have developed through caring for their child which causes role conflicts between families and nurses when the child is hospitalized.

The question of parental competency and resulting conflicts with nurses were also discussed by Robinson (1985) who analysed unstructured interviews with nine families. Parents' competency, Robinson argued, places them in a 'double bind' situation: the family must release control to nurses whilst their child is in hospital and play a passive role but resume confident, competent care of the child at home after discharge. This analysis rests on a conception of care that is highly functional: the quality of the parents' relationships with the child is not addressed, nor are the particular meanings of events to the parents. There is a danger that Robinson's level of analysis is superficial and that care is viewed in functional terms, with nursing and parental care indistinguishable from one another.

Control

Where Robinson's (1985) contribution is particularly useful is in her analysis of the relationships between nurses and parents in terms of the balance of power and the control of care. Implicit in the decision of a parent to take a child to hospital is some degree of relinquishment of control. This phenomenon has been examined within the framework of attribution theory by Strube & Berry (1985).

The option to negotiate

The call for nurses to negotiate care and roles with parents is a recurring feature of the literature of parental participation (Ferraro & Longo 1985, Knafl & Dixon 1984, Robinson 1985). However, it is not known whether nurses do attempt to negotiate with parents or whether they use other modes of attaining the desired ends (Strauss 1978) such as education.

It is clear that the nurse is in a much stronger position than the parent of a hospitalized child. The nurse is on familiar territory whereas the parent is removed from home; the nurse has the usual stresses of her occupation whereas the parent may have novel and peculiar stresses; the nurse has no special emotional anxieties concerning the child whereas the parent has; the nurse may control information whereas the parent is uncertain and dependent on others for information; the nurse's competence is a means to fulfil her role whereas the parent's competence is a source of conflict. Thus, the nurse is in a position to control the relationship, and it is only the nurse who has the power to relinquish control and to choose to negotiate with the parent about roles or about care. If the nurse does not wish to negotiate, the parent is not in a strong position to take the initiative.

Whether nurses choose to educate parents about their role in the care of their own children in hospital, or to negotiate with parents as to what their role should be, is a question the literature does not answer. It is a question that is of great importance if the relations between nurses and the parents of hospitalized children are to be understood.

The study

Some methodological problems in the study of negotiation

The problem of whether nurses choose to negotiate roles with the parents of hospitalized children raises at least two groups of methodological problems. One group is general to the study of negotiation, whilst the other arises from the context of the nurse–parent relationship.

Problems general to the study of negotiation

The nature of negotiation creates difficulty for the investigator of negotiation as a phenomenon.

An approach to the problem of method might be to place the definition of negotiation in the hands of participants; for example, simply to ask nurses, 'Do you choose to negotiate roles with the parents of hospitalized children?' The analysis of data thus collected would be highly problematic: a range of definitions of negotiation exists and it would not be possible to make comparison between individual answers based on different definitions.

The critical incident technique

The critical incident technique is a method which enables the participants in the relationships of interest to act as observers and data collectors. Thus, the problems associated with introducing a participant observer into a relationship are avoided. In addition, the participant is able to describe her or his own perception of events, so that the participant's own construction of events as negotiation or otherwise is available in the data. However, the participant is not relied on to define 'negotiation'. Flanagan (1954) defined the term 'critical incident':

> By an incident is meant any observable human activity that is sufficiently complete in itself to permit inferences and predictions to be made about the person performing the act. To be critical, an incident must occur in a situation where the purpose or intent of the act seems fairly clear to the observer and where its consequences are sufficiently definite to leave little doubt concerning its effects.

Occupational description has been the predominant use of the technique in nursing. Sims (1976) and Long (1976) described ward sisters' expectations of student nurses, and Cormack (1983) used the critical incident technique in order to describe the role of the psychiatric nurse, while Benner (1984) used critical incidents to describe excellence in nursing practice.

Nurses were approached in small groups in a room on their ward where there was not likely to be interruption, in order to maximize the response rate. The nurses were invited to participate once the study had been explained to them and were promised confidentiality. Participants were then asked to describe two incidents, one where they felt that a parent had wanted more involvement in the care of a child and one where they felt a parent wanted less involvement. Participants wrote descriptions of these incidents on prepared forms.

The sample

Included in the population was any nurse except for students who was involved in the care of children on a children's ward. The term 'nurse' was used broadly to include unqualified assistants and nursery nurses, provided they were involved in the nursing care of children. No distinction was made between nurses holding a general qualification and those specifically qualified in children's nursing because the size of the sample limited the number of variables that could be subjected to comparison.

Results

A total of 64 nurses was invited to participate in the study, none of whom refused: 112 critical incidents were received from these participants giving an overall response rate of 87.5%. Four participants returned both forms blank; eight others returned one form without a description of an incident.

At the first level of analysis two categories of non-negotiation responses were identified: 'encouragement' and 'explanation and/or advice' in addition to the category of 'negotiation'. In addition, a category of 'insufficient evidence for categorization' was identified.

The second level of categorization was more specific than the first. Three sub-categories were identified for each category, plus a further sub-category 'insufficient evidence for sub-categorization'. The categorization system which resulted is described next.

Categories and sub-categories

In this section, a description is given of each category and its sub-categories. After the description of each, a quotation from a response from the appropriate sub-category is given.

Encouragement

Encouragement refers to responses where the nurse encouraged the parent(s) to do something, whether this was something the parent showed reluctance to do, or something that the parent was doing which the nurse reinforced with encouragement. The nurse had expectations of how the parent should behave. The use of encouragement was intended to make the parent behave according to the nurse's expectations. The word 'encouragement' commonly appeared in incidents thus categorized, but its use did not automatically categorize an incident as 'encouragement'. Sub-categories of 'encouragement' follow.

(a) 'Encouragement' as reinforcement The nurse reinforced the behaviour of the parent by giving encouragement. The following serves to illustrate this.

> Encouraged parents to familiarize themselves with the ward, e.g. kitchen area, linen rooms, and talked to parents, constantly reassuring and encouraging them to try and carry out his care as they would at home . . .

(b) Reluctant parent encouraged This refers to responses where a parent was encouraged to behave in a way that the parent had shown reluctance to behave in. For example,

> We had a girl on our ward that was involved in a road traffic accident . . . Her mother was very reluctant to be fully involved in her care . . . The mother was encouraged to participate in her daughter's care by being asked if she would like to change her, but obviously at first with some assistance from the nurse so that mother could see what her daughter could actually do for herself. Other members of the rehabilitation team were involved in encouraging mother to assist in lifting techniques.

(c) Parent encouraged to be less involved in care The responses in this sub-category were similar to those in the sub-category 'reluctant parent encouraged' except that where more involvement was encouraged in that sub-category, less involvement was encouraged in this sub-category.

> . . . tactfully encouraged her to try and get some rest, told her there was adequate staff to look after her son whilst in hospital, and reassure her we were happy to care for him and did not think badly of her for going . . .

Explanation and/or advice

Explanation or advice refers to responses where the nurse either explained why a parent should behave in a certain way or advised the parent to behave in a certain way. The nurse had expectations of how the parent should behave and gave explanation and/or advice about how the parent should behave. The words 'explanation' and/or 'advice' occurred commonly in this category but their presence did not automatically categorize a response.

(a) Explanation or advice of the nurse's view of what is best for the child or parent The nurse either gave an explanation or advice of what she (the nurse) believed was the most appropriate behaviour by the parent in the best interests of the child or parent. For example,

> . . . [I] explained the importance and significance of the mother's continued involvement in the child's care in view of the child's age (3 years) and because she has to continue to manage the situation at home in the future . . .

(b) Explanation or advice about policy There were expectations of how the parent should behave inherent in the policy of the ward, the hospital or of another professional(s). These expectations were explained or advised to the parent.

> I told the mother that she would need to get special permission from the anaesthetist and that she would need to change into theatre

> clothing. I also explained the procedure in the anaesthetic room to check she would be able to cope . . .

(c) Explanation or advice to reassure an anxious parent The nurse provided explanation or advice to a parent who appeared to be anxious or distressed.

> . . . [I] sat down and explained about febrile convulsions, let her read the cooling chart and how to deal with febrile convulsions. Also explained that the child was not seriously ill and could be treated normally . . .

Negotiation

Negotiation categorizes responses where the nurse attempted to come to an agreement with the parent(s) about how the parent(s) should behave. The nurse may have had expectations about how the parent should behave but she did not seek to impose these. The nurse may have been prepared to alter her expectations during negotiation.

(a) Negotiate skills to be learnt The nurse attempted to come to an agreement with the parent(s) about whether or not a skill should be learnt and/or when it should be learnt by the parent(s).

> After 2 days the mother was obviously more relaxed about her daughter and began to ask about simple nursing duties; how to do them, is it alright for her to do them (mainly in the giving of IV medications).
>
> Basic hygiene needs required no new skills for mum but it was discussed with her and medical staff and she was supervised and taught how to give IV medications until it was felt she was at a level competent enough to give them at home without supervision.

(b) Negotiation of the distribution of work/responsibility The nurse attempted to come to an agreement with the parent(s) about how the work and/or responsibility should be distributed between parent and nurse.

> . . . [I] introduced myself as the nurse who was looking after the child and asked her if she would like to assist me in washing and changing him, as this was necessary . . .

(c) Negotiation of care The nurse attempted to come to an agreement with the parent(s) about the nature of the care to be given.

> Ward policy was to clean Hickman line with Mediswabs when giving IV drugs. Parents expressed verbally they preferred using Ind. Meths 70% spray as well and seemed uneasy if nurses used Mediswabs . . . When giving IV drugs parents were asked to spray line as they preferred and to clean the line before nurse gave IV drugs. . .

Table 29.1 Distribution of categories by grade of staff responding

	Category		
Grade of staff	*Encouragement*	*Explanation/advice*	*Negotiation*
Sister	3	6	14
Staff nurse	13	18	12
SEN	10	5	11

Insufficient evidence

Incidents were placed in the category 'insufficient evidence' where it was not possible to place the response in a category, either because so little information was given about the response that speculation was required in order to categorize the response, or because the information that was provided was too vague and inconclusive to enable the response to be categorized.

> Whenever the parents were approached, and were given advice, they said they knew the answer as this was not their first child.
> [What did you do?]
> Try and build a relationship with both parents, not talking about medical conditions, but talked on a lighter subject.
> [What happened then?]
> The parents seemed to drop the barrier. I felt they both felt guilty and inadequate as the child was in hospital, thinking it was their fault.

Table 29.1 shows the distribution of categories of response by the grade of the nurse responding. The null hypothesis, 'The distribution of categories of response will not differ between grades of qualified nurses', can be subjected to the chi-square test. In this case, chi-squared equals 9.91, which is significant at the 5% level with 4 degrees of freedom. Thus, the trends shown in Table 29.1 for sisters' responses to be categorized more often as 'negotiation' and less often as 'encouragement', for staff nurses' responses to be categorized more often as 'explanation/advice' and less often as 'negotiation', and for SENs' responses to be categorized more often as 'encouragement' and less often as 'explanation/advice' are statistically significant.

Discussion

The response rate obtained, which was 88% overall, compares favourably with previous studies that have employed the critical incident technique (Cormack 1983, Rimon 1979, Sims 1976). The response rate illustrates that the critical incident technique is an economic method of data collection: data can be obtained in a relatively short period of time with an acceptable response rate, despite the complexity of the subject investigated.

The percentage agreement on categorization varied widely between wards, 55% to 88% at category level. It is possible that this variation was caused by the quality of data varying between wards. 'Negotiation' was the category with the lowest inter-rater agreement. This might be partly explained by the nature of the categorization system. The second rater was not a person involved in or knowledgeable about nursing and it is possible that this made the task of categorizing more difficult. In particular, the category 'negotiation' provided the rater with fewer semantic clues; the word 'negotiate' does not appear in the data whilst the words 'encourage', 'advise' and 'explain' frequently do. It is also possible that the categorization of responses as 'negotiation' demands some familiarity with children's nursing.

An alternative explanation is that the category 'negotiation' was not clearly present to the second rater in the data, and thus there is a potential source of bias in the first rater's categorization of data as 'negotiation'.

The pattern of responses from different grades of staff

There is evidence of a pattern of categories of response related to the grade of the respondent. These results suggest a stratification of responses, moving from a tendency for enrolled nurses to describe themselves as responding to parents with encouragement, through staff nurses to describe themselves responding to parents with explanation or advice, to sisters who more frequently described themselves as responding to parents by negotiating.

Whether these relationships are a function of the roles of these different grades of staff or of their characteristics is unclear. However, the direction of movement from encouragement through explanation and/or advice to negotiation would appear logical: the movement is from a more rigid set of expectations of parents to a less rigid one. The movement also appears to imply an increasing respect for parents' own decision-making capabilities with increasing rank. It is necessary to restate the caution with which these results must be treated. However, the results are suggestive and further work in a larger study could examine the existence of these trends. In addition, the patterns associated with unqualified staff and the differences between nurses trained in sick children's nursing and those trained in general nursing could be explored.

Implications for nursing

Implications for nursing practice

The increased participation of parents in the care of their children is widely considered to have improved the quality of care of hospitalized children. However, it would be surprising if such fundamental changes in roles were entirely unproblematic. Where difficulties have been identified in the literature, it has been suggested that negotiation of roles could reduce the potential for conflict and prevent problems that have been encountered in practice. It is clear that the choice of whether to negotiate or to adopt alternative approaches such as coercion or education is largely in the hands of nurses. The balance of power in the nurse–parent relationship is weighted in the nurse's favour: it is the nurse who has greater control over the territory of the hospital ward and over information in a climate of uncertainty, whilst in contrast the parent has greater anxiety and stress with which to cope, due both to the fact that the child is ill and to the change in parenting role that is required.

The evidence of this study suggests that there may be differences amongst grades of staff in whether they choose to negotiate or to adopt the alternative approaches of encouraging or advising. It is only possible to speculate as to why this should be the case. It might be that the apparent differences in approach of enrolled nurses, staff nurses and sisters can be explained by the division of responsibility and authority in wards. The non-negotiation approaches of more junior staff could have been a response to a lack of authority whereas sisters were able to respond by negotiation because they had sufficient authority to do so. Presumably a more widespread use of primary nursing could redistribute authority and responsibility and enable more junior staff to choose to negotiate.

Implications for nursing education

There may also be implications for nurse educators. Is special preparation in the particular skills of negotiation required if nurses are to negotiate effectively with parents?

Implications for future research

There are important questions related to the effect of participation on the parents of hospitalized children. Is anxiety increased or decreased by participation? What are the implications of participation for parental control and autonomy?

The question of whether nurses choose to negotiate or to adopt alternative approaches has not been answered definitively. In particular, further work is necessary to establish whether the stratification of responses found in this study, where sisters tended to describe themselves negotiating with parents while more junior grades of staff tended to describe the alternative approaches of advising and encouraging, reflects actual differences in practice.

These are not only issues of parochial concern to children's nurses: similar concerns have emerged in other areas of nursing when patient and family participation have been promoted. It has been suggested that there is a danger of coercing adult patients who may be 'reluctant collaborators' (Waterworth & Luker 1990). The question of how nurses and clients negotiate their roles when there is a stress on participation is therefore one of interest in many areas of nursing and further work is required if these relationships are to be better understood.

Acknowledgement

The authors gratefully acknowledge the generous co-operation of the nurses who took part in this study.

References

Anderson, E.R. (1973) *The Role of the Nurse*, Royal College of Nursing, London.

Benner, P. (1984) *From Novice to Expert*, Addison-Wesley, Menlo Park, California.

Bishop, J. (1988) 'Sharing the caring', *Nursing Times*, **84**(30), 60–61.

Cormack, D. (1983) *Psychiatric Nursing Described*, Churchill Livingstone, Edinburgh.

Cormack, D. (1984) 'Flanagan's critical incident technique', in *The Research Process in Nursing* (Cormack D. ed.), Blackwell Scientific, Oxford.

Druckman, E. (ed.) (1977) *Negotiations: Psychosocial Perspectives*, Sage, Beverly Hills.

Ferraro, R. & Longo, D.C. (1985) 'Nursing care of the family with a chronically ill, hospitalized child: an alternative approach', *Image*, **17**(3), 77–81.

Flanagan, J.C. (1954) 'The critical incident technique', *Psychological Bulletins*, **51**, 327–358.

Goodwin, P. (1988) 'I know you're busy, but . . .', *Nursing Times*, **84**(30), 62.

Hayes, V. & Knox, J.E. (1984) 'The experience of stress in parents of children hospitalized with long-term disabilities', *Journal of Advanced Nursing*, **9**(4), 333–341.

Knafl, K.A. & Dixon, D. (1984) 'The participation of fathers in their children's hospitalization', *Issues in Comprehensive Paediatric Nursing*, **7**(4–5), 269–281.

Long, P. (1976) 'Judging and reporting on student nurse clinical performance: some problems for the ward sister', *International Journal of Nursing Studies*, **13**, 115–121.

Mishel, M.H. (1983) 'Parents' perception of uncertainty concerning their hospitalised child', *Nursing Research*, **32**(6), 324–330.

OUP (1971) *The Oxford English Dictionary*, Oxford University Press, Oxford.

Rimon, D. (1979) 'Nurses' perception of their psychological role in treating rehabilitation patients: a study employing the critical incident technique', *Journal of Advanced Nursing*, **4**, 403–413.

Robinson, C.A. (1985) 'Parents of hospitalized chronically ill children: competency in question', *Nursing Papers*, **17**(2), 59–68.

Rubin, J.Z. & Brown, B.R. (1975) *The Social Psychology of Bargaining and Negotiations*, Academic Press, New York.

Sims, A. (1976) 'The critical incident technique in evaluating student nurse performance', *International Journal of Nursing Studies*, **13**(2), 123–130.

Strauss, A. (1978) *Negotiation: Varieties, Contexts, Processes and Social Order*, Jossey-Bass, San Francisco.

Strube, M.J. & Berry, J.M. (1985) 'Attributional and emotional concomitants of control relinquishment', *Basic and Applied Social Psychology*, **6**(3), 205–220.

Stull, M.K. & Deatrick, J.A. (1986) 'Measuring parental participation: Part I', *Issues in Comprehensive Paediatric Nursing*, **9**, 157–165.

Teichman, Y., Ben Rafael, M. & Lerman, M. (1986) 'Anxiety reaction of hospitalised children', *British Journal of Medical Psychology*, **59**, 375–382.

Waterworth, S. & Luker, K.A. (1990) 'Reluctant collaborators: do patients want to be involved in decisions concerning care?', *Journal of Advanced Nursing*, **15**(8), 971–976.

Your Family Under Five (1987) Children in hospital. *Your Family Under Five*, **49**, 22–29.

30

A Partnership with Child and Family*

ANNE CASEY

Nursing models are intended to provide logical descriptions of nursing[1]. These can then form the basis of nursing practice, education and research. Many nurses find it difficult to see the usefulness of models in their everyday working lives. Each nurse probably already has a working model of her own—one which may not be consciously thought out. Nurses who work together should try to discuss and develop their ideas of what nursing is, so that their approach is consistent.

The paediatric nursing model described below began as an attempt to describe practice. Through discussion and research it is continuing to develop into a useful tool. The model expresses beliefs and facts about nursing children. It is already leading to better use of the nursing process in children's wards and forms the basis of an RSCN curriculum plan.

Building a model

The first step in building a nursing model is to make a simple statement of philosophy—what are your beliefs related to your particular field of nursing? To build an appropriate model, it is necessary to collect together the *concepts* or main ideas related to nursing. By defining these concepts and identifying the *relationships* between them, you end up with your own framework or model of nursing.

Any one of the existing nursing models that happens to match this description can be adopted in its entirety. Unfortunately however, it is difficult to find a model which is concise and suits everyone. This is the case in paediatric nursing—there did not appear to be a model which adequately reflected my philosophy:

> The care of children, well or sick, is best carried out by their families, with varying degrees of assistance from members of a suitably qualified health care team whenever necessary.

*This article was first published in *Senior Nurse*, Vol. 8, No. 4, pp. 8–9, 1988.

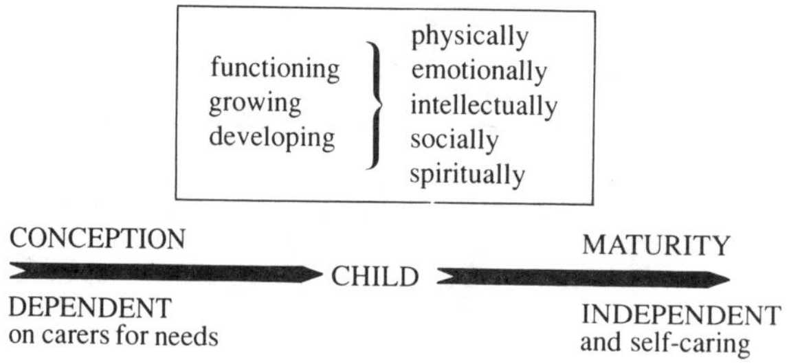

Figure 30.1 The child

In order to build a model suited to children's nursing, I began by defining concepts. The four main concepts usually associated with nursing are: Person, Health, Environment and Nursing. Because of the nature of children's nursing it is best to divide 'Person' into 'Child' and 'Family'. This does not mean that the family is another focus of nursing care (as it is in health visiting) rather that the family's central importance to the child is recognised.

The Child: The child is a unique entity: a developing human being who has rights in law. Because he is immature, his rights may differ from those of adults. The child is functioning, growing and developing—physically, emotionally, socially, intellectually, and spiritually. In order to do this, he needs care in the form of protection, sustenance, stimulation and love.

From birth the healthy child is able to meet some of his own functional needs—he breathes, expresses discomfort, digests food, eliminates waste, sleeps and moves. All the child's other needs are initially met by his family. As he grows and develops he is able to assume more of his own care. From complete dependence at birth he learns self-care until he is independent and considered mature (Figure 30.1).

Health: good health in its broadest sense is taken to mean optimum physical and mental well-being. The developing child who is healthy and well-cared for will have the best opportunity to achieve his full potential.

The way each child and his family view his state of health at any given time could be expressed on a continuum from wellness to illness.

Ill health affects growth and development, and can occur as a result of physical, social or psychological dysfunction. This dysfunction could be the result of disease, injury, congenital problem, or failure of care. Health is often significantly affected by the child's environment.

The Environment: this can be defined as 'all the stimuli from external sources which are absorbed and processed by the child'[2]. A safe and suitable environment needs to be provided in order for the child to flourish.

Influences on environment can be ethnic, social, psychological or physical. Thus a family's race or their religious convictions will affect the way their child is raised. He will be influenced not only by social contacts but also by the family's socio-economic position. The child needs to feel secure in order to develop normally. He needs to trust his carers and receive consistent handling. The physical environment does not only consist of the air we breathe and the things we eat and drink. It is also affected by the laws and lifestyles which influence our physical surroundings.

From the time of conception, the child's family will mediate between him and his environment.

The Family: even sociologists have difficulty defining the family. However, it is usually considered as a group which carries out certain social and biological functions[3]. The structure and function of families is continually being influenced by changing economic and social forces.

For the purposes of this article *family* is taken to mean parents and others who significantly influence the continuing care of the child—ie the group which takes responsibility for meeting the child's needs.

The paediatric nurse is concerned with the structure of the family, the relationships within it and the forces affecting it—but only so far as they affect the family's ability to care for the child.

The paediatric nurse complements parental care by doing things for the child, or his parents, to meet the child's needs. This care may take the form of *family care* (the usual care given to meet everyday needs) or it may be *nursing care* (that extra care given in relation to health needs). Depending on his age and ability the child may perform some of this care himself. Parents are often both able and willing to carry out nursing care of their child—but they may need help, in the form of support and teaching, to do so.

So, the nurse supports the child and his family. Creating a supportive environment may be the only nursing action necessary to assist the parents in caring for their sick child. The nurse also teaches the child and his family, furnishing them with appropriate knowledge, skills and attitudes which will promote their independence.

The process of nursing is carried out in partnership with the child and his family. An example of what this means in practice is the way that assessment is carried out. During her initial assessment of the child, the nurse attempts to establish:

- what *family care* the child routinely receives;
- the child's present condition (psychological as well as physical);
- what *nursing care* the child needs in relation to his medical diagnosis, treatment or other health needs;
- the ability of the child and/or his parents to participate in his care.

Even in the intensive care unit it is important to maintain the child's usual pattern of daily care. This consistency helps the hospitalised child to retain some sense of normality. Assessing the child's condition does not only mean measuring his weight and temperature. It means looking at the whole child. Where is he in terms of development? What does he understand about his illness or the reason for his visit to hospital? How is he reacting to these changes in his life?

Assessing the ability of the child and his parents to care also means finding out whether the parents can be present, and whether they are able to cope with being involved.

The model may seem incomplete because it does not give a list of needs to be assessed. It was decided not to attempt to condense the infinite number of a child's needs into a checklist. The reason for this decision is that within paediatric nursing there are many specialities which will have different priorities. A school nurse may wish to emphasise developmental and preventive health needs in her assessment. A nurse in the intensive care unit will want to concentrate initially on physical and emotional needs. As the patient recovers she could then start to prioritise behavioural needs—assistance with activities of living, for example.

This apparent lack of structure to the model can be seen as an advantage in that the model gives an 'umbrella' description of paediatric nursing. Under this umbrella, nurses in a particular speciality can identify and list the priority needs of their patients. The use of more rigidly defined models may mean that a single patient needs to be nursed using different models at different stages of his illness. This may be because nurses concentrate only on checklists rather than on the underlying philosophy of the model used.

The definitions of child, health, environment, family and paediatric nursing, include some indication of the relationships between them. Further illustrations of the interaction between the child, his family and the nurse are given in the following examples.

In most circumstances the family require little or no help from the health care team. Figure 30.2 illustrates the contact a clinic nurse has with the child and mother when routine immunisation is offered. The nurse gives the baby the injection, but most of her care is directed at the mother. She offers information and reassurance about side-effects, advises about feeding, and provides emotional support to help the mother hold her child for the injection.

At the opposite end of the spectrum Figure 30.3 represents the relationship in intensive care. Provision of all the child's needs, including breathing and circulation control, may be taken over by the nurse. Even here the family can be supported to enable them to participate in their child's physical and emotional care. The benefit to child and parent is difficult to measure, but instead of feeling completely helpless in the face of their child's severe illness, and the daunting competence of the professional, the parents can have a genuine place in the caring team.

There is a considerable body of research to confirm that parents are willing and able to nurse their children[4,5].

Discussion and formal research are continuing to try to validate the key statements made about concepts and relationships in paediatric nursing. This work will never be completed because the model should develop, just as our ideas about nursing develop over time. It would be encouraging if nurses feel that this description of paediatric nursing is concise and familiar. Familiarity further validates the work as a realistic model of paediatric nursing (Figure 30.4).

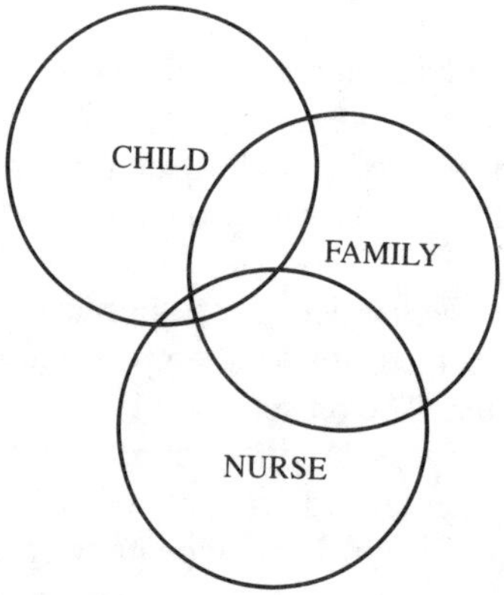

Figure 30.2 Supportive/educative nursing

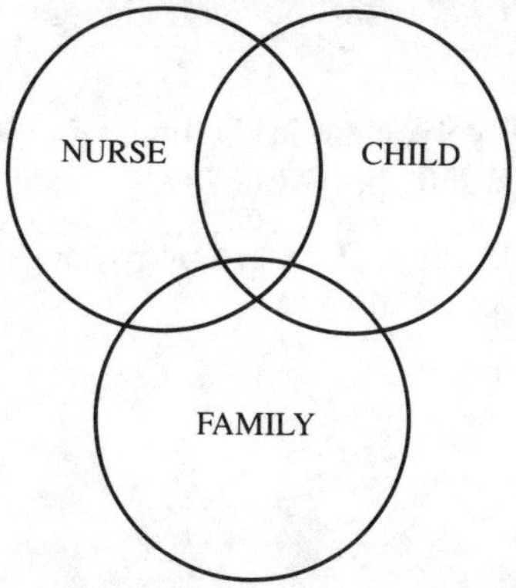

Figure 30.3 Intensive care

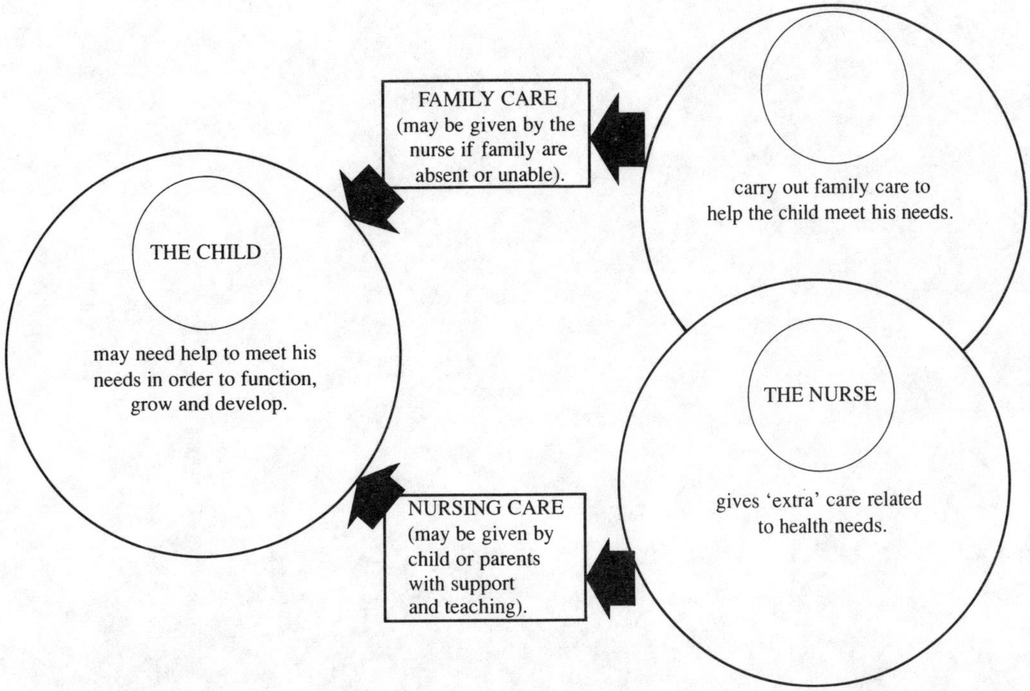

Figure 30.4 Summary of the partnership model of paediatric nursing

Notes

1. Kershaw, B. and Salvage, J. (eds), *Models for Nursing*, John Wiley, Chichester, 1986.

2. Weiczorek, R. and Natapoff, J. *A Conceptual Approach to the Nursing of Children*, J.B. Lippincott, Philadelphia, 1981.

3. Harris, C. *The Family and Industrial Society*, George Allen and Unwin, London, 1983.

4. Cleary, J. *et al.* 'Parental involvement in the lives of children in hospital', *Archives of Disease in Childhood*, **61**, 1986, pp. 779–787.

5. Webb, N., Hull, D. and Madeley, R. 'Care by parent in hospital', *British Medical Journal*, **291**, July 20, 1985, pp. 176–177.

31

Towards a Partnership in Pain Management*

ANNETTE DEARMUN

A review of recent literature indicates that the notion of negotiation and partnership between nurses and parents remains pertinent in the 1990s.[1–5] In particular, the issues of 'balance of power and control'[1] and the extent of 'partnership caring'[4] are highlighted. Increasingly, clinical areas are adopting philosophies and nursing models[3,6] which incorporate partnership in child care and there is an emphasis on defining the nurse's role within this child–parent–nurse partnership.[6]

If one believes that partnership is an essential component of children's nursing, it is appropriate to examine the potential for parents to contribute to the total care of their child. For the child experiencing surgery, this total care will include measures to avoid pain and discomfort.

This article will present some of the arguments for involving parents in the pain management of children. It will suggest some of the ways in which parents can be more formally involved in the assessment, evaluation and management of their child's pain pre and post-surgery and it will look at some of the wider implications of this for nursing practice and education.

There are some persuasive arguments for working with parents wherever possible to avoid pain during the post-operative period. Firstly, since pain is a common feature of many minor childhood illnesses, it follows that parents will often have had some experience of their child in pain at home, will know how the child reacts and the most successful comforting tactics. Despite the acute nature of surgery, with support they should be able to draw upon their knowledge and skills when in hospital.

Arguably, parents should also be the most sensitive to and aware of the actions and reactions of the child to pain and therefore best able to interpret them accurately. This is supported by Elander *et al.*,[7] who discovered that parents demonstrated the same level of awareness as nurses to signs that their child was in pain. Not only could they interpret non-verbal cues, but they were able to distinguish these from expressions of hunger or other distress.

Secondly, it has been noted that parents want to stay with their children during difficult situations or painful procedures in order to comfort them.[2,8,9] Caty *et al.*[10] provided evidence that parents were able to help their children in coping, commonly using strategies such as giving information and explaining events.

---

*This article was first published in *Paediatric Nursing*, Vol. 5, No. 5, pp. 8–10, 1993.

Thirdly, providing parents with information about what to expect, involving them in care, and thereby enabling them to feel they have some control over events in hospital, may reduce their anxiety.[11,12] This is an important feature of care because parents generally spend much time with their children post-operatively and it has been reported that they find it especially difficult to observe their child in discomfort if they do not know what to do to help.[13]

Prior knowledge and preparation are both helpful in relieving anxiety.[12] Other researchers[14–16] have found that when parents perceived they were in control of the situation, they were better able to come to terms with their child's illness.

It should therefore follow that involving parents in measures to reduce pain and increase comfort pre and post-operatively will help to reduce their anxiety. This awareness is important because pain and anxiety are interlinked[17,18] and parental anxiety can be communicated to the child with a potentially detrimental effect on the speed of the child's recovery.[19] Finally, parents need to be helped to refine their skills so they can continue post-operative care at home. The average period of hospitalisation for children who have had surgery is now only four days.[20] There is increasing national support for the setting up of paediatric day wards. The *Just for the Day* report[21] provided a blueprint for the children's day ward opened at the John Radcliffe Hospital, Oxford, in August 1992. This, together with the use of laparoscopic surgery for children,[22] promises to reduce the length of stay in hospital for the child, but may increase the likelihood of some post-operative pain or discomfort at home.[23]

It does therefore appear that there is sufficient evidence to support the view that parents should be involved in pain management.

Assessment and evaluation

Comprehensive literature reviews have suggested that pain assessment presents a major challenge.[24–26] It appears to rely largely upon the judgement of others and a combination of accurate observation and/or self report by the child, where age permits. Such judgement is dependent upon someone actually being present and on their ability to recognise the child's signs of distress. Although parents often accompany their child, O'Brien and Konsler[27] reported that nurses rarely relied upon their contribution when assessing a child's pain level. With appropriate support, parents could be involved in a more formal way to speed the recognition of pain and the better interpretation of its severity.

It could be argued that the reliability of pain assessment may be greatly enhanced by the use of assessment tools.[28] Several are available and are identified in the literature.[24–26] However, in order to gain the co-operation to use these tools effectively, it is usually necessary to spend considerable time building up rapport and trust with the child. As parents usually have this relationship already, why should they not be given the relevant information, preparation and support to enable them to assess their child's pain or educate their child to use the assessment tool?

Alleviating pain

There is evidence that pain is undertreated in children.[26] There may be reasons for this, not least myths and misconceptions related to the adverse effects of opiates in children leading to insufficient amounts being given.[29,30] Cohen[31] suggests that much of the responsibility for the comfort of the child rests with the nurse, who must assess the child's pain, make an appropriate decision about whether to give the analgesic, which one to give, what dose to use, and at what time to administer it. This profile of the nurse's responsibilities could be extended to include communicating this knowledge to parents so they can extend their range of skills in caring for their child.

The increasing use of oral, rectal and patient-controlled analgesia (PCA)[26,32] can offer opportunities for parents to take a more direct role in giving medication, for example dispensing regular paracetamol and or delivering PCA. This has the advantage of enabling the parents to medicate earlier and may free them from having to rely upon the availability of the nurse.

Gadish *et al.*[33] reported that nurses significantly chose to medicate the children rather than select other interventions. However, there may be a range of complementary therapies available which could be very effective when used in conjunction with more traditional methods and in some cases may minimise the need for narcotic analgesia and thus reduce the amount of time spent in hospital.[34] Parents could be introduced to, or encouraged to use, a range of complementary pain control methods, such as relaxation, distraction, play therapy,[35] guided imagery, breathing techniques and massage. The play specialist may advise parents about play and preparation. Any of these techniques learnt in hospital could then be applied at home.

It is also important to remember the aesthetic elements of pain management and caring, for example, providing a friendly, child-centred environment, enabling parents to accompany their children to the anaesthetic room, comfortable positioning, gentle lifting, the application of warmth, reduction in environmental stressors such as excess light and noise, and in general anticipating both physical and psychological needs. Parents and paediatric nurses can work together to enhance these aspects of quality care.

It may be seen that parents have a valuable contribution to make in the alleviation of their child's pain, but it is unwise to assume this. Their involvement should be fully negotiated, not foisted on them through expediency or lack of nursing resources.

Implications

The new educational pathways now available emphasise the supportive, educative and advisory role of paediatric nurses and aim to promote their reflective skills. This may bring new levels of critical analysis to pain management and new skills in the act of empowerment. This is necessary if partnership or empowerment are not to become more than rhetoric. By reflecting upon the knowledge and skills they use in pain assessment and management nurses will be able to share this with parents.

Watt-Watson[36] reported that many parents were given insufficient information on their possible contribution to their child's care. This problem may be partially addressed. Enhanced communication between community and ward nurses ensures appropriate exchange of information and enables them all to give support to parents pre and post-surgery. Preparation literature and aftercare advice includes a comprehensive section on parents' contribution to care and post-operative pain management.

The information-giving process can begin in the outpatient department, the GP surgery or at home. These ideas provide the foundation for some of the new initiatives on the paediatric surgical ward at the John Radcliffe Hospital. In December 1992, I appointed an experienced paediatric nurse to liaise between the ward and surgical outpatients. She is fully involved in the outpatient consultation, using the opportunity to offer advice, suggest appropriate reading material and provide information regarding the total hospital experience, including post-surgery pain assessment and management.

There are several district-wide initiatives to increase collaboration between acute and community services, for example, a group is being co-ordinated to consider the specific issues relating to liaison with the community regarding children undergoing surgery. There is also a 'twinning' system whereby community and ward nurses have the opportunity to visit and work in each other's areas. This leads to an increased awareness on both sides and anticipated improved information and support offered to parents.

It is important to keep abreast of new or complementary pain management therapies and critically to review their use and effectiveness in children. Nurses with knowledge of both pharmacological and non-pharmacological approaches to pain management will be in a better position to advise parents on various and optimal methods. A nursing-led 'pain interest group' has been set up. This has the support of the consultant paediatric surgeons and anaesthetists and enables a sharing of skills, expertise and resources.

Much of the evidence supporting parents' usefulness in pain management is largely anecdotal. There are very few published British studies which systematically explore the views of parents and nurses or evaluate the benefits and limitations of parental involvement in this aspect of care. There are many areas that would be worthy of further research, including the extent of parental contribution to pain assessment and the overall effectiveness of complementary therapies when used by parents.

Partnership between parents and nurses in pain management may be dependent upon several factors, not least a recognition and acceptance by nurses of the potential for parents to make an effective contribution to this aspect of care, and the adoption of nursing approaches to enhance parents' knowledge and skills and hence empower and enable them to become full partners in care.

Notes

1. Callery, P., Smith, L. 'A study of role negotiation between nurses and parents of hospitalised children', *Journal of Advanced Nursing*, 1991, **16**, 772–781.

2. Deamun, A. 'Perceptions of parental participation', *Paediatric Nursing*, 1992, **4**(7), 6–10.

3. Farrell, M. 'Partnership in care: paediatric nursing model', *British Journal of Nursing*, 1992, **1**(4), 175–176.

4. Stower, S. 'Partnership caring', *Journal of Clinical Nursing*, 1992, **1**, 67–72.

5. Palmer, S. 'Care of sick children by parents: a meaningful role', *Journal of Advanced Nursing*, 1993, **18**, 185–191.

6. Casey, A. 'A partnership with child and family', *Senior Nurse*, 1988, **8**(4), 8–9.

7. Elander, G. *et al.* 'Pain relief in infants after major surgery: a descriptive study', *Journal of Paediatric Surgery*, 1991, **26**(2), 128–131.

8. Webb, N. *et al.* 'Care by parents in hospital', *British Medical Journal*, 1986, **291**, 176–177.

9. Stull, M., Deatrick, J. 'Measuring parental participation: Part 1', *Issues of Comprehensive Pediatric Nursing*, 1986, **9**, 157–165.

10. Caty, S. *et al.* 'Mothers' perceptions of coping behaviours in hospitalised preschool children', *Journal of Pediatric Nursing*, **4**(6), 403–410.

11. Eberly, T. *et al.* 'Parental stress after the unexpected admission of a child to the intensive care unit', *Critical Care Quarterly*, 1985, **8**, 57–65.

12. Wolfer, J., Visintainer, M. 'Pediatric surgical patients' and parents' stress responses and adjustment', *Nursing Research*, 1975, **24**, 244–255.

13. Miles, M., Carter, M. 'Coping strategies used by parents during their child's hospitalisation on an intensive care unit', *Children's Health Care*, 1985, **14**(1), 14–21.

14. Schepp, K. 'Factors influencing the coping effort of mothers of hospitalised children', *Nursing Research*, 1991, **40**(1), 42–46.

15. Worchel, F. *et al.* 'Control-related coping strategies in pediatric oncology patients', *Journal of Pediatric Psychology*, 1987, **12**(1), 25–38.

16. Algren, C. 'Role perception of mothers who have hospitalised children', *Children's Health Care*, 1985, **14**, 6–9.

17. Booker, P., Nightingale, D. 'Post-operative analgesia for children', in Dodson, M. (ed.), *The Management of Post-operative Pain*, London, Edward Arnold, 1985.

18. Williams, J. 'Managing paediatric pain', *Nursing Times*, 1987, **83**(36), 36–39.

19. Bates, T., Broome, M. 'Preparation of children for hospitalisation and surgery: a review of the literature', *Journal of Pediatric Nursing*, 1986, **1**, 230–239.

20. OPCS, *In-Patient Enquiry 1983*, London, HMSO, 1985.

21. Thornes, R. *Just for the Day*, London, Caring for Children in the Health Services/NAWCH, 1991.

22. Miller, S. 'Laparoscopic operations in paediatric surgery', *British Journal of Surgery*, 1992, **79**, 986–987.

23. While, A., Crawford, J. 'Day surgery: expediency or quality care', *Paediatric Nursing*, 1992, **4**(3), 18–21.

24. Price, S. 'Pain: Its experience, assessment and management in children', *Nursing Times*, 1990, **86**(9), 42–45.

25. Gillis, M. 'Post-operative pain in children: A review of the literature', *Journal of Clinical Nursing*, 1993, **1**(2), 5–10.

26. Lloyd-Thomas, A. 'Pain management in paediatric patients', *British Journal of Anaesthesia*, 1990, **64**, 85–104.

27. O'Brien, S., Konsler, G. 'Alleviating children's post-operative pain', *Maternal–Child Nursing*, 1988, **13**(3), 183–186.

28. Carter, B. *Paediatric Intensive Care Manual*, London, Chapman and Hall, 1993.

29. Burokas, L. 'Factors affecting nurses' decisions to medicate pediatric patients after surgery', *Heart and Lung*, 1985, **14**(4), 373–378.

30. Beyer, J., Byers, M. 'Knowledge of pediatric pain: the state of the art', *Child Health Care*, 1985, **13**(4), 150–159.

31. Cohen, F. 'Post-surgical pain relief: Patients' status and nurses' medication choice', *Pain*, 1980, **9**, 265–274.

32. Raven, K., Ho, M. 'Children's use of PCA after spinal surgery', *Pediatric Nursing*, 1989, **15**(6), 589–593.

33. Gadish, H. *et al.* 'Factors affecting nurses' decisions to administer pediatric pain medication post-operatively', *Journal of Pediatric Nursing*, 1988, **3**(6), 383–390.

34. Spencer, K. 'Post-operative pain: the alternatives to analgesia', *The Professional Nurse*, 1989, 479–480, July.

35. Vessey, J., Mahon, M. 'Therapeutic play and the hospitalised child', *Journal of Pediatric Nursing*, 1990, **5**(5), 328–333.

36. Watt-Watson, J. *et al.* 'Parents' perceptions of their child's acute pain experience', *Journal of Pediatric Nursing*, 1990, **5**(5), 344–349.

32

A Family Nursing Approach to the Care of a Child with a Chronic Illness*

DOROTHY A. WHYTE

Introduction

This paper presents an analysis of four case studies of families caring for a child with cystic fibrosis, in order to illuminate the area of nursing practice referred to as 'providing support'. The opportunity to study this nursing situation arose from practice, spanning a 5-year period during which the author was providing community care for these families in the fulfillment of an honorary appointment with the local health board. A family profile drawn from the study was presented elsewhere (Whyte 1990).

The aim here is to report and discuss some aspects of the families' own accounts of their experience and to examine some theoretical perspectives which arose from analysis of the data. The research method will first be described.

Research method

The exploratory phase

A literature search and early fieldwork with the families clarified the fact that insight into the effect on the family as a whole and on its individual members was needed.

Exploratory work helped the author to conceptualize the main areas of concern. Following directly from this conceptualization came the formulation of the research questions:

1 How do family members respond to the genetic implications of cystic fibrosis (CF)?
2 How do families respond to the life-threatening nature of CF?
3 What events precipitate crises and what constitutes the chronic burden of care in the lives of families caring for a child with CF?

---

*This is an abridged version of an article first published in *Journal of Advanced Nursing*, Vol. 17, No. 3, pp. 317–327, 1992.

4 How does caring for a child with CF affect interaction and the coping response of families?

The exploratory phase provided rich insights into the family experience and it was clear that an ethnographic approach would be much more effective in providing the data which could inform nursing practice than would a more structured approach.

Ethnography (Hammersley & Atkinson; 1983) is a method which enables the researcher to study the ways in which people make sense of everyday life. Its central aim is the generation and testing of theory. Field & Morse (1985) included observation, interviews, genealogy, demography and life histories in the multiple methods of data collection which may be used by the ethnographer. In support of its usefulness in nursing research, they suggested that the knowledge gained was derived from the subject's view of the experience, rather than a view enforced, at least partly, by the researcher, as can be a pitfall when predetermined research tools are used.

The qualitative approach

Melia (1982) suggested that, as relative newcomers to research wishing to gain academic respectability, nurses may have been attracted to the 'hard' data of survey methods and objective measurements amenable to statistical analysis. Qualitative methodologists favour the understanding of behaviour. Benoliel (1984) wrote of qualitative approaches as:

> modes of systematic inquiry concerned with understanding human beings and the nature of their transactions with themselves and their surroundings.

Benoliel (1984) suggested that people's adaptation to critical life experiences such as chronic illness was one of the broad areas in which this approach offered a valuable expansion of knowledge.

Validity

Those favouring quantitative methods might question the validity of the data collected during this study, since it was all collected by one person, who was furthermore involved in professional practice with the families being studied. Hammersley & Atkinson (1983) argued, however, that, far from limiting the validity of the study, the involvement of the researcher, once recognized, could be exploited to yield additional insights into the field study. Reflexivity is the essential character of social research; the researcher becomes the research instrument par excellence. This capitalizes the opportunity to develop a nursing perspective through ongoing involvement with the families. A further decision which was important was the choice of the case study approach.

The case study

Case study research is intensive observation of a single subject, which may be an individual, a group, or an organization (Meier & Pugh 1986). Case study research can clarify questions, indicate approaches and make a substantial contribution to the study of behaviour. A grounded theory approach to the analysis of such data facilitates theory development.

Grounded theory

Glaser & Strauss (1967) elegantly demonstrated their strategy for handling data in their work with dying patients, from which awareness theory emerged. Their central thesis was the fact that the theory explicated was systematically obtained from the data, by inductive analysis, not by logical deduction from a priori assumptions. In the view of Hammersley & Atkinson (1983), it is the function of developing and testing theory which distinguishes social research from journalism and literature.

Data collection

The exploratory phase of the study involved introduction to the families and discussion with them of the author's role in providing a link between hospital and home, with a concern for the welfare of the whole family. During the initial interview, she made an assessment of the child's health status, using the Roper *et al.* (1980) Activities of Living Model. The author took notes as her questions were answered, but in future visits did not take notes until she had left the house.

The frequency of contacts varied according to the severity of the child's illness and the family's need for support. The smallest number of interactions was 18, the largest 101. Careful notes were made following each interaction with a family member, whether during a home visit, at the clinic or in a hospital ward, or an informal meeting through the Cystic Fibrosis Research Trust. Telephone conversations were also noted during or immediately after the event. Medical and nursing documentation was also consulted and, in one instance, the diary kept by a play leader was utilized.

The final methodological note relates to the use of a life history approach to an in-depth tape-recorded interview with each member of three of the families, and the mother in the fourth, towards the end of the period of study.

Life history interviews

The life history was defined by Denzin (1978) as presenting:

> the experience and definitions held by one person, one group, or one organization as this person, group or organization interprets those experiences.

There were three reasons for incorporating a life history interview into the case study approach. The first was that the main informant over the 5-year period of the study was in each case the mother of the affected child. Since the author was keen to gain insight into the perspective of each family member, it made sense to ask to interview each individual.

The second reason was to add depth to the data already gathered. Since the contacts with the families were in the context of a supportive relationship, rather than a research interview, another approach was needed which could frankly draw out information, thoughts and feelings from the informants.

The third reason reflects thinking from Becker's (1978) discussion in which he recommended the life history for those times when an area of study has grown stagnant; by the end of 4 years of accumulating field notes, it was necessary to take a fresh approach which would provide re-orientation to the field.

The interviews were arranged in advance. The author explained that the research she had mentioned earlier was near completion and that she would like to speak to each member of the family individually, to learn how CF had affected their lives. In each case, permission to tape-record the interview was asked for and given. Confidentiality was assured.

Data analysis

In ethnographic research the data analysis begins at the earliest stage with the formulation and clarification of research problems and continues right through to the writing-up phase (Hammersley & Atkinson 1983). There is a characteristic 'funnel' structure whereby the stages of a research project become progressively focused over time.

In this study, the analysis began in the early stages of the project as information was assimilated about CF and the family experience, and as the author tried to focus her thinking sufficiently to formulate the research questions. It continued informally to prompt questions during interaction with family members and more formally when analysis of the tape-recorded interviews was undertaken.

Editing and interpreting of the interviews and field notes resulted in family profiles. Further analysis led to the development of theoretical perspectives on nursing.

Cystic fibrosis

Cystic fibrosis is the commonest serious inherited disorder affecting the Caucasian population. It is estimated that around 400 new CF cases are diagnosed each year in the United Kingdom (Capewell 1986).

While the basic defect is one of molecular transport across cell membranes, the manifestations of the disease are diverse. The principal effects, however, are seen in the lungs and respiratory tract, the digestive system and the sweat. It is the susceptibility to respiratory infections which becomes debilitating and life-threatening, and which is associated with cardiovascular complications.

The essential characteristics of cystic fibrosis are of an inherited, pathological condition which can be treated but not cured, which is long-term with a varying course, which requires intensive daily therapy in order to maintain a reasonable quality as well as quantity of life—and which is ultimately life-threatening. It accords well with Mattsson's (1972) definition of chronic illness:

> Chronic illness refers to a disorder with a protracted course which can be progressive and fatal or associated with a relatively normal life span

> despite impaired physical and mental functioning. Such a disease frequently shows periods of acute exacerbations requiring intensive medical attention.

Adaptation was seen as a concept central to the family's adjustment to chronic illness. Roy (1983) defined adaptation as:

> the individual's response to the environment that promotes the person's general goals, including survival, growth, reproduction, and mastery or, more simply, it is behaviour that maintains the integrity of the individual.

Roy (1983) saw adaptation as freeing energy from inadequate or inappropriate coping attempts, thereby promoting health. This freedom to restructure and reorganize, incorporating the child's illness and treatment as part of the reality of family life, is the meaning of the term 'adaptation' as it is used in this study.

Question 1: How do family members respond to the genetic implications of cystic fibrosis?

Assault to self-image

The genetic implications came close to the dire prognosis in their painful impact on parents. Three of the couples spoke of the difficulties they experienced, but one father expressed it most vividly:

> I really felt as if you were going about with two horns growing out of your head, there was a physical abnormality about you, and even talking to the family, you felt as if they knew there was something wrong with you . . . . I was 22, roughly, and I felt as though I was in the prime of life, and basically you'd been hit below the belt by this—how could you say—brand on you.

This reaction illustrates the effect on self-image and self-esteem. Human sexuality is such an integral part of self-image and involves such deep emotions that the information suggesting an inability to produce healthy children can be devastating. The personal pain in reaction to the information about the genetic aspects of CF is compounded by the fact that family and others become aware of what is perceived as a grave defect. For many years one mother smarted under the comment, 'Nobody on my side's had it' from her mother-in-law. Even more painful was the suggestion that the birth of a fourth child suffering from an inherited disease, while the first three were unaffected, implied infidelity.

Frustration of generativity

A prime concern of the healthy developing adult is 'the establishing and guiding of the next generation' (Erikson 1977). Information which strikes at that aspiration strikes at something fundamental to emotional integrity.

The implications for future child-bearing were keenly felt. The advice not to have any more children cut right across natural drives and inclinations. As one father said, 'Everything was for a family'. After the loss of their first child, aged 17 months, with cystic fibrosis, his wife became pregnant, but was advised to have [a] termination. After much agonizing, they decided to go ahead with the pregnancy. She explained:

> I just wanted to take the chance, whether or not she had CF I just wanted another child. I was not caring if it had two heads; I mean that was the way I looked at it.

To produce a damaged child seemed much more acceptable than to have no child.

Difficult decisions

The knowledge gained through prenatal diagnosis, while having the potential to provide relief from the fear of having a child with CF, can also present an agonizing dilemma if the test is positive. Added to the inherent difficulty of such a decision is the sense that, where there is already an affected child, the choice to terminate a pregnancy because the fetus has the same disease may be seen as devaluing the affected child. One of the children said to his mother, 'Does that mean you wouldn't have had me?'

Genetic counselling is arguably the most sensitive of counselling areas. From each of the families there were appreciative comments on the way this aspect had been handled by medical staff, although there was not agreement all of the time with the advice given. The most helpful characteristics mentioned were the ability to listen while the couple talked through their thoughts and feelings, to provide information and to affirm the decision finally reached by the couple.

Question 2: How do families respond to the life-threatening nature of CF?

Suffering

For a parent, loss of a child is a threat to self, since so much self, physically and emotionally, is bound up in the life of the child. The situation meets Kahn & Stevens' (1986) theoretical definition of suffering as an experience in which 'some crucial aspect of one's own self, being or existence is threatened'. Finding meaning in the experience was seen to strengthen coping, but this aspect will not be taken further in this paper.

Fear was mentioned by all the couples. One father expressed it clearly:

> I got to the stage where I didn't want to ask at the hospital, ken, what was wrong. I was feared they would turn round and say, 'Well we reckon we're going to lose him' or something like that.

A spectrum of denial was shown by the families. This ranged from the response of the father just mentioned, whose denial of the gravity of his son's condition for months after the diagnosis was seriously maladaptive in terms of family functioning, to that of his son, who, at 9 years of age, told me,

> You just don't think about it and play and do everything, because it doesn't stop you. Just fight it.

Another mother, after the diagnosis of CF had been withdrawn following 5 years of treatment, looked back on their situation and commented,

> I don't think anyone can think about it in that situation. You just can't think about it or you couldn't get on with day-to-day life. That'd be the first way to a nervous breakdown.

The adaptive strength of denial is seen, reducing the stress for parents by blocking out the fearsome future and allowing them to concentrate on day-to-day life and the considerable demands of care. It is clear that it is the life-threatening nature of the diagnosis that colours the caring experience, rendering the families vulnerable to crisis.

Anger is a common reaction to a threatening situation, and when displaced on to the spouse erupts in verbal or physical abuse, reported by two of the couples. This obviously adds greatly to the stress of the situation and threatens the stability of the marriage and hence the welfare of the children. When the anger is expressed in irritation with the well siblings, it is followed by feelings of extreme guilt.

Facing the facts

The comprehension by the parents of the grim prognosis does not always synchronize with the initial interview. One cannot say with certainty how much this relates to the information given, the way in which it is given or the person who gives it. What seems clear is that comprehension depends to some extent on the preparedness of the parent to hear such news, both in terms of the child's health status and the parent's defence mechanisms. Where there has been long-term anxiety about the child's health, there is a degree of relief to have a diagnosis and treatment, mingled with the shock of the poor outlook. One mother said:

> I was relieved . . . to have a name . . . to say to somebody, he's got cystic fibrosis. I mean, I thought Willie was dying. I could have kissed the doctor.

The bleak outlook was comprehended, but at that time took second place to the fact that there was treatment available. Although faced with the same facts of experience, her husband's coping repertoire prepared him less well to deal with the threat of the situation.

The difficulty which modern Western society has in dealing with the subject of death—particularly the untimely loss of a child—intensifies the pain for parents who are living in the shadow of death. The question, 'Will he not grow out of it?' caused extreme frustration to one family. Denial was no longer an option for them as they watched their son's condition deteriorate, and they were acutely sensitive to the reactions of others.

Question 3: What events precipitate crises in the lives of families caring for a child with CF?

The chronic burden of care

The crises experienced have to be seen in the context of the daily burden of care. There is the daily demand of physiotherapy sessions—and at times of illness medical advice is sometimes to give four sessions a day. When the secretions are thick a session can take over an hour, so the investment of time and energy is very considerable. The children are not invariably co-operative with regard to physiotherapy and, coupled with the potential for conflict between partners about sharing the tasks, this is one of the major sources of intra-family conflict. Supervision of enzyme replacement, vitamin supplements and diet, along with monitoring of appetite, stools and weight gain, requires constant effort and militates against normalization.

Added to this chronic burden of care directly related to CF are the stresses of ordinary family life, of bereavements, unruly teenagers, redundancy and unemployment, health problems and anxieties about the healthy children's progress at school and the effect that family stress is having on them. Financial difficulties contributed to the cumulative burden of all the families. It is hardly surprising, when all this is taken into account, that quite minor events can cause distress of crisis proportions.

The state of crisis

Golan's (1969) description of emotional crisis identified four components: the hazardous event, the vulnerable state, the precipitating factor and the state of active crisis. The hazardous event which rendered all the families vulnerable was the diagnosis of CF. Precipitating factors included illness in the child, death of a known child, comments and reactions of peers, and societal attitudes.

The event which appeared consistently and predictably in all four case studies was an episode of illness in the child with CF. Two parents mentioned the clutching fear—'Is this it?'—which so intensified normal parental anxiety surrounding illness of a child. An important aspect of the parents' experience in relation to these episodes is the responsibility which they have to carry in relation to the ill child. There were decisions about how soon to call for medical help, and occasions when parents had to assert their view against the medical opinion. When the stakes are so high such decision making is extremely stressful. If both parents are pulling together at such times the burden is considerably eased.

It is worth noting that none of the families in the study had the level of education which would have made it easy for them to challenge a medical opinion, but their knowledge of their own child and their commitment to his or her well-being gave them the confidence to assert parental authority.

The news of death of a child with CF has reverberations right round the community of CF families. A number of parents attend the funeral. Others view such events as reasons to avoid contact with other CF families as much as possible, not only to protect themselves from pain but also to shield their child from confrontation with the threat to his own life. One older sibling went to the funeral of a family friend who had died of CF, and when she came home she tried to hide from her young brother that she had been crying. When she had to admit that she had been crying, just a bit, for Michael,

Willie was alright and then asked a lot of questions about the funeral. He asked if Michael's parents were upset, and would Michael be happy in heaven? There would seem to be a positive aspect to this crisis event in that it can provide a learning experience for siblings or for CF children and can allow them to voice anxieties usually suppressed.

The cruel teasing of peers, e.g: 'You'll be dead by the time you're 13', caused shock waves as parents and siblings shared the distress of the affected child. Strategies to deal with the offending children and to reassure their own child have to be worked out.

Finally, there were several instances where societal attitudes contributed to family stress. Although there has been a great deal of public education about CF in recent years, parents still encounter seemingly unreasonable resistance to inclusion of the child in some activities, e.g. camps and school trips. That resistance probably stems partly from fear, knowing the grim prognosis of CF but having insufficient knowledge to predict risks to the particular child and therefore being unwilling to take responsibility for his welfare. Coupled with that is evidence from two of the studies of the importance of revulsion for sputum as an irrational but significant factor in the decision-making of the person in authority.

Question 4: How does caring for a child with CF affect interaction patterns and the coping response of families?

Synchrony between partners

What seems to be crucial for family functioning is the synchrony with which partners move through the transition from seeing themselves as a normal healthy family to accepting themselves as a family with a health problem. When the wife comes to terms with the situation before her husband, there is extreme strain on the relationship. One mother in this situation said:

> I felt as if I'd two invalids at first. Bill was terrible, drinking . . . I couldn't have went to the shops and left Bill to feed him. He'd have fed him, but he wouldn't have given him the tablets. He'd have said, 'What for? He doesn't need it.' I can understand it now, I couldn't then. I really hated him then.

Where the partners have never established a complementary communication pattern, and one prefers not to know about difficult issues in family coping, they are poorly prepared to cope with a threat such as serious illness in their child. It seems that the avoidance reaction, even though seen to be maladaptive, becomes 'set' and is repeated in the face of successive threats. It is as if the couple is locked in to an interaction pattern which bars disclosure of painful feelings.

Even in partnerships displaying many more strengths than weaknesses, there are times when their resources are exhausted, communication is impeded and tension mounts. The intervention of a sensitive third party at such times can provide the needed catalyst to re-establish communication and free the couple to move forward together again.

Parents and children

Where the parents are not travelling together through the process of adaptation, the effect on the family system is likely to be dire. This was shown very clearly by the oldest sibling in one family:

> We were a close family, then something like this. It did change life . . . You felt sorry for Willie. It's hard to explain, it did change, it changed a hell of a lot, from just the three of us, then Willie coming along, then something wrong; it was a right let down. But that's how it was, you can't change it . . . I really felt sorry for my Mum and Dad but I couldn't say that. There again, whenever they gave him a row, I thought 'You're a bitch' or if it was my Dad I'd scream at him, 'Leave him alone'. If he didn't have CF and he'd done something wrong, I'd have smacked him for it, but I felt that's a shame, he's got CF, you shouldn't be doing that to him.

The youngest of the sisters said,

> My Dad wouldn't believe that he had cystic fibrosis, like it was his first laddie and he couldn't take it in. That's when I realized what was going on . . . my Dad saying there was nothing wrong with him and my Mum giving him all the tablets, like who do you believe? . . . Like before Willie was born I was the youngest, then when he was born he got all the attention.

For the healthy siblings in this family there was sympathy for the parents mixed with confusion, blame and anger, resentment at the loss of attention and over-protection of their brother.

In another family, where the child's condition was deteriorating, the mother explained,

> As soon as you see the sputum building up, that starts the stress again . . . When I moan at him, he moans at the kids—so it comes back to it's my fault.

This illustrates the cybernetic effect of stress on family interaction (Figure 32.1).

Nursing support

The aspects of nursing which were mentioned by the families were in relation to giving information, explaining the meaning of investigations, answering questions, listening, providing a link between the clinic and the home and between the home and the school, and providing help with child care.

Giving of information relates to answering the many questions which parents need to ask around the time of diagnosis in order to fully appraise the situation and mobilize coping resources. Having opportunity to raise these questions in the relaxed

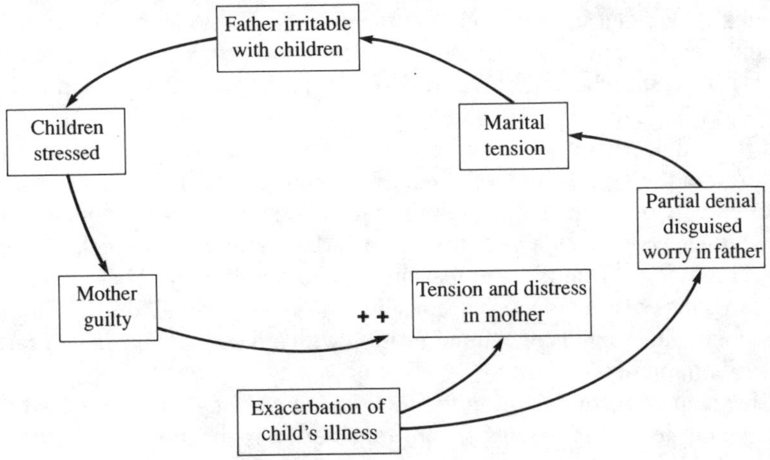

Figure 32.1 The cybernetic nature of family stress in response to the child's illness

environment of their own home and at their own time is felt to be beneficial. For fathers there may be no other opportunity to question health care staff and clarify their understanding of the condition.

The importance of listening while the many difficult areas are worked through was evident in the study. There is a need for a highly skilled level of counselling here so that the interaction can move from exploration of the problems to confrontation of difficult issues, the development of understanding and, where appropriate, the setting of goals. The approach used during the fieldwork was non-directive and there were few occasions when there was an explicit setting of goals. In the context of a long-term relationship this seems an appropriate strategy, but there is potential for purposeful intervention. Since the emphasis is on including the whole family in the focus of care, an ability to work with individuals of all ages and with the family as a group is required.

Early contact

It is particularly useful for the nurse to make early contact with each member of the family and to make it clear that she is available to answer questions or listen to problems. The concept of synchrony, or of 'travelling together' should be kept in mind as the nurse makes an assessment of the functioning of the family system. If it is apparent that one partner is opting out of care, or if there is obvious conflict in the marriage, it is especially important to investigate the problem sooner rather than later. It is clear that intervention at the peak of disequilibrium, that is, crisis intervention, is likely to be more effective than trying to change a maladaptive response which has become established. The intervention cannot be prescribed, but allowing each partner to express disappointment, fear, anger—and encouraging acceptance of one another's position and stage of acceptance—can help to clear the blocks in communication and understanding.

A key factor for the nurse is maintaining neutrality, that is, avoiding taking sides in family conflict; as Wright & Leahey (1984) stated, being 'allied with everyone and no one at the same time'. There is also a place for encouraging contact with another worker in the health care team who may be able to offer skills particularly appropriate to a specific situation, e.g. marriage counselling.

The need for a link person working between hospital and home has to some extent been recognized in the establishing of paediatric community nursing. This study highlights the complexity of the area and the importance of the nurse being equipped to help families make their way through very testing experiences in a way which protects and respects the needs of each family member and of the family unit. That being the first priority of care, it is also evident that considerable interpersonal skill is required to establish and maintain channels of communication with members of the health care team and the wider community.

The need for help with child care, in the form of baby-sitting by someone who could give physiotherapy to let the parents go out together, was mentioned by two mothers and a sibling. While in some situations the important task may be to convince parents that they can safely leave the child in someone else's care, at times when the child's condition is deteriorating there is an understandable reluctance to pass the responsibility to friends or family. The extra needs of the child are not trivial, and the parents are aware that they have acquired nursing and physiotherapy skills. These cannot readily be relinquished to leave the child in unskilled hands. At such a time the expert presence of a trained nurse would contribute greatly to the parents' peace of mind. Further, this could help to prevent social isolation and to promote healthy family functioning. The author is unaware of any scheme providing this kind of support, but it is an organizational issue which merits further investigation.

Theoretical perspectives

The family as unit of care

There has been an increasing recognition in recent years of the significance of levels of analysis other than the individual. Family-nursing literature helps to articulate this shift of focus. Hanson (1987) gave the following definition:

> Family health is defined as a dynamic, relative state of well-being. Five dimensions—the biological, psychological, sociological, spiritual, and cultural—all combine into the holistic human system. The purpose of family nursing is to promote, maintain, and restore family health; it is concerned with the interaction between the family and society and among the family and individual family members.

The study showed that the health and illness of a child with CF profoundly influenced the well-being of the parents and the siblings. The biological dimension was seen in the physical illness and the treatment regime, with the suggestion that the child's illness is at times reflected in the physical ill-health of a parent. The psychological dimension is multifaceted, encompassing the growth and development of the children, the perceptions of each family member and the dynamics of interpersonal relationships. The sociological dimension was evidenced in the availability of helpful and supportive relationships outwith the immediate family, and the interface between the family and such social systems as the school and the health care team.

The importance of finding meaning in illness and of prayer revealed the significance of the spiritual dimension for some parents. The cultural dimension was not explored in depth, but the sharing of the tasks of caring, the patterns of intra-familial interaction and the attitudes to the health care team all have a cultural basis. The five dimensions were seen to overlap with and impinge upon one another.

Systems thinking as a framework for family nursing

Systems thinking has been found to provide a helpful theoretical base for family therapy, and has been utilized by Wright & Leahey (1984) in their work on family nursing. The findings of this study confirm the theoretical perspectives of systems thinking as applicable to families caring for a child with chronic illness and the relevant nursing involvement.

In systems thinking the concept of wholeness is important, not just holistic care of the child who has the illness, but a holistic view of the family and the relationship of its parts.

A distinction which needs to be made is between viewing the child as the focus of nursing, accepting the importance of the family context, and viewing the whole family system as the unit of care. There is much talk of 'partnership with parents' in modern paediatric care, but in reality this can stop short at teaching the parents how to care for their sick child, in preparation for discharge home. The effect on family functioning of the chronic burden of care is not always appreciated. It is essential to recognize the impact of long-term childhood illness on the family system. Two of the families showed very clearly how an exacerbation of illness in the child could set off a chain reaction from the mother's initial response, the father's failure to react, to the subsequent conflict which affected healthy siblings. The whole family's stability was threatened.

It is not hard to appreciate the toll that can be placed on the marriage relationship when such events recur with increasing frequency, with little hope of a satisfactory resolution. Nurses working with such families need an awareness of family dynamics and to make it clear that their professional commitment extends to family health. It may be that using the term 'family nursing' would reinforce this important concept.

The human relationship

The relational element in family nursing is both costly and enriching for the nurse. In Griffin's (1983) fascinating analysis of caring, it is suggested that a nurse's response to a patient's need has several layers:

> There is the clinical assessment of what is required, the cognitive and moral recognition of the importance of the patient as a person and significantly, the emotional element, motivating and energizing the act, and licencing (sic) us to call it caring.

The enrichment and the demands which characterized the author's involvement with the families in the study were not peculiar to her own experience. As one paediatric community nurse said, 'You know there's going to be a breakthrough. You're working so hard for them, because of the ones you've lost. You're doing it for them too.'

Essentially family nursing requires a relationship between equals. Both parties are committed to the welfare of the affected child but also to the well-being of the family as a whole. It must be a reciprocal relationship, in which the family can consult the nurse to talk through a problem and come to a decision, and the nurse can alert the family to a problem which she perceives.

It is not, however, a problem-driven relationship; an important part of the nurse's function is to affirm and encourage the family in its coping. It is a relationship which the nurse is required to enter to meet her professional responsibilities, regardless of her own feelings. Yet to develop and nurture the kind of relationship which will help to sustain the family through the transition from seeing themselves as a healthy family to accepting the reality of a long-term health problem and its genetic implications, through the suffering of awareness of the advancing threat of death of the child, through the crisis experiences which such families meet and to help them find meaning in it all—to do this without the energizing effect of emotional involvement would not be possible.

Conclusion

This study has shown family nursing to be integral to the role of paediatric community nurses who have a commitment to promoting the health and integrity of families caring for children with cystic fibrosis. Similar studies examining family experience and nursing response in relation to other long-term conditions in various age groups would strengthen the knowledge base for practice.

The thesis presented is that nursing support involves a complex blend of information-giving, befriending, family counselling and advocacy as the nurse moves in and out of the family system and links the family with support networks in the social system. The reality of the shift in focus of paediatric nursing practice from the ill child to the whole family as a unit of care must be recognized.

References

Becker, H.S. (1978) 'The relevance of life histories', in *Sociological Methods: A Source Book* (Denzin, N.K. ed.), McGraw-Hill, New York.

Benoliel, J.Q. (1984) 'Advancing nursing science: qualitative approaches', *Western Journal of Nursing Research*, **6**, 1–8.

Capewell, G. (1986) *Cystic Fibrosis*, Office of Health Economics, London.

Denzin, N.K. (1978) *The Research Act: A Theoretical Introduction to Sociological Methods*, McGraw-Hill, New York.

Erikson, E.H. (1977) *Childhood and Society*, Triad/Paladin, St Albans, Hertfordshire.

Field, P.A. & Morse, J.M. (1985) *Nursing Research: The Application of Qualitative Approaches*, Croom Helm, London.

Glaser, B.G. & Strauss, A.L. (1967) *The Discovery of Grounded Theory: Strategies for Qualitative Research*, Aldine, Chicago.

Golan, N. (1969) 'When is a client in crisis?' *Social Casework*, July, 389–394.

Griffin, A.P. (1983) 'A philosophical analysis of caring in nursing', *Journal of Advanced Nursing*, **8**, 289–295.

Hammersley, M. & Atkinson, P. (1983) *Ethnography: Principles in Practice*, Tavistock, London.

Hanson, S.M.H. (1987) 'Family nursing and chronic illness', in *Families and Chronic Illness* (Wright, L. & Leahey, M. eds), Springhouse, Pennsylvania.

Kahn, D.L. & Stevens, R.H. (1986) 'The experience of suffering: conceptual clarification and theoretical definition', *Journal of Advanced Nursing*, **11**, 623–631.

Mattsson, A. (1972) 'Long-term physical illness in childhood: a challenge to psychosocial adaptation', *Pediatrics*, **50**, 5.

Meier, P. & Pugh, E.J. (1986) 'The case study: a viable approach to clinical research', *Research in Nursing and Health*, **9**, 195–202.

Melia, K.M. (1982) '"Tell it as it is"—qualitative methodology and nursing research: understanding the student nurses' world', *Journal of Advanced Nursing*, **7**, 327–335.

Roper, N., Logan, W. & Tierney, A. (1980) *The Elements of Nursing*, Churchill Livingstone, Edinburgh.

Roy, C. Sr. (1983) 'Roy Adaptation Model', in *Family Health: A Theoretical Approach to Nursing Care* (Clements, I. & Roberts, F. eds), John Wiley & Sons, New York.

Whyte, D.A. (1990) 'The family with a chronically-ill child', *Paediatric Nursing*, **2**(8), 20–23; **2**(9), 21–23.

Wright, L. & Leahey, M. (1984) *Nurses and Families*, F.A. Davis, Philadelphia.

33

A Description of Stressors and Coping Strategies Among Parents of Critically Ill Children—a Preliminary Study*

F.A. CARNEVALE

Introduction

The purpose of this study was to examine systematically how parents cope with the critical illness of their child.

Descriptions of stressors confronted by parents in the paediatric intensive care unit (PICU) have been documented. Descriptions of parental coping are essentially limited to anecdotal reports. Some papers describe intervention programmes to assist parental coping, although little is understood about the latter.

A qualitative investigation of parental coping in this context will help explain how parents cope with the critical illness of their child. This will help identify personal and situational factors that are related to the types of coping strategies utilised by parents. The findings of this study will, it is hoped, contribute significantly to (1) the development of research-based clinical interventions, (2) the development of evaluation research studies to examine the efficacy of various ways of coping, and (3) the evaluation of the appropriateness of qualitative methodology for the investigation of coping.

Research questions

This study is designed to examine the following questions:

1 What are the principal sources of stress (stressors) described by parents of critically ill children?
2 What are the coping strategies utilised by parents of critically ill children to cope with these stressors?

*This is an abridged version of an article first published in *Intensive Care Nursing*, Vol. 6, No. 1, pp. 4–11, 1990.

Selected review of literature

Conceptual framework

Lazarus and his associates have provided a highly cohesive and supported framework for understanding stress and coping (Lazarus & Folkman, 1984). Stress is described as a particular relationship between the person and the environment that is appraised by the person as taxing or exceeding his or her resources and endangering his or her well-being. A stressor is a demand upon a person's resources that is appraised as stressful. The perception of stress is dependent upon the person's cognitive appraisal of the situation in terms of 'what is at stake?' This appraisal is affected by several personal and situational factors. Coping refers to cognitive and behavioural efforts to manage stressors.

Parental stress in the PICU

The largest proportion of reports relating to the experience of parents of critically ill children focus on stress or stressors among parents in the PICU setting.

Critical illness in children has been described as a highly stressful experience for parents. Rothstein (1979, 1980) identified patterns of parental reactions to acute illness in children. Most parents experienced overwhelming shock, helplessness, and guilt.

In another report, families described unsatisfied needs regarding information conveyed to them, although expert technical care was provided (Carnevale et al, 1983). Waller et al (1979) reported extreme denial and hostility as a coping response by parents of critically ill children.

Bereaved parents of critically ill children have described their lack of understanding in the situation and inability to care for their child as major sources of stress (Carnevale, 1982).

There is a small amount of qualitative research on parents' needs and roles in the PICU. Rennick (1987) conducted a qualitative study of parental needs among 16 parents in a PICU. The five principal needs identified included the need to know, the need to be respected, the need to comfort, the need to be comforted, and the need to trust. Similarly Kasper and Nyamethi (1988) qualitatively examined the needs of 15 parents in a PICU. Thirty-seven types of physical, psychological, and sociological needs were identified. Parental role needs were predominant. Further research is necessary to examine the relationship between parental needs and parental stress, how adequately these needs are satisfied, and in which ways.

In a qualitative study of the mother's parental role in the PICU by Snowdon (1988) six parental roles were observed. These included vigilant parent, nurturer-comforter, medical parent, caregiver, entertainer, and protector.

Miles (1979) examined the impact of a child's hospitalisation in a PICU on the parents. Three principal groups of stressors were outlined: (1) concern about the child's condition; (2) the strange, new environment; and (3) parental role alteration. Miles and her associates (Carter & Miles, 1982) have developed the Parental Stressor Scale:PICU (PSS:PICU), a self-report instrument to measure parental stress in the PICU. This scale focuses predominantly on physical and interpersonal factors in the environment as sources of stress.

Numerous studies have used the PSS:PICU to examine parental stress in relation to the parent's sex (Miles et al, 1984), suddenness of admission (Carter et al, 1985; Eberly et al, 1985), and in relation to nursing staff perceptions of parental stress (Johnson et al, 1988).

Parental coping in the PICU

Parental coping in the PICU has received very little research attention. Miles and Carter (1983) have provided a theoretical paper which describes how Lazarus' model of coping could be related to parental coping in the PICU. Although the paper offers a model for clinical nursing, the authors emphasise the importance of further research into parental coping.

Intervention programmes

Although parental coping has been subjected to minimal scientific investigation, several papers outline nursing intervention programmes for assisting parental coping.

Jay (1977) has emphasised the importance of parental involvement in the care of children in the PICU. An association between individualised visiting policies and decreased anxiety levels among mothers in the PICU has been described by Proctor (1987).

A quasi-experimental evaluation of the influence of a responsive nursing intervention programme upon the experience of sixty-five parents in the PICU was conducted by Carnevale (1983). Statistically significant favourable outcomes were observed in relation to parental stress, coping, control, social support, and anxiety. A detailed operational definition of this nursing approach has been documented (Carnevale, 1985).

Curley (1988) reported on how a Nursing Mutual Participation Model of Care helped to alleviate stress among thirty-three parents in the PICU. Stress was measured with the PSS:PICU.

Analysis

The needs and stresses of parents of critically ill children represent the most extensively researched dimension of these parents' experience (Etzler, 1984).

Parental coping has been investigated in relation to the parent's general stress of having a child in the intensive care unit. This approach to the study of coping does not build on the current conceptualisation of coping advanced by Lazarus and his associates. Cognitive appraisal processes contribute to wide inter-individual variation in coping responses to similar situations. It seems necessary to examine coping in relation to specific relevant stressors (Carnevale et al, 1987).

A qualitative examination of parental stress and coping appears methodologically appropriate in this context. This method enables the investigator to observe coping in relation to specific stressors relevant to the respondent.

There has been no systematic study of cognitive appraisal processes in parents of critically ill children reported to date. A qualitative research method can assist in obtaining descriptions of the meanings parents attribute to different stresses.

Table 33.1 Sample characteristics

Parent	Child
Parent 1	Child A
Father, 39 years	Boy, 8 years
Self employed	Motor vehicle accident
Parent 2	Paraplegia incurred
Mother, 38 years	5 week stay in PICU
Housewife	2 older sisters
Parent 3	Child B
Father, 36 years	Girl, 2 weeks old
Radio producer	Apnoea, vomiting
Parent 4	3 months in PICU
Mother, 34 years	No siblings
Housewife, former nurse	Child C
Parent 5	Girl, 1 month old
Mother, 29 years	Sepsis
Nurse	1 month in PICU
	No siblings

Methodology

Design

An exploratory descriptive research design was utilised for this study. Subjects were interviewed using a client-centred phenomenological approach (Rogers, 1951; Field & Morse, 1985). This aims to explore the qualitative experience of the subjects.

Sample

The study was conducted within a ten bed PICU of a metropolitan university teaching children's hospital.

A purposive sampling technique was used to ensure the inclusion of parents encountering varying circumstances. Five parents participated in this preliminary study. Four of these consisted of two married couples. The characteristics of the subjects are detailed in Table 33.1.

Procedure

Parents were asked to participate in the study twenty-four hours after admission at a time when the child's condition had stabilised. The parents were interviewed during the first week following the transfer of their child out of the PICU. All interviews were conducted in the investigator's office.

Although subjects were asked to be interviewed individually, each married couple wished to participate jointly. This wish was respected.

The client-centred phenomenological interview method was used in this study to examine cognitive appraisal among parents. The aim of the interview was to obtain descriptions of how parents are perceiving the situation, 'what is it like' to have a child in the PICU? Exploratory questions are outlined in Appendix A. All interviews were audio tape-recorded. These recordings were transcribed and content analysed.

Data analysis

The tape recorded interviews were transcribed and content analysed by the investigator. The principal units of analysis were the themes that emerged in relation to stressors and coping strategies. Respective lists of stressors and coping strategies were developed, using the respondents' own words as much as possible. Similar items were grouped in an attempt to identify categories.

Findings

Stressors

Seventeen different themes emerged from the interviews relating to sources of stress or stressors. They were grouped into five categories of stressors including (1) parental role conflict, (2) concern for child, (3) the environment, (4) friends, and (5) the child's siblings. Every parent referred to their role as a parent in the PICU as a significant source of stress while four out of five referred to this as a greatest source of stress.

Stressor categories are defined below along with actual statements illustrating respective stressors.

(1) *Parental role conflict* refers to thoughts and feelings pertaining to an inability to parent. These were largely related to situational constraints (predominantly staff related). One mother said,

> I should have had her on my body. Especially after a week, I felt, I had to badger people to hold her. People were friendly but they didn't understand that I wanted to hold her all of the time. I wanted to get into bed with the kid and stay there for days and days.

A father stated

> My feelings were so complicated. My baby was a kind of a hostage. They were giving intensive care. The quality of that care is important. You're in a certain sense dependent. So that's one practical reason for not wanting to put people against you. Then there's the human feelings of wanting to get along, not wanting to be conspicuous, a trouble-maker, here comes 'them', a lot of paranoia. What is the role of parents in decision making. This is where I feel we got absolutely no satisfaction. The doctor respected our intelligence in speaking with us

> but was completely unbending when it came to having a say in decisions.

(2) *Concern for child* refers to concern for the child's well-being. This included concern for the child's physical condition as well as the child's feelings.

(3) *Environment* involves the level of activity, noise, lights, and people in the environment. This also included significant changes in the environment such as transfer to a ward.

> The transfer to a ward was really hard. It's so quiet. It's like going from an amusement park to a morgue. There isn't enough staff for someone to stay with your kid.

(4) *Friends* refers to the particular behaviours of friends that caused distress.

> Your friends don't know what to do. They look the other way. People that you know well. They don't know how to handle it. A close friend took a long time to say 'Hi, how's it going?' I know he cared but, it really hurt.

(5) *Siblings* includes the feelings and perceptions of other children in relation to the situation.

> My other kids heard all kinds of stories. That their brother was in a coma, a vegetable, or dead. We didn't bring them in at first. We sat down with them and told them exactly what was happening, every night.
>
> When we came to visit the first time, the little one started shaking, she really was shaking. We went out to the parent's room and talked about it. Then she wanted to go back and she was fine.
>
> That's a good thing about letting brothers and sisters in ICU. They know what to expect. They see for themselves. It's real.

Coping strategies

Thirty-four different themes related to coping strategies were identified. These were grouped into five categories including (1) things you think about (cognitive), (2) actions directed toward other people (interpersonal), (3) drawing on support from others (social support), (4) things you do (direct action), and (5) drawing from the environment. Coping strategies are defined below, and illustrative examples are provided.

(1) Things you think about to deal with the situation.

> It was really scary. You're constantly looking at the machines. Everyone tells you to forget the machines and look at the child, but they're all looking at the machines.

After a while you begin to tune out the other kids and focus on yours.

I was very bitter and resentful because you don't have control over your child at all and you can't assume responsibility for the kid. I was very, very . . . quite angry at times. But I knew the system and you can't fight it.

I ended up resigning myself to just waiting it out until they decided that she could go home. I hated that place. Nobody cared.

(2) Actions directed towards other people such as staff, family, and friends.

We were lungeing, trying to get in on decisions. Always edgy, alert, trying to figure out how we could get a grip on our child's life.

Parents having control has no solid basis. Hospitals are the territory of nurses and doctors. They have made a choice to be there but the parents have not. Therefore they have not prepared themselves and cannot catch up with the medical team. One of the things you try to do quickly as a parent is learn things quickly and sometimes make pathetic efforts to speak knowledgeably when . . . You try to sound smart, to sound sensible. But you can never manage it.

When your child is in a crisis, you try to make that place your community. A centre of your world. All the people are your community. You contact with these people, begin to have personal interests in staff, their personalities.

(3) Drawing on support from others. This included family and friends.

My husband was very good, a total support, and was there all the time. We planned together, went together, went out of our way to find out about her, he was calm, he listened, he took care of her too, he held her, he went out of his way to be with her. He was fantastic. He was the only one there.

(4) Things you do refers to particular behaviours that alter the environment favourably.

We read the chart all the time. It was pretty dramatic at some points when a nurse would ask if we really should be reading the chart. They're trying to hide something from me. They don't want to tell us something. Why wouldn't they tell you? This is my son!

It was written down, so it was tangible.

(5) Drawing on aspects of the environment that helped you deal with the situation. This refers to having private space, a telephone, etc.

There was no consistent relationship between types of stressors and the strategies used to cope with these. A variety of strategies were used to cope with each stressor. It is interesting to note that three of the parents coped with parental role conflict with the staff by resigning themselves to the way things were and waiting to get their child out of the unit.

Limitations of the study

The principal potential limitation of the study lies in the validity of self-report data as a methodology for observing coping. Pearlin and Schooler (1978), Hymovitch (1984), and Graydon (1984) utilised self-report methods in describing coping and reported no significant problems with validity. Obviously use of the findings from a preliminary study of five parents is limited. However it does provide the basis for development of the research.

Discussion

The findings of this preliminary study have highlighted problems in the literature relating to stress and coping among parents in the PICU.

Miles alone (1979) and with her associates (Miles, et al, 1983, 1984, 1985) have made the most rigorous contribution to knowledge in this area. They have focused on the PICU environment as a major source of stress for parents. This study suggests that issues surrounding the parental role are likely to be the most consistent and principal stressors. Also, the three types of stressors described by Miles, i.e. (1) child's condition, (2) PICU environment, and (3) parental role, do not seem to be exhaustive. Parents in this study have also described friends, the child's feelings, and the siblings' feelings as sources of stress.

Miles and Carter (1983) have offered the only documented attempt to measure coping in this context. The findings of the preliminary study raise questions regarding the content validity of the Miles and Carter instrument. Several of the themes identified in this study are not included in the Miles and Carter scale. Some of these include 'I resigned myself', 'I tried to get in on decisions', 'I avoided friends,' and 'I read the chart'. Indeed some of the strategies described in this report have not been emphasised in the literature at all.

Implications for clinical practice

The findings of this study, although preliminary at present, can help caregivers attain an understanding of the experience of parents in the PICU and develop supportive strategies. It is interesting to note that parental role conflict with professional staff has emerged as a principal source of stress. Conventionally, the child's condition and the PICU environment have received considerable attention as stressors. These are difficult to manage as the extent to which they can be altered is limited.

It seems regrettable that parental role conflict should emerge as a major source of stress, as this is a problem that could be managed by parents and staff. Some parents reported attempts to resolve this such as 'I tried to get in on decisions, always on the alert, on the edge', or 'I tried pathetically to speak knowledgeably, sound smart and sensible so staff would tell me things'. On many occasions, parents felt that assertive strategies like these served only to further alienate them from staff, 'So I just had to deal with this as the way I was going to be treated in order for my baby to get medical care. I couldn't wait to take her home.'

It seems necessary for caregivers in this setting to consider strategies that can help to resolve these conflicts between staff and parents. These can include a review of existing practices and behaviour toward families, meeting with families to discuss roles and the implementation of educational programmes to help caregivers develop their knowledge and skills in working with parents.

Appendix A

Interview guide

Introduction: I would like to talk with you about what it is like to have (*child's name*) in an ICU.

1. What are some of the things you have found hard to deal with while your child was in the ICU? (identify stressors).
2. (Focus on what appears to be most significant stressor) When you were having trouble with (*stressor*), what things did you think about? How did you feel? (cognitive appraisal)
3. What types of things did you do or think about that helped you deal with (*stressor*)? (identify coping responses)
4. What are some of the things that made it easier for you to deal with (*stressor*)? (identify coping resources)
5. What things did other people do or say that made it easier for you to deal with (*stressor*)? (social support)

References

Carnevale, F.A. (1982) 'Child death in hospital: the survivor's perspective', *Focus on Critical Care*, **9**(4), 7–9.

Carnevale, F.A. (1983) 'The influence of a complemental nursing approach upon the experience of parents within the pediatric intensive care unit', Unpublished Masters research report, McGill University, Montreal.

Carnevale, F.A. (1985) 'Nursing the critically ill child: A responsive approach', *Focus on Critical Care*, **2**(5), 10–13.

Carnevale, F.A., Annibale, F., Crenier, A., Guy, E., Ottoni, L. (1987) 'Nursing in the ICU: Stress without distress', *Canadian Critical Care Nursing Journal*, **4**(2), 16–18.

Carnevale, F.A., Espinosa, P.S., Fortin-Berrardino, L., Guy, E.R., Harvie-Carbonneau, S.E., Powell, M.A., Tetreault, E., Veneziano, A. (1983) 'Induced paralysis', *The Canadian Nurse*, **79**(10), 45–51.

Carter, M.C., Miles, M.A. (1982) 'Parental stressor scale: Pediatric intensive care unit', *Nursing Research*, **31**, 121.

Carter, M.C., Miles, M.S., Buford, T.H., Hassanein, R.S. (1985) 'Parental environmental stress in pediatric intensive care units', *Dimensions of Critical Care Nursing*, **4**, 180–188.

Curley, M.A.Q. (1988) 'Effects of the nursing mutual participation model of care on parental stress in the pediatric intensive care unit', *Heart and Lung*, **17**, 682–688.

Eberly, T.W., Miles, M.S., Carter, M.C., Hennessey, J., Riddle, I. (1985) 'Parental stress after the unexpected admission of a child to the intensive care unit', *Critical Care Quarterly*, **8**, 57–65.

Etzler, C.A. (1984) 'Parents' reactions to pediatric critical care settings: A review of the literature', *Issues in Comprehensive Pediatric Nursing*, **7**, 319–331.

Field, P.A., Morse, J.M. (1985) *Nursing research: The application of qualitative approaches*, London, Croom Helm.

Graydon, J.E. (1984) 'Measuring patient coping', *Nursing Papers*, **16**(2), 3–12.

Hymovich, D.P. (1984) 'Development of the chronicity impact and coping instrument: Parent questionnaire', *Nursing Research*, **33**(4), 218–222.

Jay, S.S. (1977) 'Pediatric intensive care: Involving parents in the care of their child', *Maternal-Child Nursing Journal*, **6**(3), 195–204.

Johnson, P.A., Nelson, G.L., Brunnquell, D.V. (1988) 'Parent and nurse perceptions of parent stressors in the pediatric intensive care unit', *Children's Health Care*, **17**, 98–105.

Kasper, I.W., Nyamathi, A.M. (1988) 'Parents of children in the pediatric intensive care unit: What are their needs?' *Heart and Lung*, **17**, 574–581.

Lazarus, R.S., Folkman, S. (1984) *Stress, appraisal, and coping*, New York, Springer Publishing.

Miles, M.S. (1979) 'Impact of the intensive care unit on parents', *Issues in Comprehensive Pediatric Nursing*, **3**, 72–90.

Miles, M.S., Carter, M.C. (1983) 'Assessing parental stress in the intensive care unit', *Journal of Maternal Child Nursing*, **8**, 354–359.

Miles, M.S., Carter, M.C., Spicher, C., Hassanein, R.S. (1984) 'Paternal and maternal stress reactions in the pediatric ICU', *Issues in Comprehensive Pediatric Nursing*, **7**, 333–342.

Pearlin, L.I., Schooler, C. (1978) 'The structure of coping', *Journal of Health and Social Behaviour*, **19**(3), 2–21.

Proctor, D.L. (1987) 'Relationship between visitation policy in a pediatric intensive care unit and parental anxiety', *Children's Health Care*, **16**, 13–17.

Rennick, J.E. (1987) *The needs of parents with a child in a pediatric intensive care unit*, Masters thesis, Nursing Faculty, University of Toronto.

Rogers, C.R. (1951) *Client-centered therapy*, Boston, Houghton Mifflin.

Rothstein, P. (1979) 'Family reaction to acute overwhelming illness in children', *Critical Care Medicine*, **7**(3), 130.

Rothstein, P. (1980) 'Psychological stress in families of children in a pediatric intensive care unit', *Pediatric Clinics of North America*, **27**, 613–632.

Snowdon, A.W. (1988) *The maternal role in the pediatric intensive care unit and hospital ward*, Masters thesis, School of Nursing, McGill University, Montreal.

Waller, D.A., Todres, I.D., Cassem, N.H., Anderten, A. (1979) 'Coping with poor prognosis in the pediatric intensive care unit', *American Journal of Diseases in Children*, **133**(Nov), 1121–1125.

34

Strategies for Family-Centered Care in the Critical Care Setting*

CINDY HYLTON RUSHTON

In the past two decades, systems of care for children and their families have evolved into a family-centered care (FCC) model. This 'new' philosophy of care has emerged in response to the changing health care needs of infants and children and in recognition of the integral role of the family in providing comprehensive care (Shelton, Jeppson, & Johnson, 1987; Koop, 1987). Many professionals agree that respect for families and involvement of them in the care of their children is the foundation of quality pediatric health care. Yet when specific attitudes, policies, and practices concerning families are examined, both subtle and overt actions do not seem to reflect commitment to such respect and involvement. Furthermore, while it may be possible to achieve FCC during routine health care encounters, many nurses and other health care professionals wonder if it is REALLY possible to achieve a family-centered care in the critical care setting.

The meaning of FCC in the clinical setting is often based on intuition and untested assumptions with few empirically based guidelines to direct family-centered interventions. However, the Association for the Care of Children's Health (ACCH) has identified eight elements that are thought to be essential for implementing family-centered care (Shelton, et al, 1987) (see Table 34.1). These elements can be used as the basis of care delivery for infants, children, and their families in all health care settings. This article will explore the application of the elements of FCC in the neonatal or pediatric critical care unit and suggest strategies for successful implementation.

Family-centered care in the critical care setting

Critical care nurses and other professionals caring for ill or injured infants and children struggle to balance the effects of technology with caring. Creating a caring, family-centered atmosphere in the critical care setting is often hampered by the rapid changes in the child's condition, the high tech nature of the setting, staff shortages, professional attitudes, and institutional priorities.

*This article was first published in *Pediatric Nursing*, Vol. 16, No. 2, pp. 195–199, 1990.

Table 34.1 Elements of family-centered care (Shelton, Jeppson & Johnson, 1987)

1	Recognition that the family is the constant in the child's life while the service systems and personnel within those systems fluctuate
2	Facilitation of parent/professional collaboration at all levels of health care
3	Sharing of unbiased and complete information with parents about their child's care on an ongoing basis in an appropriate and supportive manner
4	Implementation of appropriate policies and programs that are comprehensive and provide emotional and financial support to meet the needs of families
5	Recognition of family strengths and individuality and respect for different methods of coping
6	Understanding and incorporating the developmental and emotional needs of infants, children, and adolescents and their families into health care delivery systems
7	Encouragement and facilitation of parent to parent support
8	Assurance that the design of health care delivery systems is flexible, accessible, and responsive to family needs

Moreover, a child's critical illness threatens family stability and the resources and coping abilities of parents (Broome, 1985). Parents are confronted with unfamiliar people and technology as well as life saving interventions that are often painful and frightening. Parents and caregivers commonly experience powerful emotions and stress that accompany an encounter with life threatening illness or injury, particularly when infants and young children are involved.

Despite the potential barriers to FCC in the critical care setting, many nurses and other health care professionals have successfully implemented FCC in their intensive care units. To do so, barriers must be identified and used to guide the development of specific goals, objectives, and evaluation criteria for the delivery of FCC. Institutional and unit changes do not occur quickly or without compromise. Changes must be deliberate, well planned and supported by a network of committed professionals and parents. Professionals must skillfully elicit the support of the consumers of critical care services—parents—to enhance their efforts to successfully implement FCC in the intensive care unit (ICU). Together, parents and professionals can realize the true impact of their partnerships on the outcomes of quality care on critically ill or injured infants and children.

Elements of family-centered care

The elements of FCC (AACH, 1987) provide the framework for implementation strategies in the critical care setting. Each element will be addressed individually and specific strategies for implementation identified.

Element no. 1

Recognition that the family is the constant in the child's life while the service systems and personnel within those systems fluctuate

The family has the ultimate responsibility for responding to the child's emotional, social, developmental, and health care needs. To treat the critically ill child respectfully is to acknowledge and value who they are outside of the medical context in addition to the relationships that are central to their lives. This means making the family the unit of care instead of isolating the child's needs from those of the family.

Strategies

1 Create partnerships with parents from admission through discharge. Viewing parents as equal partners from the beginning sets the stage for parental confidence and competence in meeting their child's needs after the critical care experience.
2 Affirm the unique roles of parents and professionals in providing care for the critically ill infant or child. The critical nature of their child's illness or injury requires parents to temporarily relinquish much of their parenting role to others. The goal of critical care interventions should focus on providing specialized care commensurate with the child's physiologic needs and assisting parents to resume or adapt their parenting roles following their child's critical illness (Rennick, 1986).
3 Delineate the roles and responsibilities of parents and professionals for providing care. Ask parents how they would like to participate in their child's care and be involved in decision making. Offer opportunities for active participation based on individual parental readiness and encourage participation in ways that are personally rewarding (Curley, 1988). Devise policies that define and support parental involvement.
4 Avoid portraying the nurse as the 'expert' caregiver at the expense of parental self-esteem. When nurses and others replace parents as primary caregivers and advocates for their child, parental involvement often becomes supplanted. Parents begin to believe that they cannot contribute to their child's recovery in a meaningful way. Therefore nurses can assist parents to identify ways to revise their parenting roles by offering suggestions regarding ways to comfort the child, to provide diversional activities, and to engage in direct caregiving during the child's ICU stay.
5 Keep the critical care experience in perspective. Nurses and other professionals must be mindful of the short duration of professional involvement in the lives of critically ill infants and children and of the impact of their interventions on future family functioning.

Element no. 2

Facilitation of parent/professional collaboration at all levels of health care

The cornerstone of successful collaboration between parents and professionals is mutual respect for the unique perspectives and contributions each has to offer the health care relationship. Traditionally, the relationship has been dominated by professionals who determine the extent of parental involvement. This shift to a collaborative partnership between parents and professionals may be particularly challenging in the critical care setting, where professionals have been exclusively responsible for providing intensive care, making rapid decisions, and controlling the flow of information to families. A partnership cannot occur without deliberate assessment of the attitudes and expectations of both and a mutual commitment of each to the new relationship.

Strategies

1 Before professionals can collaborate with families, they must become skillful in collaborating with each other. Evaluate the climate of collaboration within the critical care unit and the institution. This can be accomplished by examining authority and decision-making structures, methods for resolving conflict, tolerance of plurality of views, and the degree of stress, job satisfaction and staff turnover.
2 Explore professional attitudes about the role of families in the critical care setting. In doing so, define and articulate beliefs about the family's role in the provision of critical care as a basis for a conceptual framework and a philosophy of care.
3 Implement a collaborative care delivery model, such as primary nursing or case management, that empowers parents to advocate on their child's behalf and that creates equal partnerships with professionals (Mancini & Phillips, 1984; Bethea, 1985). Devise formal and informal mechanisms for parent/professional collaboration. Establish standards that support mutual care planning and include parents in patient care conferences.
4 Throughout the critical care experience, seek and value parental values, preferences, and suggestions regarding ways to enhance their child's care. Parents know their child best and provide a valuable perspective regarding the responses of the child to critical care interventions.
5 Identify sources of inequality in the decision-making process. Determine if parents are afforded appropriate opportunities and enough information to make informed decisions and if appropriate weight is given to parental views in the decision-making process. Determine if there are decisions made without family input. If so, under what circumstances and for what reasons.

Element no. 3

Sharing of unbiased and complete information with parents about their child's care on an ongoing basis in an appropriate and supportive manner

Sharing information between parents and professionals is the first step toward establishing a collaborative relationship. During a child's critical illness, opportunities for optimal communication and information sharing may be deficient or inadequate. Parents cannot fully participate in decision making or care if they do not have access to adequate information or if they fail to understand what they are told. The crisis and stress created by the child's critical illness or injury and the nature of the critical care environment may impose additional barriers to good communication.

Strategies

1 Assist parents to gain access to information about their child's condition, treatment options, and support systems. Assign consistent nurses and physicians to facilitate a consistent, ongoing flow of information. Help the parents to interpret the professional unit and institutional hierarchy in order to ensure optimal access to appropriate personnel.
2 Engage in honest, straightforward discussions of the child's condition and prognosis. The ambiguity of uncertain outcomes and the unpredictability of their child's course may create significant anxiety for parents (Mischel, 1983). Recognize the potential impact of uncertainty on parental decision making and emotional state. Determine the degree of diagnostic and prognostic certainty needed for parents to make decisions. This should be compared with professional expectations of their diagnostic and prognostic capabilities and disparities between them addressed.
3 Provide opportunities for parents to voice their concerns, feelings, fears and to sort out conflicting emotional and cognitive issues. Be a good listener! Validate and clarify parental perceptions and knowledge base by determining what parents understand and repeatedly reinforcing information.
4 Enhance communication by establishing eye contact, admitting the limits of one's knowledge, avoiding jargon, using simple words and conveying an understanding of parental concerns and feelings.
5 Avoid delays in giving important information to parents. Important or distressing information may need to be repeated over several sessions. Assure consistency in information and terminology since parents may attach significance to certain terms that may result in an overly optimistic or pessimistic interpretation. Recognize that as parental anxiety increases, they may resort to searching for a more positive version of the situation from different health care team members (Rothstein, 1980).
6 Allow adequate time, consider the timing of disclosures and titrate information sessions to parental tolerance. Mobilize support systems when distressing news is given. When possible, schedule regular family meetings to relay information and discuss treatment goals and prognosis (Lust, 1984).

Element no. 4

Implementation of appropriate policies and programs that are comprehensive and provide emotional and financial support to meet the needs of families

A child's critical illness, injury, and potential disability will have an impact on the child, parents, siblings, extended family and on finances, career goals, and marriage. Support needs are multi-dimensional, varied, and change over time. Thus, policies and programs must be comprehensive and responsive to the changing needs of the child and family during the critical care experience and beyond.

Strategies

1 Assess the support needs of the child and family. During a child's critical illness support needs may include: crisis intervention, food and lodging, transportation,

sibling and parent to parent support, mental health services, financial assistance, and arrangements for child care. Develop individual strategies to address identified needs.

2 Involve support personnel such as clinical nurse specialists, social workers, patient representatives, and psychiatric liasions to provide appropriate services during the child's critical illness.

3 When possible, anticipate parental needs instead of waiting for a request for help. Parents may be hesitant to verbalize their own needs when their child is critically ill and may welcome unsolicited professional assistance.

4 When time constraints seem to prohibit developing optimal supportive relationships with parents, human touch and a caring attitude can convey concern and understanding. Use touch to build a sense of trust in the ability of the nurse to care for their child in a sensitive manner. However, nurses must be sensitive to the family's personal and cultural norms regarding touch and personal boundaries. Human presence, just standing nearby, can also be reassuring to parents. Even when caring for another patient, let parents know who is available to respond to their child's needs and how they can access them. Sometimes, standing close by without saying anything can be a powerful source of support.

5 Examine unit and institutional policies, including family and sibling visitation, to assure that family relationships are maintained and the role of parents supported during the critical care admission (Heater, 1985). Most critical care units have general visiting hours but may still have restrictions about when parents and brothers and sisters can visit (Roberts, Maieron, & Collier, 1988). Determine if policies are consistently followed or if individuals interpret policies inconsistently based on their personal philosophy instead of established standards.

6 Examine the role of siblings in the care of the critically ill infant or child. Develop strategies to encourage participation by siblings in the care of the critically ill child. A formal sibling program including preparation of siblings for their visit, follow-up contact, individual or group activities in the waiting room, or a sibling library can be facilitated through a collaborative effort among nurses, child life specialists or volunteers (Rushton & Booth, 1986).

7 Devise mechanisms for parental input into the development of critical care policies and services that directly impact on family functioning. Establishing a parent advisory board and developing parent satisfaction surveys can facilitate a family focus in the critical care setting.

Element no. 5

Recognition of family strengths and individuality and respect for different methods of coping

The entire family system will be affected during a child's critical illness (Hedenkamp, 1980). Each family member will interpret and respond to the situation differently. Recognizing the child's and the family's individual strengths is an important prerequisite for respecting their unique coping strategies. Nurses are in a pivotal role to recognize the coping strategies and the methods of adaptation of family members to the child's illness and disability and to intervene appropriately (Philichi, 1989).

Strategies

1 Appreciate the variation in parental responses to their child's critical illness including: crisis reactions, information seeking behaviors and mourning reactions (Etzler, 1984). Parental perceptions of the critical care environment and their child's diagnosis and illness trajectory may also influence their reactions.

2 Identify potential stressors that parents may experience when their child is admitted to a critical care setting. These stressors may be influenced by: (a) environmental factors associated with the critical care environment; (b) situational factors related to the severity of their child's illness, uncertainty of outcomes, feelings of helplessness, alterations in the parenting role created by lack of information, loss of control, imposed separation; staff behaviors and communication patterns; and (c) personal/family factors related to the parent's personality, current and past life experiences (Miles, 1979; Lewandowski, 1980; Stevens, 1981; Miles & Carter, 1982; Miles & Carter, 1983).

3 Identify the strengths and resources of both the child and family. Emphasize strengths instead of focusing on weaknesses or needs.

4 Document an ongoing assessment of family strengths, coping and functioning. Obtain a complete assessment of the family constellation upon admission to the critical care unit. Respect cultural, religious and family values in addition to socioeconomic differences. Assist families to evaluate how they are affected by their child's critical illness or injury. Ascertain how the family was functioning prior to their child's critical illness. An already disorganized family may experience severe disruption as a result of a crisis event such as a child's critical illness or injury (Fife, 1985). An assessment of previous parental roles and relationships with the child, communication patterns, parental perceptions and understanding of the illness or injury, feelings engendered by the child's illness and unmet parental needs should also be made (Miles, 1979).

5 Avoid making assumptions about the parents' state of mind, knowledge or commitment. Refrain from subjective labeling of parents as noncompliant, uninterested, emotionally unstable or uncaring. Observe and document parental behaviors and validate and clarify impressions with the family. Explore various rationale for behaviors and attitudes that parents may exhibit.

6 Separate facts from feelings when interpreting information. Often there are strong emotions attached to the situation surrounding the child's critical illness that may influence parental interpretation of their child's condition or the behavior of professionals.

7 Recognize that the nurse or other professionals may be the target of parental emotions and anger. Often parents fear that their child's care will be compromised by their behavior. Thus professionals must create a supportive environment that promotes positive parent coping and trust between parents and caregivers (Fletcher & Sarin, 1988).

Element no. 6

Understanding and incorporating the developmental and emotional needs of infants, children, and adolescents and their families into health care delivery systems

A comprehensive, family-centered approach to critical care involves devising strategies to address the physiologic, social, emotional, and developmental needs of the child. At times, the critical care environment may preclude optimal attention to the child's developmental issues. Critical care interventions typically focus on restoring the child to optimal physiologic condition, often at the expense of developmental considerations. Moreover, critical care professionals may be unfamiliar with normal developmental patterns and with interventions to facilitate or restore developmental progress.

Strategies

1 Be knowledgeable of normal developmental patterns and the impact of critical illness on achieving developmental milestones (Green, 1983). The nature and severity of the child's illness, the impact of the unfamiliar and stimulating ICU environment, the effect of altered sleep cycles, and stress created by imposed separation for family members are important considerations (Stevens, 1981).

2 Document baseline physiologic functioning, typical signs of stress or decompensation, responses to interventions, and coping strategies. Recognize typical coping strategies employed by the critically ill child based on developmental stage, such as regressive behaviors. Collaborate with parents to devise supportive interventions to restore the child to their previous developmental level without reinforcing regressive or inappropriate patterns of behavior.

3 Incorporate developmentally appropriate interventions into the plan of care for critically ill children including play and therapeutic interventions to prepare children for procedures or surgery (Stevens, 1981; Betz & Poster, 1984; Wilson & Broome, 1989). When feasible, provide preadmission programs to the ICU for planned admissions.

4 Use multidisciplinary programs to meet the developmental needs of critically ill children. Devise comprehensive developmental plans through collaborative efforts among the child, family, nurses, therapists, child life specialists, and volunteers. Communicate goals and activities to parents and all members of the health care team. Explore ways to enhance parental participation. Recruit volunteers, foster grandparents or parent substitutes when parents are unavailable to visit to enhance support for developmental activities.

5 Consider creative strategies for enhancing developmental goals, particularly for infants and children requiring prolonged ICU admissions. Designate a regular part of the child's schedule for developmental activities. Use specialized developmental care plans and activity diaries to encourage communication and document progress (Rushton, 1986; Nugent, 1989). Conduct weekly multidisciplinary developmental rounds to update goals and revise activities.

6 Adapt technology and care routines to allow greater opportunity for developmental activities. For example, use a portable ventilator for the ventilator-dependent child

or lengthen ventilator and oxygen tubing to enhance mobility or promote group activities based on age and developmental stage. For older children, make referrals to hospital school programs or tutors to maintain skills.

Element no. 7

Encouragement of parent to parent support

Support by professionals should be augmented with parent to parent support (Winch & Christoph, 1988). Recognizing the role of other parents as 'veterans' of the ICU experience can help to reduce isolation by creating a social network. Support groups can provide mutual support and friendship, information gathering/sharing, problem solving and exploring ways to improve the systems of care (Nathanson, 1986).

Strategies

1 Become familiar with established parent support groups such as: Parent to Parent, Sick Kids Need Involved People (SKIP), Candelighters or Compassionate Friends. Additionally there are a variety of parent support groups that are targeted to parents of children with specific conditions such as cardiac disorders, cancer, AIDS, genetic disorders, or diabetes. Provide information and as appropriate, refer parents to specific groups.

2 Develop a roster of parents who are willing to provide parent to parent support to parents of critically ill infants and childen. Determine what qualifications and preparation, if any, are necessary for parents to provide support to others. Establish a mechanism to notify parents of the support needs of parents with children in the ICU.

3 Explore the feasibility of establishing a parent support group for the parents of critically ill infants and children. Periodic meetings of parent support groups can informally address the needs of parents during their child's critical illness. Encourage parents who have previously experienced their child's critical illness, nurses, social workers, clergy, and other health care team members to participate in group organization. Identify sources of institutional and financial support to ensure the group's viability and success (Nathanson, 1986).

Element no. 8

Assure that the design of health care delivery systems is flexible, accessible, and responsive to family needs

To make FCC a reality in the critical care setting it will be necessary for parents, professionals, and administrators to collaborate to redesign the services and the care delivery system to ensure optimal responsiveness to the needs of children and their families.

Strategies

1 Examine the structure of the care delivery system and the degree of unit and institutional commitment to FCC. Identify the goals and outcomes of critical care services. Explore alternative care delivery models that enhance continuity of care and support family integrity. For example, consider the feasibility of implementing primary nursing or case management in the critical care setting.
2 Avoid fragmentation of services when multiple consultants and health care providers are involved in a child's care. A primary nurse or case manager can be a valuable asset in coordinating services and information and maintaining continuity of care. Furthermore, assigning a consistent attending physician for infants and children with long ICU admissions can avoid disrupting continuity and patient care goals when physician coverage rotates.
3 Identify physical barriers of the critical care setting that prohibit successful implementation of FCC. Survey the critical care facilities to assess the appropriateness and accessibility of: (a) lodging and sleeping facilities within the institution or nearby; (b) places for parents to take care of personal needs; (c) waiting rooms that are easily accessible to unit staff; (d) places for private conversations with staff or family members; (e) facilities for families to 'room-in,' and (f) methods of providing privacy within the critical care setting such as curtains and privacy screens should be explored (Olds & Daniel, 1987).

A priority for the 1990s

As the critical care setting becomes increasingly dominated by technology and the health care systems restructure to meet the needs of sicker patients, successful implementation of FCC will become crucial. Providing family-centered care for ill or injured infants and children and their families must be a priority for nurses and other health care professionals in the 1990s. Critical care nurses can be instrumental in advancing the goals of FCC by assuming the leadership to ensure that care is provided in a comprehensive, developmentally appropriate and family-centered manner to all critically ill children and their families.

References

Bethea, S.W. (1985) 'Primary nursing in the infant special care unit', *JOGN*, **14**, 202–208.

Betz, C.L. & Poster, E.C. (1984) 'Incorporating play into the care of the hospitalized child', *Issues in Comprehensive Pediatric Nursing*, **8**, 343–355.

Broome, M.E. (1985) 'Working with the family of a critically ill child', *Heart & Lung*, **14**, 368–372.

Curley, M. (1988) 'Effects of the nursing mutual participation model of care on parental stress in the pediatric intensive care unit', *Heart & Lung*, **17**, 682–688.

Etzler, C. (1984) 'Parents' reactions to pediatric critical care settings: A review of the literature', *Issues in Comprehensive Pediatric Nursing*, **7**, 319–331.

Fife, B. (1985) 'A model for predicting the adaptation of families to medical crisis: An analysis of role integration', *Image*, **17**, 108–112.

Fletcher, A.B. & Sarin, A.V. (1988) 'Communicating with parents of high risk infants', *Pediatric Annals*, **17**, 477–480.

Green, E.C. (1983) 'Normalization: meeting growth and development needs of children in a pediatric intensive care unit', *Children's Health Care*, **12**, 43–44.

Hedenkamp, E. (1980) 'Humanizing the intensive care unit for children', *Critical Care Quarterly*, **3**, 63–73.

Heater, B.S. (1985) 'Nursing responsibilities in changing visiting restrictions in the intensive care unit', *Heart & Lung*, **14**, 181–186.

Johnson, B. (1989, May 12) 'The nurse as advocate for the hospitalized child', Paper presented at *Pediatric Nursing '89*, Health and Education Council, Baltimore, MD.

Koop, C.E. (1987) *Children with special health care needs—Campaign 87*, Washington, DC: U.S. Dept. of Health and Human Services.

Lewandowski, L. (1980) 'Stresses and coping styles of parents of children undergoing open-heart surgery', *Critical Care Quarterly*, **3**, 75–84.

Lust, B. (1984) 'The patient in the ICU: A family experience', *Critical Care Quarterly*, **7**, 49–57.

Mancini, M.R. & Phillips, K.M. (1984) 'Critical care calls for primary nursing', *Nursing Management*, **15**, 42C–42J.

Miles, M. (1979) 'Impact of the intensive care unit on parents', *Issues in Comprehensive Pediatric Nursing*, **3**, 72–90.

Miles, M. & Carter, M. (1982) 'Sources of parental stress in pediatric intensive care units', *Children's Health Care*, **11**, 65–69.

Miles, M. & Carter, M. (1983) 'A conceptual model for assessing parental stress in intensive care units', *American Journal of Maternal-Child Nursing*, **8**, 354–359.

Mischel, M. (1983) 'Parents' perceptions of uncertainty concerning their hospitalized child', *Nursing Research*, **32**, 324–330.

Nathanson, M. (1986) *Organizing and maintaining support groups for parents of children with chronic illness and handicapping conditions*, Washington, DC: Association for the Care of Children's Health.

Nugent, K. (1989) 'Routine care: Promoting development in hospitalized infants', *American Journal of Maternal-Child Nursing*, **14**, 318–321.

Olds, A. & Daniel, P. (1987) *Child health care facilities: Design guidelines—Literature outline*, Washington, DC: Association for the Care of Children's Health.

Philichi, L. (1989) 'Family adaptation during a pediatric intensive care hospitalization', *Journal of Pediatric Nursing*, **4**, 268–276.

Rennick, J. (1986) 'Re-establishing the parental role in the pediatric intensive care unit', *Journal of Pediatric Nursing*, **1**, 40–44.

Roberts, M.C., Maieron, M.J. & Collier, J. (1988) *Directory of hospital psychosocial policies and programs*, Washington, D.C.: Association for the Care of Children's Health.

Rothstein, P. (1980) 'Psychological stress in families of children in a pediatric intensive care unit', *Pediatric Clinics of North America*, **27**, 613–620.

Rushton, C. (1986) 'Promoting normal growth and development in the hospital environment', *Neonatal Network*, **4**, 21–30.

Rushton, C. & Booth, P. (1986) *The role of siblings during pediatric hospitalization*, Presented at 21st Annual ACCH Conference, San Francisco, CA.

Shelton, T., Jeppson, E. & Johnson, B. (1987) *Family-centered care for children with special health care needs*, Washington, DC: Association for the Care of Children's Health.

Stevens, K.R. (1981) 'Humanistic nursing care for critically ill children', *Nursing Clinics of North America*, **16**, 611–622.

Wilson, T. & Broome, M. (1989) 'Promoting the young child's development in the intensive care unit', *Heart & Lung*, **18**, 274–280.

Winch, A.E. & Christoph, J.M. (1988) 'Parent-to-parent links: Building networks for parents of hospitalized children', *Children's Health Care*, **17**, 93–97.

SECTION 7

Organizing for Change

Introduction

The theme of this section covers areas of practice in which there has been innovation. Change can be threatening to anyone involved in it, but it need not be. Providing that those initiating and managing the change understand the change process and that they prepare those who have to make changes adequately, then innovation in practice can be an exciting and satisfying aspect of professional life. The papers in this section look at specific areas of children's nursing in which attention has been focused and in which nurses have made changes in practice.

The way in which the nursing team is organized has been an area of research for more than a decade. In the first paper in this section a comparison of team and primary nursing is made. The systems are considered in the way they affect decision-making and accountability. Rafferty gives a balanced overview of each method of delivering care and in the concluding section stresses that whichever system is chosen, nurses must both understand and share the philosophy on which it is built.

It has been known for some years that preparation of children before admission reduces the trauma associated with that experience. However, pre-admission programmes were very slow to develop as Glasper and Stradling point out in their paper. They describe the pre-admission programme in Southampton and explain the stress inoculation theory which underpins these programmes. Details of the costs involved are included along with many details of the way that the service was designed and initiated.

The paper by Broome focuses on a particular area of pain management, preparing children for painful procedures. The author points out that despite 20 years of research very little has been achieved in translating the research findings into clinical protocols for the preparation of children. To redress this, Broome has surveyed the literature and gives a comprehensive account of a variety of preparation strategies which can be employed. The range of coping skills which can be taught to children are also described, and recommendations of age appropriated examples are included. In the concluding section of the paper, methods of evaluating the effectiveness of pain management programmes are detailed.

The final paper in this section discusses the issue of how stress affects neonatal nurses. The intensity of the work and the constant possibility of death produce a work area which is widely known to produce relatively high rates of staff 'burnout'. Hannon describes the many factors which contribute towards the unrelenting stressful nature of the work and suggests ways in which staff cope with these stresses. Intervention to reduce stress is advocated, including methods which increase staff skills through continuing professional education. Finally the author describes how managers of units can be proactive in establishing support mechanisms and the necessary skill mix to deal with stress as it arises.

35

Team and Primary Nursing*

DAWN RAFFERTY

The method by which nursing care is delivered is influenced by the beliefs and values which nurses hold, the nature of the organisations in which they function, and the profession itself. Organisation of care, thus, has a philosophical base.

The nature of the care system used will determine the extent to which individual nurses take responsibility for the care which they give and the extent to which they exercise freedom to practice. Here, let us look at the relationship among styles of nursing and the professional issues of autonomy, accountability and the values which underpin nursing.

Historical perspective

To understand these two methods of care it is necessary to consider them in evolutionary context. Until the 1930s nursing was primarily centred on the 'case method', patient assignment was on a one-to-one basis and nurses met the total nursing needs of the patient. Because of the expanse of the hospital system, economic pressures and a shortage of registered nurses, this system gave way to a task-orientated, routinised and ritualistic mode of care. Tasks were delegated down through a rigid hierarchical structure. This system led to a high level of dependency on rules, regulations and rituals which were counter-productive to nurses' decision-making role and which, therefore, militated against professional development.[1] Rhodes refers to the ethos of this structure as the 'bureaucratic ideology'.[2] While elements of this approach have been retained, the decade of the 1960s witnessed the emergence and progressive influence of humanistic values espoused in the philosophical system of humanistic existentialism.[3]

The system takes account of the whole person and recognises the human being's uniqueness and capacity for self-direction. Priority is placed on the therapeutic value of care through the interpersonal relationship between nurses and patients. During the 1970s the nursing process became increasingly popular, and it was necessary to seek

---

*This is an abridged version of an article first published in *Senior Nurse*, Vol. 12, No. 1, pp. 31–34, 39, 1992.

an appropriate mode of care in which a more individualised and problem-solving approach could be used.

A brief description

Total patient care systems and humanistic values, then, were factors which influenced change from task-allocation to team nursing which was seen as a way of providing better patient care with available resources. The ward team is broken down into subgroups, which, under the leadership of a registered nurse, provide care for groups of patients, utilising the available skills within the team. Team members share responsibility for assessing and planning care. This method is now the most popular way of delivering care in the UK, however, primary nursing continues to gain momentum, as with the case method the focus is on the one-to-one nurse/patient relationship. Like team nursing, the ward team is subdivided into smaller groups of care-givers but with the primary nurse taking individual responsibility for a 'case load'. In his or her absence, responsibility is delegated to an associate nurse who maintains the prescribed care initiated by the primary nurse.

Philosophy of care

Thora Kron, one of the pioneers of team nursing, describes the concept as a philosophy rather than a method of patient assignment. She identifies two fundamental beliefs; the patient's right to be provided with a high standard of care and the carer's right to be given help to produce such standards.[4]

Primary nursing, popularised by Manthey[5] in the USA, is a method of organisation of care and a philosophy of care which has professional patient-centred practice at its core.

The philosophies of both systems appear to subscribe to humanistic values. Team nursing looks to fulfil the ideal of 'best possible care' through enhanced interaction between patients and staff; patients relate to a small number of nurses rather than to the total ward staff. The method assumes the premiss that nurses working in small groups with a leader provide better care than when working as individuals.[4] However, team nursing is open to wide interpretation; the time-span of allocation may vary from the duration of a shift to permanent allocation to a group of patients. The mode of care within the team may vary too, from task-allocation to almost a primary-nursing situation. Therefore, continuity of care may vary as may the degree of patient-centredness. In primary nursing a high priority is placed on the individual nature of the care which is realised through the one-to-one nurse/patient relationship and which is maintained throughout the duration of care. Reed identifies discrepancies in the beliefs underpinning team nursing and also highlights philosophical differences between the two modes of care. Reed found that when compared with each other, team nurses had dissimilar philosophies about care, whereas primary nurses held similar beliefs. Also, team nurses identified aspects of direct physical care as being most important, whereas primary nurses placed a higher value on psychological components of care.[6]

The second major philosophical difference is concerned with Kron's statement about nurses' rights to receive help in order to achieve a high standard of care. The team system is very much a supportive and collegiate one; the team leader formulates a plan of care and evaluates outcomes of care, but team members also participate in these activities. In fact, some sources, such as Pearson[7] who quotes Barrett[8], view this team planning as the heart of team nursing. Conversely, in primary nursing the primary nurses exercise their individual professional judgement to assess, plan and evaluate care. They carry out much of the direct care themselves and in their absence the key areas of their prescribed plan are maintained by associate nurses. It appears then that the philosophy of team nursing is less coherent or explicit than that of primary nursing and whereas team nursing depends on shared judgement, primary nursing advocates the professional judgement of the individual.

Accountability and autonomy

Professional dimension

While the two systems are similar in terms of creating small, functional units within a larger unit, primary nursing attempts to sever the ties with bureaucratic ideology whereas team nursing only loosens them. Primary nursing mirrors the Griffiths style ethos of decentralisation: that is, large unwieldy organisations are divided into self-governing units in which individuals can be more readily called to account.[9] Team nursing does not represent this ethos as it retains the notions of a hierarchical structure, group cohesion and shared responsibilities. In management terms, primary nursing with its clear lines of responsibility, appears more structured and as each nurse is individually responsible for the care which she or he gives, individual performance can be measured.[10]

While this is desirable from the point of view of professionalism and for promotion of standards, it may be stressful for the individual practitioners.[6] It is vital, therefore, for primary nurses to be adequately prepared for the role and also that there is an effective support system through nurse managers and continuing education. Quality assurance systems should be used to determine staffing ratios and skill mix. It is important that such tools are used effectively to limit management's cost-cutting activities which could overburden the primary nurse with too high a case-load and, consequently, compromise standards.

In light of the preceding discussion, this tends to suggest that primary nursing is more likely to fulfil the criteria of professionalism than is team nursing. To substantiate or refute this assumption, it is necessary to explore the degree to which each system provides scope for the professional dimensions of responsibility, authority and accountability.

Rye[1] sees accountability as the basis of professional standards and relates the degree of accountability to the degree of authority vested in the individual. It is this authority which gives the practitioner autonomy in his or her work. Chapman associates autonomy with professionalism: 'the greater the autonomy of decision-making by the individual, the greater the right to be called a professional'.[11]

According to Copp[12] (p42) accountability has become an increasingly important issue in nursing. Professor Rebecca Bergman of Tel Aviv University identifies several

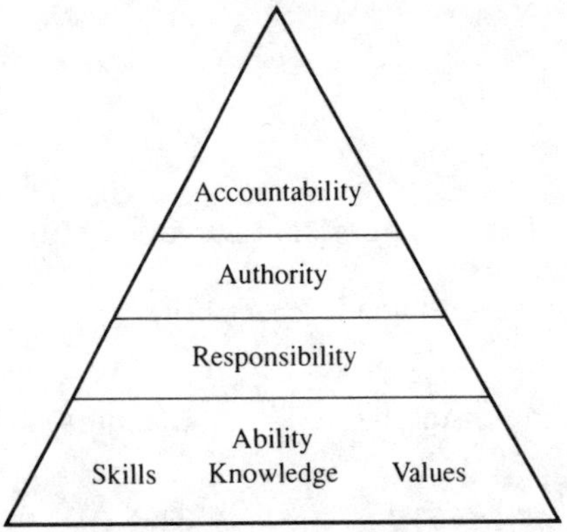

Figure 35.1 Bergman's model

reasons for this, two of which are pertinent to this discussion:

- the problem-solving approach which requires analysis and accounting to oneself and others;
- the increased responsibility associated with primary nursing[13] (p54).

Bergman's model (Figure 35.1) identifies the preconditions leading to accountability. The model assumes a hierarchical approach, that is, the 'wider-order' issues need to be achieved before progressing up the pyramid. To what extent do team nurses and nurses in the primary system achieve these preconditions?

The skills and knowledge requirements for team leaders and primary nurses may be considered comparable since exponents of both systems recommend that these positions should be held by registered nurses. In relation to team nursing, this prerequisite is often qualified by reference to an 'appropriately skilled registered nurse',[4] and, in the case of the primary nurse, a minimum of one year's experience with 'adequate preparation for the role' is recommended.

The degree of responsibility concomitant with the staff nurse role is affected by the role assumed by other key workers, for example, the ward sister/charge nurse. The team-nursing system maintains the tradition of centralised decision-making, and, therefore, team leaders retain some dependency on the ward sister/charge nurse in respect of clinical decisions. Primary nursing, in which the power base is decentralised, allows the primary practitioner rather than the ward sister/charge nurse to set priorities of care. In this way, both roles have potential for development. The ward sister/charge nurse is relieved of direct responsibility for planning, implementing and evaluating care and is thus able to develop skills in teaching quality control and care consultancy.

Some sources express concern regarding the potential reduction of clinical authority and responsibility of the ward sister/charge nurse.[10] However, for the primary nurse there is clear allocation of responsibility. She or he undertakes the management of care of a small number of patients in collaboration with the families of those patients. Responsibility is 24 hours a day, 7 days a week. The primary nurse accepts responsibility according to her or his job description and is given authority for decision-making

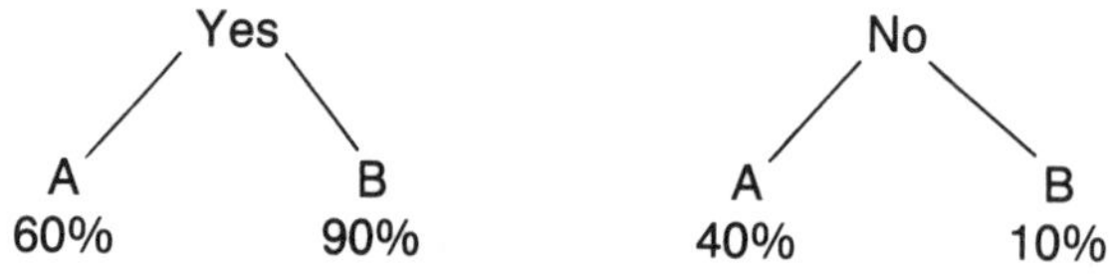

Extracts from staff survey[17] (p10)

Figure 35.2 Do you feel you have 24-hour accountability?

	Strongly agrees	Agrees	Disagree	Not sure
A	20%	66%	6%	8%
B	5%	88%	7%	0%

Figure 35.3 Under primary nursing I have found that I am more accountable for certain patients than I was under team nursing

and is answerable for decisions and actions which she or he takes. Primary nursing then does endeavour to provide staff nurses with a high level of autonomy.[14]

In team nursing, individual responsibility is much less explicit. The team leader assumes a leadership/supervisory role in assessing planning and evaluating care, but this responsibility may only be for the duration of a shift and it is shared by team members. Waters[15] (p8) states that 'it is crucial to the effective practice of team nursing that there are no strict boundaries of responsibility'. This aspect of shared responsibility is seen as a major disadvantage by some critics, because it is difficult to hold anybody accountable for anything.[6]

Other writers view this in a more favourable light. Salvage[16] for example, criticises the idea of individualised responsibility in nursing and feels that it is unfair to hold the bedside nurse responsible because she or he has no control over material and human resources.

Based on the preconditions to accountability, as identified in Bergman's model, the primary nurse has more responsibility and authority and hence is more accountable in the clinical role than is her or his counterpart in the team-nursing system with its somewhat grey area of shared responsibility. This conclusion is verified to some extent by empirical study. Wilson and Dawson, for example, carried out a comparative study between primary nursing and team nursing in two long stay elderly care units in Canada.[17] Responses were recorded after 6 months (A) and 1 year (B) respectively of implementing primary nursing. Favourable responses were returned in relationship to accountability in primary nursing (see Figures 35.2 and 35.3).

Although the validity of such responses is open to question (it may have been useful, for example, to have conducted a questionnaire while team nursing was still operational rather than making comparisons in retrospect), the figures for these two items are consistently favourable in relating primary nursing with accountability. It could be argued that the positive responses after the first six months may have been due to the change itself and a desire for the new system to be successful, but the sustained trend in positive responses after one year tends to militate against this.

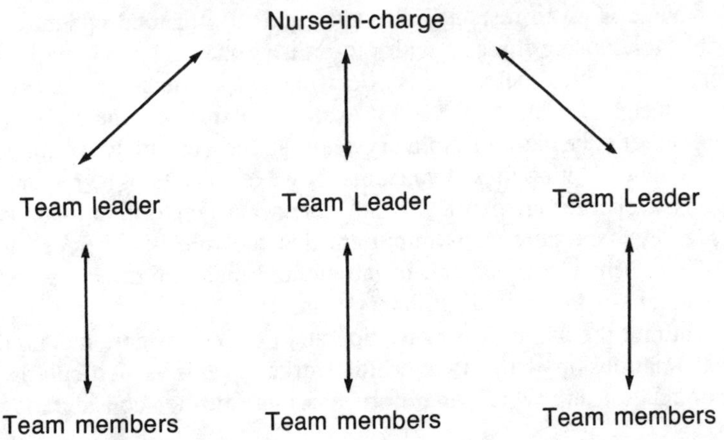

Figure 35.4 Structure of team nursing

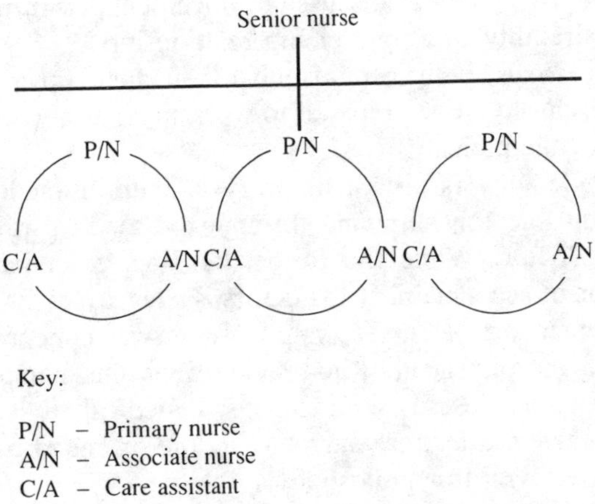

Figure 35.5 Linear structure (adapted from Wright[20] (p26))

Organisational dimension

Accountability and autonomy of nurses affects and is affected by the communication system within the ward unit. According to Waters[15] (p9), critics of the team nursing system suggest that it promotes a traditional and hierarchical communication system (see Figure 35.4).

Hunt[19] (p37) describes this as a pyramidal communication system and contrasts it with the linear structure (see Figure 35.5).

The communication and reporting system in the team-nursing structure may be complicated with team members reporting to [a] team leader who reports to the ward sister/charge nurse, and vice versa. Communication with other professionals is directed through the ward sister/charge nurse. The reporting system in the linear structure is care-giver to care-giver which is likely to strengthen personal accountability. Also, as the primary nurse is given responsibility and authority for total patient care she or he is responsible for liaising directly with other disciplines.

However, some critics feel that this is detrimental to the cohesiveness of nurses as a total ward team. Bowers[10] (p17), for example, expresses the view that 'primary nursing strengthens the multidisciplinary team at the cost of weakening the nursing team'. Cohesiveness within these two teams, however, need not be mutually exclusive. The ward sister/charge nurse role, which changes when primary nursing is implemented, is a key issue here. It is important that the role is developed to coordinate activities of the primary groups and to initiate and maintain effective communication between members of the multidisciplinary team.

It is evident that the mode of organisation and delivery of care has implications for professional relationship with other health workers. This is particularly true of the nurse/doctor relationship which, therefore, warrants further consideration.

The nurse/doctor relationship

The Royal College of Nursing discussion document *Towards Standards* makes reference to the desirability of a partnership relationship.

'Doctors and nurses must both recognise that their goals for a patient may differ or even conflict. But each should be prepared to work in a partnership to achieve the best possible outcome for the patient'[19] (p8).

This partnership ideology is a contemporary one; traditionally, nurses have seen themselves as responsible for following through the medical prescription and being accountable to the doctor. While the former remains essential, the latter is inappropriate. The notion of accountability to doctors is a legacy of the philosophical period of Romanticism,[3] when part of nurses' value system was concerned with dependence and subservience to the physician. Rhodes describes this perspective as the 'Paramedical ideology'[2] which describes nursing as a medical division of labour. (It is interesting that the current dilemmas surrounding the extended role of the nurse have implications associated with this philosophy.)

What are the doctor/nurse relationship implications of the two styles of nursing in question? Work by Roberts[14] reveals that primary nurses were less satisfied with the relationship than were team nurses. Salvage[16] expresses the view that such conflict relates directly to the autonomous status of the primary nurses. A review of the literature reveals no such conflict with team-nursing systems. Perhaps, it may be concluded from this that the autonomous nature of primary nursing is implicated. However, as the lines of communication within the team-nursing system can be complex, this potentially affects interpersonal relationships. It is likely that some adjustment is required by both nurses and doctors.

Primary nursing brings about a redistribution of power which necessitates professionals taking responsibility for their own work. Some authors associate relationship problems with doctors who feel threatened because they are not in charge of nurses.[15] While this may be true in some situations, it is more likely that negative reactions are the result of doctors not being aware of changes which have been implemented. When change has implications for the role of others, it is vital that all staff are given adequate information before that change is instigated. For their part, nurses need the confidence to be creative and less concerned about whether their ideas are always approved by the medical staff.[10] Although some sources do report increased collaboration when primary nursing is used,[20,21] accountability to doctors is still a view which is widely held[2] and nurses may find it difficult to step aside from the perceived safety of the paramedical ideology.

Conclusion—a general perspective

Organisational methods of care must be based on a shared and known philosophy which promotes individualised care and which takes account of the whole person. For nursing to develop on a professional basis, nursing systems must enhance autonomy and accountability for the individual practitioners and facilitate partnership/collaborative roles with other disciplines, particularly doctors. It is important that nurses recognise their unique function and distinguish their role from that of others. This will allow nursing to expand and avoid the extension of the nursing role with functions of other professionals.

On balance, primary nursing appears to identify more closely with these values than does team nursing. However, primary practitioners must be adequately prepared for their role and given proper support. The development of the ward sister/charge nurse role as coordinator, clinical resource person and quality controller is important for the retention of a clinical career structure and to facilitate cohesion of the ward and the multidisciplinary teams. While primary nursing is likely to be a popular choice with managers, it is essential that the system is properly staffed and that the temptation to cut costs by diluting the skill mix or increasing caseloads *must* be avoided, for any system is only as good as the weakest link.

Notes

1. Rye, D. (1982) 'Accountability in nursing', *Nursing Focus*, April, 90, 91, 110.

2. Rhodes, B. (1983) 'Accountability in nursing: alternative perspectives', *Nursing Times*, September 7, 65–6.

3. Bevis, E. (1982) *Curriculum Building in Nursing—A Process, 3rd edition*, St Louis MO, CV Mosby.

4. Kron, T. (1981) *The Measurement of Patient Care, 5th edition*, Eastbourne, W B Saunders, pp. 30–6.

5. Manthey, M. (1973) 'Primary nursing is alive and well in the hospital', *American Journal of Nursing*, **73**(1), 83–7.

6. Reed, S. (1988) 'A comparison of nurse-related behaviour, philosophy of care and job satisfaction in team and primary nursing', *Journal of Advanced Nursing*, **13**, 383–95.

7. Pearson, A. (1983) *The Clinical Nursing Unit*, London, Heinemann.

8. Barrett, A. (1968) *The Head Nurse—Her Changing Role, 2nd edition*, Norwalk CT, Appleton-Century-Crofts.

9. Griffiths, R. (1983) *NHS Management Inquiry*, London, Department of Health and Social Services.

10. Bowers, L. (1989) 'The significance of primary nursing', *Journal of Advanced Nursing*, **14**, 13–9.

11. Chapman, C. (1980) 'Janforum. Professionalism and nursing. What does professionalism mean?' *Journal of Advanced Nursing*, **5**, 103–12.

12. Copp, G. (1988) 'Professional accountability: The conflict', *Nursing Times*, October 26, **84**(43), 42.

13. Bergman, R. (1981) 'Accountability—Definition and Dimensions', *International Nursing Review*, **28**(2), 53–9.

14. Roberts, L. (1980) 'Primary nursing. Do patients like it? Are nurses satisfied? Does it cost more?' *Canadian Nurse*, **76**(2), 20–3.

15. Waters, K. (1985) 'Organising nursing care. Team nursing', *Nursing Practice*, **1**, 7–15.

16. Salvage, J. (1985) *The Politics of Nursing*, London, Heinemann.

17. Wilson, N., Dawson, P. (1989) 'A comparison of primary nursing and team nursing in a geriatric long-term care setting', *International Journal of Nursing Studies*, **26**(1), 1–13.

18. Hunt, J. (1988) 'Primary nursing. The next challenge', *Nursing Times*, December 7, **84**, 49.

19. RCN (1981) *Towards Standards*, London, Royal College of Nursing.

20. Wright, S. (1987) 'Primary nursing. Patient-centred practice', *Nursing Times*, September 23, **83**, 38.

21. Tucker, F., Deaver, L. (1986) 'Implementation of primary nursing in one emergency department', *Journal of Emergency Nursing*, **12**(3), 157–62.

36

Preparing Children for Admission*

ALAN GLASPER and PAULINE STRADLING

The Department of Health has endorsed the concept that modern child health care requires a service integrated between hospital and community and one that provides for the child as a whole. Such a service should aim to meet the social, emotional and spiritual needs of children and their families.

The growth of paediatric pre-admission programmes throughout the UK represents one facet of this integrated service. Paediatric nurses have a long history of endeavouring to improve the care of their patients and families. Innoculating children against the stresses of hospital admission may be partially helped through the provision of pre-admission programmes.

Traditionally, the role of parents has been undermined during a child's illness which requires hospital admission. In some instances nurses have taken over care completely, leaving parents to feel helpless and inadequate. Care-by-parent schemes which encourage active involvement of the parent(s) can be initiated during a pre-admission programme where the role of the family can be explored. Such family-centred care ensures that parents and children receive educative, psychological and social support from the hospital personnel.

Before planning and implementing a pre-admission programme for children and their parents in Southampton, we decided first to ascertain the opinion of parents. Maddison[1] has highlighted the importance of seeking the opinion of consumers, as she believes that parental opinion is most valid in that it reflects that of the child. The results of a parent questionnaire showed that parents were in favour of a pre-admission programme and that they would support such an innovation.

The psychological sequelae of a hospital admission during childhood can be found in the wealth of literature on this subject. There are still many procedures to which children are subject in hospital which may cause anxiety. In the absence of parents it is believed that this anxiety is exacerbated. Children dread hospital procedures: needles, tests, anaesthetics and even death may all be associated in the mind of a child with hospital. The benefits of parents may be incalculable when considering methods of reducing anxiety in children about to undergo stressful procedures. It has been suggested that children's fears change with age and level of cognitive development.[2]

*This article was first published in *Paediatric Nursing*, Vol. 1, No. 5, pp. 18–20, 1989.

Pre-school children are especially frightened by noises, strange persons or events. School children are fearful of bodily injury, disease and separation, among others.

Naturally, a hospital admission may therefore precipitate fear-evoking responses in young children. Preparing children for such fear-evoking events has been shown to be effective in clinical practice. Rodin's study[3] has indicated that preparing children for painful procedures such as venepuncture does lessen their effects, while the presence of parents can reduce anxiety further.

Visintainer and Wolfer[4] have shown that psychological preparation for children undergoing minor surgery increases cooperation, decreases upset behaviour and results in less anxiety. Many paediatric units throughout the UK support the hypothesis that preparation does result in less psychological upset as shown in the wide variety of information mailed to parents in the week before the child's admission. Colouring books and information leaflets are now used by many paediatric units.

The changes in children's behaviour after hospitalisation underpin the growth of formal pre-admission programmes for children about to be admitted to hospital. Vernon *et al.*[5] have collected data which confirms that children between six months and four years are most likely to be upset following hospitalisation. Mellish[6] has said that the criteria for surgical success should be measured not only by intact wounds and safe discharge but also by intact emotions in the child and family.

Pre-admission projects

Such programmes are intimately concerned with stress innoculation. Meng and Zastowny[7] have likened stress innoculation to medical innoculations and indicate that any pre-admission programme should have three distinct phases:

a) Education regarding the nature of stress;
b) Introduction and development of specific coping skills;
c) Practice of coping skills during exposure to stressors.

There are few paediatric centres in the UK who routinely offer pre-admission programmes for children and their families. The project at Nottingham was, until recently, the only programme available.[8] This 'Saturday Morning Project' was started in 1982, conceived by Vera Wooten and Dr William Hayne, a paediatric anaesthetist.

The emotional trauma associated with anaesthesia and surgery in children has for a long time been widely recognised.[9] Ideally any preparation for a planned hospital admission should involve the parents.

Stress innoculation can successfully be carried out in a school classroom, enabling all children to be prepared for the possibility of hospital admission.[10]

The essential message of school-based preparatory programmes is that hospital is a place of healing not hurting. Children are able to relate to hospital staff if they can learn about their functions. Health care professionals can visit the classroom and demonstrate they are real people. The work of the primary health care team, including the school nurse, must not be underestimated when such schemes are developed.

The amount of pre-operative preparation given to the parents is thought to be the most important factor in successful conquest of operation anxiety.[11] In pursuing strategies to overcome such anxieties some workers have developed specific pre-operative tools such as games.[12,13] The use of therapeutic play figures strongly in most pre-admission programmes although many such programmes have yet to be critically evaluated.

Hospital based pre-admission programmes are not without marginal costs and this may be one reason for their relatively slow growth in the UK.

The use of volunteer staff[14] may provide the key for accelerated growth, especially in the light of raised parental awareness and expectations.

Admitting children to hospital before surgery in an attempt to prepare them for what may be a stressful experience has shown positive results.[15] The recognition that post-operative recovery is enhanced if the patient's pre-operative anxiety is reduced by better preparation for the ensuing stressful situation has been addressed by some theatre personnel.[16,17] Pre-operative visits and pre-operative therapeutic play programmes represent some attempts by theatre personnel to overcome such anxieties.

The psychological sequelae of a hospital admission in early childhood are associated with an increased incidence of behavioural disturbances in adolescence.[18]

Clearly, different preparatory strategies must be employed if one is able to prepare all children and their families for such events. The differing stages of child development must be addressed. Young children especially require more than just verbal explanations. Appropriate child centred methods such as therapeutic play, story books, role play and puppet shows[19] can be successful.

Planning a programme

A major contribution of a pre-admission programme is to minimise parental contagion. Most children are dependent on their parents' emotional support for help in coping with anxieties. The simplest anxiety is that produced by contagion, shown in the child who becomes frightened when he is in close contact with frightened adults. If those whose role is one of protection become frightened themselves then this can be transmitted to the child as quickly as if it were a highly infectious disease. Thus it is important to prepare parents as well as children for stressful events.[20] Skipper and Lennard[21] have demonstrated that the quality of interaction between an authoritative person such as a nurse and a hospitalised child's mother can lower the mother's stress and produce changes in her definition of the situation. This has a demonstrable effect on the child's stress, producing a change in his social, psychological and physiological behaviour.

Inspired by the pre-admission programmes in Toronto, Canada and Nottingham, England, the staff of the Paediatric Unit in Southampton established a working party to plan and initiate a similar programme.

The course leader of the NNEB programme at the local College of Further Education was co-opted onto the working party and proved most valuable. She not only wanted to include the concept of pre-admission programmes in her teaching syllabus but also offered the use of two NNEB students per week during term time to act as helpers on Saturday mornings. The group identified three stages that should be included in the planned programme.

1. Therapeutic play session

There are considerable differences between adult and child cognitive processes. Many adults use inappropriate language when explaining aspects of treatment to children. This is especially true of hospital personnel who are often confronted with an infinite variety of children's explanations of illness. What may be an appropriate explanation for an eight year old may be wholly inappropriate for a four year old. The two to 11 year old child often gives life to inanimate objects and this trait can be usefully adapted when discussing aspects of illness. Staff should be able to offer a variety of treatment explanations that are consistent with the child's level of cognitive development.

The working party approached the Children's Unit's League of Friends to seek funding for the purchase of a range of therapeutic play materials, including specialist toys and a compact purpose-built wooden storage chest. This chest allowed all items used for the pre-admission programme to be stored neatly and unobtrusively in the foyer of the Children's Day Unit where the programme would be run.

Two anatomical dolls were also bought with the help of the Southampton Lions Organisation. These two Zaadie Dolls, one female the other male, are cloth covered rag dolls and represent one of the new generation of anatomical models developed specifically for children in hospital. Jamie and Janine, as the dolls are known, come equipped with their own weekend cases in which there are two extra faces (a sleeping face, useful for discussing anaesthesia, and a sad face complete with embroidered tear), and an extra appendix (in case one is lost). The dolls have three layers which peel apart using velcro fastenings to expose the vital organs. The sleeping face is always used when the doll is opened.

The dolls can be catheterised and the female doll is equipped with an injection site on the left thigh and is recommended for use with young diabetic children. The female doll also has a removable wig to illustrate hair loss.

With the help of the NNEB students, we transformed old nurses' uniforms and doctors' white coats into new miniature versions for children. The resulting dressing up game component of the programme is proving very popular. The medium of play knows no boundaries and if it allows children to act out their fears and fantasies it will be constrained only by imagination.

2. A narrative slide presentation

A simple format was adopted for this part of the programme consisting of sequential slides covering the hospital stay from admission to discharge. Parents of inpatients and day patients were approached and consent obtained to photograph them and their children at various stages and during various procedures.

The collection of suitable slides was complicated by the fact that two distinct client groups were scheduled to attend the planned pre-admission programme, day case and longer stay children and their families. It was eventually decided to use two collections of slides to reflect the differing experiences of both groups.

3. A tour of relevant clinical areas

The differing needs of both groups dictated that there should be two tours: prospective inpatients and their families being shown around the unit while the prospective day

Table 36.1 Costing

Plus	£5.45 gross pay per hour
	National Insurance 9%
	Saturday enhancement 30%
	Superannuation 7.5%
	46.5%
	Approximate payment per hour = £8

It was necessary to calculate the hourly rate for three hours to allow staff to set up the programme and clear away afterwards:
Therefore £8 × 3 hours = £24 per Saturday per person.
ie. £48 per Saturday for 2 staff.
It was nominally agreed to run the programme for 50 weeks of the year:
£48 × 50 weeks = £2,400 per year

patients and their families watched the appropriate slide presentation, and vice-versa. The tour was planned to incorporate a visit to the theatre complex where parents could find out about their role if they wished to accompany their children to the anaesthetic room.[22]

The harsh economic climate prevailing in the health service today presents special difficulties for nurses planning innovative programmes for specific client groups. The programme was costed in terms of staff salaries and a bid submitted to the Clinical Services Manager.

Two experienced children's nurses and one play therapist/nursery nurse were considered the minimum number of staff required to ensure the viability of the programme. Volunteer helpers would be actively encouraged to participate.

It was assumed that the playworker staff could be involved with the pre-admission programme during their normal working hours and would therefore require no extra payment. For the purposes of costing it was assumed that the maximum cost for trained staff would be at the highest incremental point on the E Scale (see Table 36.1).

The Clinical Services Manager (a physician) and the Assistant Clinical Services Manager (a sick children's nurse) fully supported the aims of the programme and monies were made available to start the programme in February 1989.

While only two families arrived for the inaugural session a redesigned invitation and better advertising has resulted in a considerable increase in the uptake of the programme.

Under the auspices of the Which Jubilee Research Grant awarded by the Consumers' Association the programme will be fully evaluated.

Notes

1. Maddison, M. 'Consumer Survey of Paediatric Wards', *Australian Nurses Journal*, **6**(1), 27–28, 1977.

2. Miller, S. 'Children's Fears—A review of the literature with implications for nursing research and practice', *Nursing Research*, July–August, **28**(4), 1979.

3. Rodin, J. *Will This Hurt?* Royal College of Nursing, London, 1983.

4. Visintainer, M., Wolfer, J. 'Psychological Preparation for Surgical Paediatric Patients. The effect on children's and parents' stress responses and adjustment', *Paediatrics*, **56**(2), August 1975.

5. Vernon, D. *et al.* 'Changes in children's behaviour after hospitalisation', *Amer. J Dis. Child*, Vol. **111**, June 1966.

6. Mellish, P. 'Preparation of a child for hospitalisation and surgery', *Pediatric Clinics of North America*, **16**(3), August 1969.

7. Meng, A. and Zastowny, T. 'Preparation for Hospitalisation: A Stress Innoculation Training Program for Parents and Children', *Maternal-Child Nursing Journal*, **2**(2), 87–94, 1982.

8. Fradd, E. 'Learning about hospital', *Nursing Times*, January 15, 1986.

9. Jackson, K. 'Psychological preparation as a method of relieving the emotional trauma of anaesthesia in children', *Anaesthesiology*, 12–293, 1951.

10. Eiser, C., Hanson, L. 'Preparing Children for Hospital: a school based intervention', *The Professional Nurse*, April 1989.

11. Sharman, W. 'Tonsillectomy Through a Child's Eyes', *Nursing Times*, December 4, 1985.

12. D'Antonio, I. 'Therapeutic Use of Play in Hospitals—Symposium on Paediatric Care; Psychosocial Aspects', *Nurse Clinics North America*, **19**(2), 351–359, June 1984.

13. Brett, A. 'Preparing Children for Hospitalisation—a classroom teaching approach', *J.O.S.H.*, **53**(9), November 1983.

14. Johnson, M. and Salazar, M. 'Preadmission programmes for rehospitalised children', *American Journal of Nursing*, August 1979.

15. Fassler, D. 'Reducing Preoperative Anxiety in Children. Information versus emotional support'. *Patient Counselling and Health Education*, January, 1980.

16. Leonard, M., Kalideen, D. 'So You're Going to Have an Operation', *Nat News*, February, 1985.

17. Bonner, M. 'Can my friend go with me?' *Nursing Times*, October 1, 1986.

18. Quinton, D., Rutter, M. 'Early Hospital Admissions and Later Disturbances of Behaviour. An attempted replication of Douglas' findings', *Dev Med Child Neurol*, **18**, 447, 1976.

19. Glasper, A., Moon, S. 'Paediatric Nursing—Canadian Style', *Southampton Medical Journal*, **1**, Spring 1987.

20. Robinson and Clarke. 'Reactions of Children to Health Care Encounter', *Hospital care of children*, Oxford University Press, Oxford, 1980.

21. Skipper, J., Lennard, C. 'Children, Stress and Hospitalisation—A field experiment', *Journal of Health and Social Behaviour*, **9**, 275–286, 1968.

22. Glasper, A. 'Parents in the Anaesthetic Room: A Blessing or a Curse?', *Professional Nurse*, **3**(4), 1988.

37

Preparation of Children for Painful Procedures*

MARION E. BROOME

The preparation of children for stressful medical procedures has been an important focus for research in nursing, medicine, and psychology for the past 20 years.

Yet findings from studies have not been translated into useful recommendations that nurses can use to promote more effective ways for children to cope with painful events. This is partially due to the fact that the phenomenon of pain in children is recognized as very complex, and researchers have only begun to examine selected variables that influence children's responses. When research in a specific area such as children's pain is in such initial stages, researchers are often hesitant to recommend direct application of preliminary results. However, there is some consistency in findings reported to date that can be used to begin developing clinical protocols for preparation of children.

What factors should nurses consider when designing a psychological intervention to decrease children's distress from acute pain? How are these interventions structured? How is the effectiveness of the intervention evaluated? Previous studies of pain management in children have used varied interventions that can be classified as cognitive, affective, or biophysical (Broome & Lillis, 1989). Although there is justification for use of biophysical management in some situations, this article focuses on the two classes of interventions designed to alter the child's cognitive perception of the pain experience and/or the child's emotional response to the event.

Who to prepare for painful experiences?

Most pediatric nurses have noted that children differ widely in their response to painful procedures. Some children exhibit little or no behavioral response and provide little verbal acknowledgement of the pain experienced while others are very active and articulate during and after the experience (Hester, 1979; Broome, Bates, Lillis & McGahee, 1990). Differences in these children are thought to be related to the way they appraise the stressfulness of the situation (Lazarus & Folkman, 1984). This appraisal is affected by a variety of variables, including previous experience, age, parental

*This is an abridged version of an article first published in *Pediatric Nursing*, Vol. 16, No. 5, pp. 537–541.

anxiety, and how the child responds to threatening or stressful events. Younger children respond to painful procedures with more distress than older children. However, there seems to be a curvilinear relationship between age and anxiety preceding a clinical procedure, with adolescent and preschool children demonstrating the most distress (Winer, 1982). Child anxiety, fear and maternal anxiety have all been found to influence the child's response during immunizations and dental procedures (Broome, 1986; Johnson & Baldwin, 1969; Wright & Alpern, 1971). Without intervention, children who are distressed during a painful procedure will increase their distress behaviors over time (Katz, Kellerman, & Siegel, 1980).

Children have been the recipients of the majority of interventions described in the literature. However, parents are often present during painful experiences and are asked to answer questions that the child has prior to and after experiencing the pain. The subject of parental presence during painful procedures remains controversial in clinical practice. Many nurses and physicians believe that the presence of a parent is upsetting to a child. This assumption is usually based on their experience with young children in particular who often exhibit more behavioral and verbal resistance if the mother is present. However, this more active response on the part of the child does not always indicate a greater perception of pain. In fact, it may be used by children as a coping mechanism to deal with the pain (Broome, *et al.*, 1989; Hester, 1979).

Research has not provided a definitive answer to whether parental presence decreases pain perception (Broome & Endsley, 1989b; Shaw & Routh, 1982; Vernon, Foley & Schulman, 1967). Some researchers of child behavior found that children were more distressed when parents were present, others found less distress, while others reported no difference. The children were not asked in any of these studies if the parents' presence was reassuring. Yet, when well children were asked what helped them most when they were in pain, 99% stated the presence of their parent (Ross & Ross, 1988). Until more studies investigate this issue, it is best to ask the child and parent what their preferences are. If parents choose to be present, they must be thoroughly prepared for the procedure including suggestions about how they can help support their child during the procedure. If they choose not to be present, the parent should be assured that someone will be available during the procedure to provide comfort for the child. The child's ability or desire to use self-control techniques independently or to rely on adults to provide additional control cues, such as a parent giving instructions to breathe, must also be considered. Some school-age children want to 'do it themselves' while others want a parent to work with them.

When parents are present, they often find that the child asks them many questions prior to and during the procedure. These questions include: How much will it hurt? How long will it last? Why does it have to hurt? When will it be over? Will they do it again? If the child alone is the primary recipient of the information and preparation, a parent may be unable to answer these questions. Both parent and child will experience increased anxiety. Therefore, parents should always be given the opportunity to be involved in preparation for the painful procedure. If they choose not to be present for the painful experience, they will be able to reinforce the nurses' teaching, correct misperceptions, and comfort the child after the procedure. Hence, preparation should be scheduled at a time when the parent is present. It is also helpful for parents to have written information that reinforces what was taught and can be referred to later.

The age of the child should influence the type of information given and when it should be provided (Bates & Broome, 1986). Infants and younger toddlers are generally not cognitively able to comprehend detailed procedural information or anticipate events. The older toddler (2+ years) can be given a simple description of what will happen immediately prior to the event. However, older children seem to benefit from preparation several days before the event, if possible. This timing allows the older child to think about how he or she will respond and what actions or behaviors can be used to cope with the experience (Flavell, 1963). Younger children who are unable to cognitively anticipate or think through behaviors will most likely become more anxious if prepared far in advance.

Structure and process of preparation

Recent research on pediatric pain management identified a variety of interventions that are effective in reducing behavioral distress, pain ratings and physiologic response to pain in children (Broome, Lillis & Smith, 1989; Broome & Lillis, 1989). Preparation programs have traditionally focused on providing the child with (a) information about what will happen and how it will feel and/or (b) what the child can do during the procedure to distract or relax and reduce the perception of pain (Broome & Lillis, 1989). The focus of most nursing research has been on the first category of preparation—provision of information. Information about what will occur during the procedure and what sensation the child will feel has been shown to be more effective in reducing distress than just the former alone (Johnson, Kirchhoff & Endress, 1975; Fernald & Corry, 1981).

Most children also benefit from being able to anticipate what will happen during a painful procedure. In a recent study of children undergoing lumbar puncture procedures (Broome, *et al.*, 1990), the children with cancer often repeatedly asked 'What are you doing now? What will you do next?' These children had all experienced the procedure before, yet still requested information about the timing of the pain stimulus during the procedure. This implies it is important to think of the timing of preparation in two ways—that given prior to the event as well as during the procedure. This may require that information provided during the procedure may be given by someone other than the nurse, perhaps the parent.

A variety of preparation strategies have been used, including books, puppets enacting the procedures, and videotaped modeling where children viewed child models experiencing and reacting to a painful procedure (Bates & Broome, 1986). Nurses responsible for preparing children should develop a technique that is most useful in their particular setting. If no video equipment is available, coloring books or hand puppets could be used. Broome, *et al.* (1989) found that the medium used to deliver the intervention, such as books or puppets, did not vary the effectiveness of the intervention.

Coping skills

There are several types of skills and techniques nurses can teach to children to help them cope with a painful procedure (Patterson & Ware, 1988). These skills include relaxation, distraction, and imagery. The purpose of these techniques is to break the cycle of tension prior to the procedure and provide competing stimuli for the pain stimulus during the procedure (Campos, 1989; McCaffery & Beebe, 1989). The primary goal of any intervention used during a painful procedure is to decrease the child's perception of the quality and quantity of pain experienced. It should not be to teach children only to control their behavior in order to increase their cooperation with the health care team. It may not be effective for some children to inhibit (control) their behavior if a decrease in pain perception is a goal (Broome, Bates, Lillis, & McGahee, 1990). Hence, interventions should be discussed with the child and parent, and past coping behaviors should be assessed.

Cognitively-focused interventions should be developmentally appropriate (Broome, *et al.*, 1989; Gedaly-Duff, 1987). The preschool child uses preoperational thought that includes representational or symbolic thought processes (Flavell, 1963). The preschooler is now capable of anticipating future events and how to respond to these. These new cognitive skills are not language oriented, as they are in the school-age child, but rather action oriented, imagistic, and concrete. Hence, the strategies used to prepare children for a painful event will require the use of objects they can manipulate and specific age-appropriate descriptions of what will happen and ways to respond. These younger children (ages 3–7) will respond best to puppets, cartoons, stories, and dolls using action-oriented, imaginative plots that explain the painful experience and provide the child with some ideas of how the characters responded (Bates & Broome, 1986; Patterson & Ware, 1988).

The school-age child has the ability to extend thought to potential possibilities from the actual situation in the present. These children can be engaged in discussion of what they think will happen, how they responded in the past, and how they would like to respond to this painful procedure now. These children often benefit from the use of a videotaped live model who experiences the pain and exhibits some realistic reactions. Verbal descriptions of what will happen, how the child may feel, and what actions to take in order to relax and be distracted are included in such preparation programs for the school-age child.

The nurse can use specific types of interventions with children for painful procedures (see Table 37.1). Cognitive strategies are those that provide factual information designed to alter the child's perception of the threat by describing what will happen during the procedure and how it will feel.

Affective strategies are designed to provide the child with coping skills and emotional support to reduce anxiety during the painful experience (Broome & Lillis, 1989, p. 77). These interventions include relaxation, parental presence and imagery. Use of these interventions necessitates the child and parent be taught prior to the procedure and, the first time they use them, will require the nurse [to] provide additional coaching and cues during the procedure unless they have had an opportunity to practice the techniques. Ideally, time should be available for the parent and child to practice the simple techniques. Patterson and Ware (1988) have developed a very useful written instruction procedure for parents who plan to help their child during a procedure. Tapes such as 'No More Fears' (Canadian Cancer Socity, 1987) are available that teach the parent and child ways to cope with the event. Most children will require continued support during the painful procedure to enable them to use the strategy.

Table 37.1 Intervention strategies for children experiencing a painful procedure

Cognitive strategies	Source
Prior to procedure	
Audiotaped sensory and procedural information	Johnson, Kirchhoff & Endress, 1975 Gedaly-Duff, 1987
Videotaped filmed preparation with models	Melamed, Weinstein, Hawes, & Katin-Borland, 1975; Vernon, 1974
Puppets or dolls	Cassell, 1975 Broome & Endsley, 1987
During procedure	
Thought-stopping	Ross, 1984
Hypnosis	Zelter & LeBaron, 1982 Kellerman, Zelter, & Ellenbury, 1983
Distraction (ie. breathing)	Broome, Lillis, Bates & Wilson, 1988 Jay, *et al.*, 1987
Music	Caire & Erikson, 1986
Positive self-talk	Nocella & Kaplan (1982)
Affective strategies	
Parental presence	Broome, & Endsley, 1989a; 1989b Frankl, Shiere & Fogels, 1962
Relaxation	Hobbie, 1989 Patterson & Ware, 1988

Evaluation of interventions

A variety of methods have been used to evaluate the effectiveness of pain management programs (Broome & Lillis, 1989). Biophysical assessments such as pulse and cortisol levels have been used. Observations of children's distress and coping behaviors have been evaluated using either videotaped segments of the painful procedure (Maikler, 1989; Broome, Lillis, Wilson, & Bates, 1988) or raters who are present at the event (Broome & Endsley, 1987; 1989a). Some of these methods are easier to implement in certain settings than others. For instance, there is a long and detailed observation tool developed by Susan Jay and colleagues (1987) that can be used to assess the degree of distress during a bone marrow or lumbar puncture. Although it works well in longer pain situations, it is time consuming and requires the observer to be trained. Most self-report measures such as the *Oucher* (Beyer, 1988) and *FACES* (Wong & Baker, 1988) are less costly to administer, are quicker, and yield valuable information (see Table 37.2).

Nurses can 'make a difference' in how children cope with painful procedures. Cognitive preparation for the event is very important but not enough. Children and parents need to be taught ways to decrease the child's perception of the pain

Table 37.2 Some methods used to evaluate effectiveness of interventions

Method	Description	Source
Self-report		
Color matching	Colors organized vertically by child to describe pain.	Eland, 1981
FACES	6 faces.	McCaffery & Beebe, 1989; Wong & Baker, 1988
VAS	10 cm line with end point descriptors of intensity of pain.	Ross & Ross, 1988
OUCHER	5 pictures of a toddler in no pain to much pain.	Beyer, 1988
Behavioral		
CHEOPS	Six types of verbal & non-verbal behaviors on 4 point scale.	McGrath, Johnson, Goodman & Unruh, 1985
Observation of Behavioral Distress	Verbal and non-verbal distress behaviors weighted by frequency.	Ross & Ross, 1988
Procedure Behavior Checklist	Check of 8 behaviors on 5 point likert scale.	LeBaron & Zelter, 1984
Physiologic		
Heart Rate		
Blood Pressure		
Palmer Sweat Index	Fingerprint impression.	Johnson & Dabbs, 1967

experienced. Nurses should be creative in the methods they use, base techniques on the child's developmental level, and carefully evaluate the effectiveness of the intervention.

References

Beyer, J. (1988) *The Oucher: A user's manual and technical report*, Denver, University of Colorado Health Science Center.

Bates, T., & Broome, M. (1986) 'Preparation of children for hospitalization and surgery: A review of the literature', *Journal of Pediatric Nursing*, **1**(4), 230–239.

Broome, M. (1986) 'The relationship between children's fears and behavior during a painful event', *Children's Health Care*, **14**, 142–145.

Broome, M. (1985) 'The child in pain: A model for assessment and intervention', *Critical Care Quarterly*, **8**(1), 47–55.

Broome, M., & Endsley, R. (1987) 'Group preparation of children as a moderator of child response to pain', *Western Journal of Nursing Research*, **9**(4), 484–502.

Broome, M., Lillis, P., Wilson, T., & Bates, T. (1988) *Effectiveness of a pain management program for pediatric oncology patients*, Funded by American Cancer Society, N No. 141, Medical College of Georgia.

Broome, M., & Endsley, R. (1989a) 'Parent and child reactions to an immunization', *Pain*, **37**(1), 85–92.

Broome, M., & Endsley, R. (1989b) 'Parent presence and childrearing practices and child response to an injection', *Research in Nursing and Health*, **12**, 229–235.

Broome, M., Lillis, P., & Smith, M.C. (1989) 'A meta-analysis of research in pain management programs in children', *Nursing Research*, **38**(3), 154–158.

Broome, M., & Lillis, P. (1989) 'A descriptive analysis of pediatric pain management research', *Journal of Applied Nursing Research*, **38**(3), 74–81.

Broome, M., Bates, T., Lillis, P., & McGahee, T. (1990) 'Medical fears, coping behaviors, and pain perceptions in children during lumbar puncture', *Oncology Nursing Forum*, **17**(3), 361–370.

Caire, J., & Erikson, S. (1986) 'Reducing distress in pediatric patients undergoing cardiac catheterization', *Children's Health Care*, **14**, 146–152.

Campos, R. (1989) 'Soothing pain elicited stress in infants with swaddling & pacifiers', *Child Development*, **60**, 781–792.

Canadian Cancer Society, (1987) *No fears, no tears*, Vancouver, B.C., Author.

Cassell, J. (1985) 'Effect of brief puppet therapy upon the emotional responses of children undergoing cardiac catheterization', *Journal of Consulting Psychology*, **29**, 1–8.

Eland, J. (1981) 'Minimizing pain associated with pre-kindergarten intermuscular injections', *Issues in Comprehensive Pediatric Nursing*, **5**, 361–372.

Fernald, C., & Corry, J. (1981) 'Empathetic vs. directive preparation of children for needles', *Children's Health Care*, **10**, 44–47.

Flavell, (1963) *The developmental psychology of Jean Piaget*, New York, Van Nostrand–Reinholdt.

Frankl, F., Shiere, F., & Fogels, H. (1962) 'Should the patient remain with the child in the operatory?' *Journal of Dentistry for Children*, **29**, 150–163.

Gedaly-Duff, V. (1987) 'Preparing young children for painful procedures', *Journal of Pediatric Nursing*, **3**(3), 169–178.

Hester, N. (1979) 'The preoperational child's reaction to an immunization', *Nursing Research*, **28**, 250–255.

Hobbie, C. (1989) 'Relaxation techniques for children and young people', *Journal of Pediatric Health Care*, **3**, 83–87.

Jay, S., Elliot, C., Katz, E., & Siegel, F. (1987) 'Cognitive, behavioral and pharmacologic interventions for children undergoing painful medical procedures', *Journal of Consulting Clinical Psychology*, **55**, 860–865.

Johnson, J., & Dabbs, J. (1967) 'Enumeration of active sweat glands: A simple physiological indicator of psychological changes', *Nursing Research*, **16**(3), 273–276.

Johnson, K., & Baldwin, D. (1969) 'Maternal anxiety and child behavior', *Journal of Dentistry for Children*, **36**, 87–92.

Johnson, J., Kirchoff, K., & Endress, M. (1975) 'Altering children's distress behavior during orthopedic cast renewal', *Nursing Research*, **24**(11), 404–411.

Katz, E., Kellerman, J., & Siegel, S. (1980) 'Behavioral distress in children undergoing medical procedures developmental procedures', *Journal of Consulting and Clinical Psychology*, **48**, 356–365.

Kendall, P. (1983) 'Stressful medical procedures', in D. Meichenbaum & M. Jaremko (eds), *Stress reduction and prevention*, New York, Plenum Press.

Kellerman, J., Zelter, R., & Ellenbury, (1983) 'Adolescents with cancer: Hypnosis for the reduction of acute pain and anxiety during medical procedures', *Journal of Adolescent Health Care*, **4**, 85–90.

Lazarus, R., & Folkman, S. (1984) *Stress, appraisal & coping*, New York, Springer.

LeBaron, S., & Zelter, L. (1984) 'Assessment of acute pain and anxiety in children and adolescents by Self-Report, Observer Reports, and the Behavioral Checklist', *Journal of Consulting & Clinical Psychology*, **52**, 729–738.

Maikler, V. (1989) *Infant's responses to varied pain stimuli*, Doctoral dissertation, University of Illinois.

McCaffery, M., & Beebe, A. (1989) '*Pain: Clinical manual for nursing practice*', St. Louis, C.V. Mosby Company.

McGrath, P., Johnson, G., Goodman, J., & Unruh, A. (1985) 'CHEOPS: A behavioural scale for rating postoperative pain in children', in H.L. Fields, R. Dubner, & F. Cervero (eds), *Advances in pain research and therapy*, Vol. 9. Proceedings of the Fourth World Congress on Pain (pp. 395–402). New York, Raven Press.

Melamed, B., Weinstein, D., Hawes, R., & Katin-Borland, M. (1975) 'Reduction of fear-related dental management problems using filmed modelling', *Journal of American Dental Association*, **90**, 822–826.

Nocella, J., & Kaplan, R. (1982) 'Training children to cope with dental treatment', *Journal of Pediatric Psychology*, **7**, 175–182.

Patterson, K., & Ware, L. (1988) 'Coping skills for children undergoing painful medical procedures', *Issues in Comprehensive Pediatric Nursing*, **11**, 113–143.

Ross, D. (1984) 'Thought stopping: A coping strategy for impending feared events' *Issues in Comprehensive Pediatric Nursing*, **7**, 83–89.

Ross, D., & Ross, S. (1988) *Childhood pain: Current issues, research and management*, Baltimore-Munich, Urban & Schwarzenberg.

Shaw, E., & Routh, D. (1982) 'Effect of mother presence on children's reaction to aversive procedures', *Journal of Pediatric Psychology*, **7**, 33–42.

Vernon, D., Schulman, J., & Foley, J. (1967) 'Effect of mother-child separation and birth order on young children's responses to two potentially stressful experiences', *Journal of Personality and Social Psychology*, **15**, 167–174.

Vernon, D. (1974) 'Modeling and birth order in responses to painful stimuli', *Journal of Personality and Social Psychology*, **29**, 794–799.

Winer, G. (1982) 'A review and analysis of children's fearful behavior in dental settings', *Child Development*, **53**, 1111–1133.

Wong, D., & Baker, C. (1988) 'Pain in children: Comparison of assessment Scales', *Pediatric Nursing*, **14**(1), 9–17.

Wright, G., & Alpern, G. (1971) 'Variables influencing children's cooperative behavior at first dental visit', *Journal of Dentistry for Children*, **38**, 60–64.

Zelter, R., & LeBaron, S. (1982) 'Hypnosis and Nonhypnotic techniques for reduction of pain and anxiety during painful procedures in children and adolescents with cancer', *Behavioral Pediatrics*, **101**, 1032–1036.

38

Support Can Reduce the Stress Factor: Stress in Neonatal Nursing*

K. MARTINA HANNON

The emotional and technological demands of working in a neonatal unit (NNU) make it extremely stressful for all health professionals involved. This article describes why stress is such an important factor in NNUs, outlines coping mechanisms currently used to overcome it and makes suggestions for change. The stresses involved in neonatal nursing originate from the environment itself and not from any inherent 'weakness' in nursing practice. It is time nurses recognised their limitations, made use of their strengths and helped each other to create an environment which makes nursing more enjoyable, less stressful and altogether more acceptable.

The intensity of work in NNUs and the fine line between life and death impose tremendous stress on medical and nursing staff. The critical condition of a large number of babies who require care in NNUs goes against all the normal expectations of a maternity unit and pregnancy in general, where outlook is positive and life for most of us begins. The environment itself can be challenging, as is expressed by Van Dias (1987):

> A special care baby unit is hot, there are masses of complicated clicking, buzzing, whirring, ringing machines and everywhere is the sense of walking a tightrope while attempting to do something natural: take care of a new born baby. The impact of such a place on staff and families can be powerful.

No matter how well neonatal nurses familiarise themselves with the technology which is essential to the health and wellbeing of the babies in their care, it is hard not to become stressed by the constant alarms ringing at varying volumes. Initially the stress is brought about by the worry of which alarm is ringing and whether it is a life-threatening problem, and culminates in the grinding on the nerves of oxygen saturation monitors ringing because a baby's saturation is reading 95 per cent while he or she is nursed in air. It is not practical, however, to turn the alarm off completely or to set

*This is an abridged version of an article first published in *Professional Nurse*, Vol. 8, No. 8, pp. 496, 498, 500, 1993.

its limits higher, as the baby may suddenly desaturate, even though he or she is reading high in air. All alarms have the essential purpose of alerting nurses to a problem.

Burnout

The repetitive and unrelenting nature of work in a unit continuing night and day can be physically and psychologically exhausting. The term most used in the literature to describe stress in NNUs is 'burnout'. Wilson (1989) explores the three stages of stress, and states:

> In its extreme form, the 'exhaustion phase' of the stress response is characterised by cynicism, withdrawal, emotional detachment from work, rigidity and inability to admit to personal needs. It is known colloquially as 'burnout' and is responsible for high rates of absenteeism and lack of job satisfaction.

Proctor (1990) describes her own personal experience of burnout in a NNU, and explores the factors both within and without the unit which led to it.

In the present economic climate, all areas of the NHS have suffered from inevitable staff shortages (Hingley and Harris, 1986). Added to this is the increased number of premature and very low birth weight babies. This has evolved from increased scientific knowledge, both in the field of assisting childless couples to conceive as a result of artificial insemination, which often results in multiple births, and in the technology necessary to keep these babies alive. The overcrowding effect this has on units, with ill babies who will be long-stay and have many time-consuming problems, however, adds to staff's feeling of being 'stretched to the limits'. Proctor also says the heavy workload means that time is at a premium, just when the babies and their parents most need time, support and attention. This gives rise to feelings of guilt among staff, lowering morale even further. Lack of time can also lead to gradual loss of contact with other members of staff at a time when nurses need to vent their fears and anxieties and gain each other's support. Mutual contact and support is vital to those working in areas of high stress.

Jacobson (1988) examined the sources of stress in intensive care units (ICUs) identified in a national survey in America: interaction among care givers; interaction with management of the unit; the nature of direct patient care; inadequate knowledge and skills; inadequacy of the physical work environment; life events and lack of administrative rewards. A more recent survey found the rank order to be compatible with earlier studies, with more emphasis on team communication, problems of patients and their families, and nurses' role conflicts (Vachon, 1987).

The concept of teamwork is a key element in the life of a NNU. The rapid turnover of junior medical staff often puts considerable strain on nurses, and more identifiably on senior nursing staff. Doctors may be constantly revising treatment and may not give nurses credit for their experience and knowledge, which will inevitably lead to tension and added stress.

An air of glamour is often associated with working in the caring profession. The media often uses the 'angel' stereotype—which the public is often quite happy to absorb—to represent nurses, and fails to portray the real-life picture of increased technology, staff shortages and low morale. The media thus encourages an idealism which, in the light of problems faced in the profession today, cannot be lived up to and becomes a major source of stress among nurses. External factors also add to nurses' stress levels: everyday life can bring with it stressors of one form or another, whether personal bereavement, marriage difficulties, mortgage problems or parental concerns.

Good versus bad stress

Hughes (1990) believes that stress is neutral: it can be good or bad for the individual depending on a host of other factors. It is, in fact, essential for living, as without it we would do very little and would certainly not survive real danger for long. Some stress (known as 'eustress') is good for us, as it acts as a stimulus for high performance. Everyone, however, has a personal 'threshold' at which further stress becomes counter-productive—when 'eustress' flips over into 'distress'. In NNUs, this becomes clearer as carers are stretched to the limit (Heywood-Jones, 1989), resulting in poor concentration, poor decision-making and excessive demands that compromise performance. The emotional stresses of working with premature or low birthweight babies combined with the unseen demands of anxious parents, demanding medical staff and impossible machinery mean it can take little to upset the balance of even the most level-headed, experienced and self-assured staff nurse.

The distinction between 'good' or 'bad' stress is not always clear, although there is some evidence to suggest nurses, in particular, can distinguish between them in their work (Bamber, 1988). It may be more important, however, to ask whether good stress has the same effect as bad stress.

Coping with stress

In view of the numerous origins of stress in NNUs and the fact that stress reactions reflect the individual's understanding of the situation and his or her ability to act accordingly, the first step in promoting adaptive stress responses lies in selecting suitable staff (Wilson, 1989). This, naturally, requires skilled interviewing techniques. Intelligence, high motivation and common sense also dictate our ability to adjust and find coping strategies to stress, such as maintaining social contact outside work and pursuing diverse interests. Multiple stressors have a cumulative effect, and candidates for these jobs who face difficult situations at home are less likely to cope with the added burden of neonatal care. Bamber (1988) suggests that often 'lack of skills' as a result of unsatisfactory training is a cause of ineffectiveness among nurses, which leads to misdiagnosis of problems and inappropriate goal setting. Continuing professional education can encourage coping skills and thus increase staff effectiveness, and is also a useful way of keeping staff in touch with new ideas and reviewing well-established ones. Educating staff in the causes and symptoms of burnout would also enable nurses to recognise these features in themselves before they become disabling.

Another aspect of neonatal nursing which harbours doubts and anxiety in the minds of many carers is the knowledge that, intentionally or non-intentionally, they inflict harm to prevent harm. Carton (1987), for example, highlights transcutaneous and oxygen saturation monitors which alert nurses to potential danger from high or low oxygen or carbon dioxide, but inflict small peripheral burns in the process.

Death is a great source of anxiety and stress to all neonatal staff. Honest discussion concerning prognosis will ease the distress of staff and families by allowing them to prepare themselves when a baby is obviously dying after a prolonged illness. It is important to try to come to terms with the exceptionally frequent encounters with death which working in NNUs entails.

Providing support

While factors contributing to stress are varied, implementing small changes in the workplace may alleviate some of the stressors. It is only by joining forces to consider and implement positive changes in working practice that neonatal nurses can help reduce some of the stress involved in their work. Leaving the specialty for other, less demanding, fields only presents a short-term answer.

One of the key factors in promoting a less stressful environment is to establish a supportive atmosphere—NNUs should be friendly places where everyone works together. More interaction with senior members of staff will mean more time and support for junior colleagues. Ward managers should try to recognise signs of stress in colleagues and allow them to work in less intensive areas for a while (Dopson, 1988). Arranging regular meetings to discuss areas that need to be looked into, problems that have arisen in the unit and ways in which to cope with them is another way of relieving stress. Skill mix is important where staff from different fields—midwives, paediatric nurses, nursery nurses—all work together. Neonatal nurses are, of course, lucky; although they work in a highly technological, busy unit, they have the advantage of promoting life—a life with shaky beginnings but, hopefully, a sound future. Only time will tell.

References

Bamber, M. (1988) 'Slant on stress', *Nursing Times*, **84**(11), 60–63.

Carton, A.S. (1987) 'Nursing problems of the previable (below 26/40) neonate', Neonatal Nurses National Conference Paper, Nottingham.

Dopson, L. (1988) 'Working in the hothouse', *Nursing Times*, **84**(8), 16–17.

Heywood Jones, I. (1989) 'Stretched to the limits', *Nursing Times*, **85**(46), 38–40.

Hingley, P. and Harris, P. (1986) 'Lowering the tension', *Nursing Times*, **82**(31), 52–53.

Hughes, J. (1990) 'Stress: scourge or stimulant', *Nursing Standard*, **5**(4), 30–33.

Jacobson, S.F. (1988) 'Coping skills for neonatal nurses', Paper presented at the Neonatal Nurses National Conference, Nottingham.

Proctor, J. (1990) 'Experience of ''burnout'' in the special care baby unit', *Midwives Chronicle*, **September**, 266–67.

Vachon, M.L.S. (1987) 'Coping skills for neonatal nurses', Paper presented at the Neonatal Nurses National Conference, Nottingham.

Van Dias, S. (1987) 'Psychotherapy in special care baby units', *Nursing Times*, **83**(23), 50–52.

Wilson, I.R.A. (1989) 'Stress related to neonatal intensive care nursing', *Midwives Chron. and Nurs. Notes*, **102**(1222), 366–68.

Bibliography

Bailey, R. (1985) *Coping With Stress in Caring*, Blackwell Scientific, Oxford.

Cooper, C. (1988) *Living with Stress*, Penguin, London.

Witrin-Lanoil, G. (1985) *Coping with Stress*, Sheldon Press, London.

These books offer an insight into how stress arises, and [how] people can adapt and live with it. Various coping mechanisms for dealing with stress are outlined.

SECTION 8

Changing Practice in Children's Nursing

Introduction

In this section we turn to the future and focus on trends in children's nursing, and on nursing at large. This Reader (and the course which it supports) should have given you a good insight and grounding in current knowledge, themes and issues in working with children and families to promote child health. The aim of the collection of papers for this final section is to motivate you to continue to maintain your interest and professional education in your chosen field of work, and to encourage you to be proactive in working for child health.

The first reading is part of the *Health For All Nursing Series*, produced by the World Health Organization Regional Office for Europe in Copenhagen. It is an edited extract of a policy strategy document and is part of the long-term 'Nursing in Action' programme. This aims at operationalizing the WHO HFA concepts and principles into patient care, through nursing actions. It recognizes nurses as a powerful force for change, and thus legitimizes working for change as a central health care activity. Skills necessary for successful management of change are identified, and nurses are encouraged to develop these. The paper finishes with an exhortation to share 'good practice', by its dissemination. This plea is especially important. Health professionals frequently invent and perform 'good practice' in the course of their day to day work. Rarely does the profession at large hear about it. Thinking and writing is a legitimate activity too! Rarely are nurses encouraged to reflect on and write about their practice: the pressure is always to get on with the (physical) job. But unless and until 'good practice' is more widely reported the theoretical knowledge base of the profession will not progress.

The first reading focuses on changing nursing practice. In some situations this is very difficult because of the health care context in which practice is enacted. Sometimes there is a need for broader, more political changes to be made. Recognizing this, we include, as the second reading, a Guide to Parliamentary Lobbying.

The final two papers in this section look to the future in child health nursing. In the first of these Williams notes the increased national emphasis on health promotion and primary health care in policy strategies. She also comments on the fact that, in the future, consumers will become more involved in health care issues and decisions about the type of health care that is required. Overspecialization is cautioned against, and the creation of a new, generic, child health nurse is advocated.

In his paper, Glasper provides a vision for child health nursing that is bright and optimistic, and offers specific guidance in the areas of education, practice, research and development. Commenting on changing patterns of research, Glasper recognizes both that unity is strength (multidisciplinary research teams), and that, if nurses are to be taken seriously by other academics, they need to compete for funding, engage in research activity, and be measured by the same criteria as are other health care researchers. Like Williams, Glasper identifies some trends in primary and secondary health care in the UK, and encourages alliances and partnerships with parents and consumers in health care delivery.

39

Changing Nursing Practice*

WORLD HEALTH ORGANIZATION

Nurses—a force for change

Nurses do not seem to have a history of managing and controlling change, yet this professional group has great potential. About 5 million people work in nursing jobs in the WHO European Region. They work in every conceivable health setting, come from a wide range of educational and social backgrounds, and in their professional and personal lives have contact with every section of the population. They already act as agents for change, often without recognizing it. Whether reviewing the way they organize their work, helping a family at home, teaching a patient with diabetes to change her lifestyle, or carrying out a quality survey—nurses are actively involved in change wherever they work and in almost everything they do. Change is so big a part of the nurse's role that its significance is often underestimated, and opportunities to improve the planning and organization of change may be missed.

To some extent this reflects a tendency in the profession to undervalue what nurses do. Dismissing nursing as caring, common sense or menial can hide its intricacy and value. Nursing becomes part of the scenery for the stage on which the grander and more exciting health acts (the technological advances and medical breakthroughs) are played out. Some writers[1–5] have argued that the fact that most nurses are women reinforces this tendency. In a male-dominated culture that gives the greatest status to the actions and values of men, women's work may be dismissed or ignored. Further, women's work is not seen to include agitation for change; as Oakley[5] says:

> Nurses, like all women, have to contend with one important obstacle to change; real women are not supposed to be revolutionaries. If we complain about our situation, or the system, we are liable to be called ill, neurotic, menopausal, premenstrual, or in need of some curative relationship with a man.

---

*This is an abridged version of *Changing Nursing Practice* (Health for All Nursing Series), Copenhagen, World Health Organization Regional Office for Europe, pp. 4–11, 14–15, 22–26, (1992).

There is no evidence to suggest that nurses always and naturally resist change. In fact, nurses appear to engender a huge amount of change despite the obstacles mentioned. The health visitor who works with a family to improve the nutrition of the children, the midwife who prepares a mother and father for the birth of their child, and the hospital nurse who helps a patient to adjust to disability are all working in their own ways to produce change. Similarly, many nurses work for change as individuals in professional, social and political organizations.

How change is introduced is important. Resistance appears to be strongest when nurses feel change is forced on them. The many examples of this in nursing's history include the development of the nursing process, which was often undermined because nurses felt that they were being pushed into change against their will.[6] Attempting change by the use of power—by those at the top upon the ranks below—is risky.

A crucial factor in avoiding resistance and creating acceptance appears to be the degree to which nurses themselves can determine the progress of change. This requires knowledge and skill, combined with the opportunity to participate in and control the change process. Unfortunately, certain knowledge and skills that nurses need to be 'change masters'[7] are not always readily available to them. Personal growth and awareness, communication skills and assertiveness are not included in all nursing education curricula. Indeed, it could be argued that the people in power in health organizations rarely encourage these qualities in nurses. Consider the implications if every nurse in Europe were an assertive, aware and skilful change agent! Bearing in mind that most of them would be women, the effects would go far beyond nursing and health care to society as a whole.

Nurses may sometimes be denied opportunities for development because certain powerful individuals and groups fear the consequences. Further, the culture of nursing itself hinders change in some respects. Oakley[5] notes that if only 'Nightingale had trained her lady pupils in assertiveness rather than obedience, perhaps nurses would be in a different place now'. Martin's research[8] emphasizes that resources, the working environment, management and leadership style, and educational opportunities have equally important parts in determining the success of nurses as change agents. Nurses have a complex position in health care and in society; the challenge is to define what they need to change their situation and to empower them to fulfil their potential in the care of others.

Managing change

Before embarking on change, nurses should reflect on their situation, to decide whether they possess the requisite knowledge, skills and resources to achieve their goals. The nurses' aim may be, for example, to help a patient to change her lifestyle by giving up smoking, to work with colleagues to reorganize care on the ward or to use the results of a patient survey to change the way a clinic offers its services. No matter [what] the aim, all proposals for change demand certain prerequisites:

(*a*) an understanding of how the organization works and who are the influential people in it;
(*b*) a knowledge of what resources are needed and how to obtain them;
(*c*) teaching, communicating and teamworking skills;

(*d*) awareness of personal abilities, strengths, limitations and knowledge;
(*e*) awareness of the practicalities of the work situation and organizational priorities;
(*f*) time;
(*g*) a knowledge of how change is achieved and the different strategies that can be used;
(*h*) managerial and educational support.

Even managing what appears to be the simplest of changes is therefore fraught with potential difficulties; success depends on a great many factors. This section points out some of the main elements and stages in the change process. The nurse's personal knowledge and skills are crucial. Knowledge of how change can be brought about is likely to make the management of change much easier and to lead to success. This knowledge is as important to nurses as knowing the principles of preventing cross-infection or how to deal with a cardiac arrest.

Strategies for change

A growing body of knowledge is now available to nurses about the management of change.[9–12] This literature shows three approaches to implementing change.

The first is the power coercive approach. This is a top-down method. People in authority instruct others to do things differently. It assumes that people obey the orders of higher authority, and it is usually accompanied by some sense of threat (such as loss of job or other punishment) if they do not. This approach is a common feature of military and hierarchial organizations, or those that rely heavily on bureaucratic control; in the health field, it is associated with rigid and institutionalized ways of delivering care.

Unfortunately, this approach appears to inhibit initiative and creativity in the people who receive the orders. This style also underestimates the ability of individuals and groups to resist proposed changes, or to revert to old ways of doing things once the attention of authority moves elsewhere.

Second, the rational empirical approach assumes that most people are guided by reason and self-interest, and that, given choices, they will act in the way that brings maximum benefit to all. This approach is also somewhat top-down and authoritarian. It assumes that information and instructions tend to flow in one direction, from people with knowledge and power to those without. A simple example would be a nurse providing a group of smokers with much information and all the logical knowledge on why and how they should give up the habit. The rational or empirical style would expect the smokers to desist simply because reason should prevail.

This approach leaves open the possibility that the workers in an organization can be manipulated, perhaps cynically, by people in authority. It raises the question, in health care particularly, of what happens when the interests of the staff conflict with those of clients. Whether people will always act on the basis of reason is also open to doubt. Ignorance and prejudice can influence nurses' approaches to care; witness, for example, the response of many nurses to people with AIDS.

Third is the normative re-educative approach. This style differs from the others; here change moves from the bottom up. It is based on the belief that people need to be involved in all aspects of changes that affect them, because they will accept and implement only the changes that fit into the informative culture (their values, goals and relationships). This approach accepts the premise that people can best achieve change by acting collectively, with maximum involvement of the people in the group. Because the group owns the change process and the outcome, it is more likely to accept and sustain the changes.

In the first two strategies, power lies in the hands of people with knowledge and authority. Both therefore carry the risk of resistance or rejection by people who feel that change has been forced on them. Of the three strategies, a growing body of evidence in nursing favours the normative or re-educative style; it is argued[9,13] that this is more likely to produce long-term changes in practice. The approach has been extensively used in some WHO Member States to foster changes in nursing practice, for example, in nursing development units—centres dedicated to innovation, improvement and evaluation in nursing practice. In these centres, practising nurses can determine their path of change and spread the results outward into the wider health care system.

Responses to change

Several writers have identified different roles and responses within the change process. Considering these can help nurses to predict the reaction to proposed changes in their own setting, and plan for them accordingly.

Rogers[14] describes roles and types. The leaders of innovation may at first be in a minority. Some follow the suggestions enthusiastically (the early adopters), some with a little more thought and consideration (the early majority). Another group may be somewhat sceptical, but eventually embrace the changes (the late majority). Others (the laggards) may put up considerable resistance, try to subvert the whole process and never change their practice.

While these ideas may help nurses to identify possible responses to change, they should be viewed with caution. People are rarely so predictable. Further, it is important to consider why people respond as they do. For example, the laggards may be assumed to be difficult or negative. Not all changes, however, are necessarily for the better. A nurse resisting a proposal to cut staffing levels may be seen as a heroine by some, and a laggard by others. Much depends upon the nature of the change proposed, how it is carried through and the personal beliefs and values of the people involved. Some colleagues may be set in their ways, but is this because they do not see the relevance of the change, feel excluded from the process or fear the consequences?

Keyser[15] discusses the usefulness of four strategies in different situations. He calls the first approach *telling*. This usually involves a combination of the rational empirical and power coercive approaches. Here people in authority tell the staff what to do and expect them to get on with it. Some have argued[16] that this style is acceptable for people that have 'low ability' or no willingness to change. Sometimes it is used to deliver information until the staff have accepted the change and developed confidence. Then the level of supervision and control can be reduced.

The second approach, *selling*, corresponds with the rational empirical approach. Convincing information is provided so that the new idea is more readily taken up. This is most effective where people are willing to change at the outset.

The third approach is *participating*, which is principally normative re-educative. Here the participants themselves identify the need for change and choose the direction they will take. The fourth approach, *delegating*, is an extension of the participating style. It appears to be most appropriate for individuals and groups who have already achieved a self-directed approach to change. The change agent provides some support, but only when asked by the individual or group.

This discussion shows that certain key strategies make the successful implementation of change more likely. Although the managers and educators can give valuable support to the work of the staff, it is at the level of practice, where nurses work with patients and clients, that change matters most and its effects can be most directly felt.

Planning change

Nurses can work as change agents in an enormous variety of settings, to change the behaviour of clients—individuals and groups—as well as colleagues, and not only within but also outside their immediate sphere of work. While this text focuses on the knowledge and skills that nurses need to improve nursing practice, change in any sphere is much more effective if it is planned. Success does not depend only on the bright idea and boundless enthusiasm; in fact, reliance on these alone is probably a recipe for failure. Enthusiasm and ideas need to be tempered with sober reflection and careful planning. This is not to say that planning will produce perfect results—it will not. Change by nature entails unpredictability. This can never be eradicated, even by the best-laid plans. Nevertheless, good organization and planning can help to reduce potential risks and conflicts. This is especially important when nurses pursue changes that may affect vulnerable patients or clients.

Problem-solving underpins change management, which has steps similar to those of the nursing process:

- assessing the situation;
- planning (or deciding what needs to be done);
- implementing (or putting the plan into action);
- evaluating the effects and making changes.

A change culture

Readiness is another key factor. Why should a team or hospital seem to become ripe for change? This ripeness usually results from a combination of factors, such as:

- changing expectations of society, and new laws and conventions;
- changing aspirations and outlooks of nurses and other professionals;
- changes in technology, medicine and health care;
- local organizational changes;
- local management objectives and decisions;
- new leadership patterns and the presence of change agents.

Any or all of these factors may combine to produce a climate for change. This climate does not affect all staff in the same way; some may be adventurous, others resistant. Indeed, success will depend on individuals' willingness to take stock of their own situation, and their feelings about change and the part they can play in it.[17]

Just as external events and forces may affect the climate for change, so factors affecting motives and feelings determine each individual's response. Thus each member of staff will contribute according to personal views and feelings. The question is whether the person:

- sees the need for change;
- agrees with the change;
- wishes to support colleagues;
- feels valued and supported at work;
- feels secure and supported in personal life;
- sees change not as a threat but an opportunity;
- sees possible rewards in the change, such as greater job satisfaction, better patient care or more pay.

People often see change as threatening when they feel uninvolved in decisions which affect their lives. This fact gives strong support for the bottom-up approach to change in nursing. Resistance is exacerbated when staff are unhappy at work or feel that their contribution is not valued. In addition, people with personal problems may be less willing to participate in innovation at work. Some senior staff resist change because they perceive it as criticism of past practices.

A work environment is supportive of staff when managers are helpful and accessible, learning is encouraged and staff feel reasonably rewarded for what they do. Such a climate is more likely to produce a culture that accepts change as motivating and beneficial. In such places, change becomes a way of life, a normal part of the day-to-day work that is accepted as commonplace and ordinary.

Spreading the word

Nurses often take part in exciting projects, but do little to tell others about their experiences. Nurses can thus waste much time and effort in pursuing a problem that someone else has already solved. It is important to disseminate information on work that is completed or under way. Results, good or bad, need to be shared. Nurses can share their work by:

- producing written reports for internal and external use, including texts of varying length and style for publication in journals, research bibliographies and elsewhere;
- joining a network of others with similar interests;
- joining professional organizations that offer information sharing;
- accepting invitations to speak about their projects at meetings and conferences;
- passing information to the mass media—newspapers, television and radio;
- making tape recordings, including video tapes;
- providing open days and study sessions on their projects.

Conclusion

Nurses are well placed to be major change agents in the health care system and in society as a whole. Acquiring knowledge and skill in the management of change will make them more effective in this role. Nurses have often relied on heroes/heroines for change: charismatic and forceful leaders who drive changes forward. The place for this model is limited. The thoughtful planning of change using a collective approach (with nurses working together for action), and a programme of managerial and educational support are much more likely to ensure long-term, meaningful changes in attitudes and behaviour.

Nurses need to work to seek ownership of change, to learn how to plan it, and to recognize the pitfalls and know how to overcome them. They need to share their knowledge and experience with each other, to keep up to date in their profession, to continue their own personal growth and to develop their awareness. While they may be able to do this in advance of a specific change programme, the act of change, with all its conflicts, is a great opportunity for learning and growth.

Nurses often set high standard for themselves, but they need to allow time for change to take place and to cherish achievements in the process of change, no matter how small. At the same time, nurses should also care for themselves. While being committed, energetic and passionate at work, they must also make space for their own pleasures, pastimes and friendships.

While change can be learned about, prepared for and planned, it can never be simple and straightforward. Change brings with it volatility and unpredictability. Unexpected situations can arise and people can respond irrationally. The nurse who masters change is able to use a wide range of knowledge and techniques and adapt them to many different circumstances. Such a nurse is a potent force for change in health care, and a real contributor to enhancing the quality of care for patients. Leaving aside issues of professional and personal growth, or the enhancement of the status of nursing, what really matters is that change improves the care of patients. The nurse who can change and improve practice gives valuable service to the wellbeing of others.

Notes

1. Beardshaw, V. & Robinson, R. *New for old?—Prospects for nursing in the 1990's*, London, King Edward's Hospital Fund for London, 1990 (Research report No. 8).

2. Benner, P. *From novice to expert*, London, Addison-Wesley, 1984.

3. Lawler, J. *Behind the screens*, Edinburgh, Churchill Livingstone, 1991.

4. Salvage, J. *The politics of nursing*, London, Heinemann, 1985.

5. Oakley, A. 'The importance of being a nurse', *Nursing Times*, **80**(50), 24–27, (1984).

6. Hayward, J., ed. *Report of the nursing process evaluation group*, London, King's College, 1986 (NERU Report No. 5).

7. Kanter, R. *The change masters*, London, Allen & Unwin, 1984.

8. Martin, J.P. *Hospitals in trouble*, London, Blackwell, 1984.

9. Wright, S.G. *Changing nursing practice*, London, Edward Arnold, 1989.

10. Bennis, W.G. *et al. The planning of change*, London, Holt, Reinhart & Winston, 1976.

11. *Managing change in nurse education*, London, English National Board for Nursing, Midwifery and Health Visiting, 1987.

12. Lancaster, J. & Lancaster, W. *The nurse as a change agent,* St Louis, Mosby, 1982.

13. Pearson, A., ed. *Primary nursing*, London, Croom Helm, 1988.

14. Rogers, E.M. *Diffusion of innovations*, New York, Free Press, 1962.

15. Keyser, D. 'Meeting the challenge' in: Wright, S.G. *Changing nursing practice*, London, Edward Arnold, 1989.

16. Haffer, A. Facilitating change. *Journal of Nursing Administration*, **16**(4), 18–22, (1986).

17. Plant, C. *Managing change and making it stick*, London, Fontana, 1985.

40

Guide to Parliamentary Lobbying

MARJORIE GOTT

Politics plays a major part in working for change in organisations and communities. Politics is about decision making, and is the study of who gets what, when and how.

Public policy is a planned course of action, taken to address shared issues and concerns. Policy decisions about health and welfare services are made by elected and appointed officials. Just as health workers must understand the distribution of power within a family in order to promote healthy behaviour, they need also to know the powerbrokers (or stakeholders) locally and nationally if they are to successfully influence policies to promote health. By virtue of their close understanding and expertise in the causes and effects of health and disease, health workers are in an influential position to contribute to the ongoing health debate.

One way to become familiar with current health issues and concerns is to regularly read (different) newspaper accounts of them, paying attention to who the key players are. Another way is via your professional organisation, or union. Both the RCN and the BMA for example have Parliamentary Units that exist to represent their members' (and members' clients') best interests to Parliament.

Parliament

The UK Parliament consists of the House of Commons, the House of Lords, and the Queen. All three institutions have to agree to any new law which is to be passed. The bulk of the work (and influence) resides in the House of Commons and is carried out by the 651 Members of Parliament (elected representatives) of the British people.

Britain is also subject to European Community (EC) laws. Both Houses of Parliament have committees which examine EC proposals before they become law. The likely effects of a law on Britain are, therefore, known before it is passed. Britain sometimes has to alter her laws to bring them into to line with new European laws. This usually follows debate.

Both Houses of Parliament offer debates on matters of national and international importance. Debates concerning health and welfare issues frequently occur. Members of the public can attend and listen to Parliamentary debates by either queueing at the St Stephen's entrance at the Houses of Parliament for admission to the Public Gallery, or by obtaining a ticket from the local Member of Parliament's Office. Transcripts of debates, offering a word for word attributable account, are contained in the Official Report (Hansard). Copies of Hansard are available and can be studied in major (city and university) libraries, and the libraries of professional organisations (RCN, BMA).

The House of Commons Public Information Office (Tel: 071 2194 272) offers information and guidance on when particular debates are due, and who has asked Parliamentary questions on a particular issue.

The House of Commons spends around half of its time in making laws. Both the government and the opposition have a role to play. The Government is concerned with legislation outlined in its party manifesto and the Queen's speech which is presented to Parliament as a Bill.

The opposition acts to challenge, and thus help balance or ameliorate, the effects of government policies.

The House of Lords is, ultimately, subject to the power and authority of the House of Commons. They have no financial power, and the House of Commons has the power to overturn their decisions. It is worth noting however that the Lords can be a powerful sounding board for forming popular opinion; government defeats in the House of Lords are always heavily reported in the national press.

Parliamentary bills are of two main types: public bills and private bills. Private bills affect only one particular area or organisation, so the most important type of bill is the public bill. These consist of government bills and private members bills. Both are designed to affect the public as a whole. Government bills are sponsored by the government, while private members bills are sponsored by individual back bench MPs. Bills become Acts of Parliament when they receive Royal Assent. Generally, because they are piloted through Parliament by Ministers, government bills are more successful than private members bills.

Bills generally go through several stages, all of which offer the opportunity for influence by the public, professional organisations and MPs.

- The consultative stage. This is organised by the department sponsoring the bill. Prior to the NHS reforms of 1992 the Department of Health invited professional and public comment on its 1991 Consultative Document: *The Health of the Nation* (Government White Paper).
- The 'reading' stages. The first reading informs Parliament about the government's intention: the second offers the first real opportunity for debate to occur.
- The committee stage involves detailed scrutiny and amendment of bills in the light of previous debate. Committees are formed for the purpose (ie Health Committee) by representative (political) membership of the House of Commons.
- The report stage involves reporting back to the Commons and the opportunity for final amendments.
- The third reading is the final opportunity to debate and vote on the bill in the House of Commons before it is passed on to the House of Lords.
- Lords amendments are invited by the same process outlined above. When the two Houses agree the bill proceeds to:
- Royal assent, in which the Queen signifies her assent, and the bill becomes an Act of Parliament.

Early in the Parliamentary process Green and White Papers are sometimes issued to gauge public and professional response to government intentions. A Green Paper is 'soft' and just acts to 'test the water' on issues. A White Paper is more committed as it declares the government's intention to legislate, and describes how the new law will operate.

Laws are shaped and enacted by departments, led by ministers (Secretaries of State). Because of the scale and importance of the Department of Health, the Minister is of cabinet rank, therefore at the centre of government decision making.

Lobbying

Lobbying is the term used when seeking to try to influence policy makers towards a particular course of action. To lobby effectively you need to know who is influential. Within both Houses of Parliament there are a number of key MPs and peers (lords) who lead on health policy for their political parties. Professional organisations and trade unions keep a list of these people, as do the main public libraries, and local MP's offices.

MPs are often the best people to lobby if you want information about, or want to influence a health issue, as they rely on your vote, so should be concerned about your opinion! Their interest will be enhanced if you are part of a larger action group, particularly if the group can interest the media in its concerns. The local media (newspapers, radio) are keen to have items to report, particularly local issues. They are also generally very interested in health issues. Influencing health issues is however an area where health workers may feel particularly vulnerable, so, if you do organise, you would be wise to obtain the advice and support of the local branch of your professional organisation or trade union.

Getting the most out of your MP

Before the meeting

1. Write asking for a meeting either in Parliament or in his/her constituency (remember that MPs hold regular 'surgeries' in their constituencies, and you can ask to make an appointment at one of these). Say who you are and say what you want to meet about.

   All MPs can be reached at: House of Commons, London SW1A 0AA. Tel: 071 219 3000.
2. Agree a date. Tell the local media you are meeting your MP.
3. Write to the MP confirming your agenda. Explain who will be coming, who they are and what they represent. Confirm the venue and the duration of the meeting.
4. Agree that a small representative group of not more than five people should attend.
5. Prior to the official meeting with the MP, have a 'dress rehearsal' with the group about the main points you want to get across.
6. Decide who is to lead on each item. Have all the facts and figures at your fingertips about the issue.
7. Be clear about what it is you expect the MP to do on your behalf.

8 Prepare an information pack to leave with the MP setting out your points and giving local examples.

During the meeting

1 Introduce everyone and confirm the time there is available to you. Confirm the points you wish to cover.
2 Go through the points. Ask for the MP's suggestions on every point.
3 Seek commitments from the MP to take up your case in Parliament. Clarify ways in which he might do this.
4 Make it clear that you will be reporting back to your colleagues and the local media about your meeting. Ensure that the MP knows that this will not be the last he/she will see of you.

After the meeting

1 The group should meet immediately to agree the interpretation of what took place.
2 Report to the local media any undertaking that has been given, get it on record.
3 Report back to the rest of the members.
4 Plan how to undertake any follow up agreed, or any ideas arising out of the meeting. Decide who will maintain contact with the MP, how, and when, and how progress will be reported back to the group, other colleagues and the media.

41

The Future of Paediatric Nursing*

SUE WILLIAMS

Before going forward to the future it is often important to reassess where we are currently, and what the shape of the service might be in the future, leaving aside at this stage the competing political scenarios which in themselves will impact upon the future. I would however like to make the point that what you are about to hear is my personal view and should be treated as such, no doubt those of you at the operational level may have very different ideas about the shape of the service in the future and more particularly the needs of children for health care.

However, let us start at the macro-level. What are the general trends? Recently we were presented with the first document which addressed the 'Health of the Nation' providing a clear focus on current health issues, and highlighting the need for multi-agency co-operation in improving preventative care, whilst recognising the unique role of health professionals in educating the general public in health matters. Undoubtedly the consultation that has followed its publication has sharpened the debate and the action plan that will follow will present a real challenge when planning future services. There is no doubt that more emphasis will be placed on primary care, general practitioners will expand the range of services they offer: more health promotion clinics, screening services and minor surgery. Already they are beginning to offer more specialist services for example, physiotherapy, speech therapy, counselling and some alternative therapies such as aromatherapy. The doctor's surgery you and I know is likely to look very different. The Roy Report on Community Nursing (1991) suggested new models for delivering community nursing (in its broadest sense). Many of these are currently being trialled, accelerated by the development of Community Trusts and GP Fundholders.

In the secondary care service lengths of stay have decreased rapidly over the last 10 years. Medical technology is advancing and many of the treatments/interventions which were or are familiar to you and I, will disappear or be overtaken by new methods or new drugs. Genetic engineering may eradicate some of the major problems such as cystic fibrosis. Hospital care is likely to be highly technical, very expensive, and specialist services are likely to be available only in tertiary centres where economies of scale can moderate cost, and leading consultants can continue to research and develop new treatments. A local hospital may well be an extension of the community hospital of today, offering a range of low cost treatments, rehabilitation and possibly

*This paper was presented at the Edinburgh Conference, 1992.

short stay care for acute episodes, possibly linked into a larger general hospital able to provide a greater range of services for the wider community. I wouldn't at this stage like to hazard a guess at the size of community these hospitals might serve, but the aim would be to provide a more limited range of services at each level, taking us away from the current pattern where we have aimed to provide the majority of services at the district general hospital level.

The third major influence in the future will, I feel, be the consumer. We are already seeing the power of consumer opinion; the recent Select Committee Report on Maternity Services highlights that more women want to have their babies in local, more friendly surroundings and no doubt this will stimulate again the discussions on the virtues of hospital birth versus home births. The important element however is that women's opinions are being heeded. The Patient's Charter again focuses in on Consumer rights and as people become more familiar with these rights there is no doubt they will start to challenge the system.

What does all this mean for the care of children in the future? There is no doubt in my mind that one of the areas that has changed most rapidly in this century is care of sick children. Our understanding of their needs, our ability to deal with their health problems, and the advances in treatment of both acute and chronic disorders have changed the picture substantially. I recall my first ward experience in a children's hospital: half of the cots were taken by children with TB meningitis, the remainder being mostly acute chest infections, asthmatics and epileptics. Many of those children were in hospital for months, and many such as the asthmatics were readmitted regularly. Added to that, parental visiting was restricted. A children's ward today is a very different picture, the majority of children are admitted for very short spells, parents are in evidence day and night, chronically ill children may be admitted for respite but generally are supported at home.

What then is the next step? Current changes in the service have to some extent dismantled the innovative approaches adopted by some health authorities in the form of a children's service—'seamless care' with paediatric outreach and paediatric community services providing continuity of care from acute episodes of illness through to long term support of the chronically ill child. The development of hospice services for children has tended to develop specialist care regimes which many community nurses are not able to replicate. The highly technical nature of secondary services has seen the development of 'sub-cultures' in children's nursing, paediatric intensive care, paediatric oncology and paediatric neurology to name a few!

Where is the children's nurse that I once knew—able to look after a child with any complaint in any hospital?

We can of course argue that it is a good thing that it is impossible for us to be expert at everything. If we believe that statement then there is no doubt that in secondary care we will increasingly see the development of narrow areas of specialism; already in our local hospital we are seeing the development of a liver transplant service with its attendant nurse specialist. To a large extent this will make nurses in secondary care less flexible and possibly narrow their career options. How do you make career changes when you have spent five–ten years working in a specialised haematology unit? What will be needed for retraining such individuals?

However, I have no doubt that in secondary care, particularly in tertiary services, this will be the picture. In order to have a continued understanding of the specialty nurses will have to be working continually within it, because the advances and changes are so rapid. There has been a view expressed from some sources that we should be looking for a nurse/technician, but we have to decide: is that the model we want; is that what our ill children need?

What about the remainder of the care? Community hospitals will provide many of the local services, possibly in partnership with both consultants and GPs, local OPD minor surgery, acute medical care, some investigations. Here a generalist nurse will be more important, particularly the children's nurse who has a variety of skills and knowledge. Her ability to deliver care in both the local hospital and within the local community will be crucial.

Here I would like to suggest a revolution. If we believe in 'seamless care'—'continuity of care'—'named nurse' and all the other values that we extol so readily, then we could put them into action by implementing a child health worker/nurse who takes over the care of both the well and the ill child in the community setting. This would encompass both the statutory responsibilities for the under-fives currently held by the health visitor; delivery of direct care for ill children as needed; supporting parents of chronically sick children; advising on health promotion, diet and exercise for children and possibly taking on in some instances the current role of school nurses. I see this entity as being an integral part of the primary health care team with a defined case load of children and their families, working either from a GP surgery/health centre or based in the community hospital, dependent upon local situations. No doubt different organisational models would evolve but the key factor would be to encompass both health and illness in one individual—for families with particular problems, for example severe childhood disability, chronic illness or terminal care the role of key worker could be adopted—calling in specialist advice and support as needed by the family. If this model were adopted then changes in the content of education programmes would be necessary, but, with the foundation programme of Project 2000 already established, adjustments to the branch programmes could easily be achieved.

The new role would allow the paediatric nurse to have a much greater influence on child health generally and also establish herself as an integral part of primary health care provision. There could, of course, be the argument that if we follow this model to its ultimate form, the specialism of paediatric nurse will be diluted and disparate in the future. However, the important element is to ensure that wherever children need care the appropriate skills are available for that care. In particular, we will need to build bridges between highly specialised care, and more general care. For example, when children are admitted to tertiary care services, the nurse who has been supporting that child and his family in the community or local hospital should ensure that there is an effective communication channel established with two way flow of information. Likewise when children are discharged from tertiary services there should continue to be, as now, clinical specialists who operate an outreach service not only to support the child and family, but also the staff who will be delivering any continuing care component.

The Court Report (1976) stated, 'the importance of the family must be reflected in the organisation and delivery of health services for children'.

As paediatric nurses we strongly support this philosophy. Any new organisation of services must keep this idea in the forefront. Our aim in the future should be to maintain ill children within their own family surroundings as much as possible, and only use hospital care as a last resort! Likewise we need to build trusting relationships with families and this could be more easily achieved if all health care, both prevention and intervention could be accessed through one individual: the child health nurse. This would enhance the role of the paediatric nurse and ensure a high quality of care for all children.

References

Department of Health and Social Security, Department of Education and Science, and Welsh Office (1976) *Fit for the Future: Report of the Committee on Child Health Services* (Chair: Professor Donald Court), HMSO, London.

Roy, S. (1991) *Nursing Comm: Report of the working group*. NHSME, HMSO, London.

42

Trends in Child Health Nursing: A Vision for the Future*

ALAN GLASPER

Introduction

Nursing, health care and the National Health Service are undergoing profound change. The almost Maoist upheavals within health care have important ramifications for child health nurses working in tertiary, secondary and primary health care sectors. Although some nurses have found these changes bewildering, the consequences for the future development of children's nursing are already apparent. Although children's nurses have a long history of endeavouring to improve care of their particular client group, so often this has been perceived as reactive rather than proactive. The legacy of the past is ever present and must be given due cognisance when planning future trends in health care delivery. This must be addressed on three fronts: education, practice and research and development. In an era of economic austerity, with the emphasis on economy, efficiency and effectiveness, it is not always easy to plan for the future. Darbyshire[1] argues that 'we must rediscover our passion for and about nursing as a real social force with an ethic of good immovably embedded within it'. Have child health nurses ever lost this philosophy? There is no doubt that they have been seen by their interdisciplinary peers as altruistic, well meaning and caring; after all, children are universally liked. Some professional colleagues believe that children's nurses are passive, reactive and somewhat traditional, but this does not accurately reflect the reality of children's nursing in the 1990s. The vision for the future development of this branch of the profession of nursing is both bright and optimistic.

Education

Unlike the majority of the industrialised nations of the world, the UK alone has maintained a tradition of separate registers for different branches of the profession. The commonest route to specialisation, with the advent of the Project 2000 diplomate courses, is at pre-registration level, meaning that student nurses are dedicated towards

---

*A draft version of an article to be published in two parts in *Child Health*, 1993, **1**(3): pp. 93–6 and 1994, **1**(4): pp. 160–3.

a branch of the profession from day one of the course. The logic behind this rationalisation is that individual nurses will select their area of specialisation, such as adult nursing, children's nursing, mental health nursing, mental handicap nursing or midwifery, and stay within that area for the whole of their professional working lives. As a direct consequence, the numbers of available post-registration courses leading to other parts of the register have been severely reduced. The argument against this rigid approach is that many individuals entering the profession, especially if they are young, may not have based the decision to enter a particular branch of nursing on experience, but purely on emotive grounds. The reality is, that like medical students, nurses only choose their final area of specialisation after they have experienced different clinical environments. This would mitigate against choosing a speciality too early in one's nursing career.

Generic nurse

Some members of the profession are increasingly articulating the benefits of a generic nurse. What would the ramifications be for the children's nurse of the future? The proponents of the generic nurse would argue that this would be the most cost effective way of ensuring an adequately educated and trained workforce. Given the covert discrimination against nurses holding special registration finding work in Europe, the USA, Canada and Australia, there might be considerable support for genericism among the profession.

Ramifications

Were the profession to follow the generic route, certain safeguards would have to be imposed if one was to protect the integrity of the existing specialised branches. This could be achieved through imaginative curricular design which would, for example in the case of children's nursing, allow suitable exposure to a variety of clinical experiences in both tertiary, secondary and primary care settings. Such a generic course might allow for nurse interns to practice only at a certain set level with future gradings being dependent upon post-registration education and practice. This, of course, already exists in its embryonic form through the ENB educational framework and higher award scheme which is closely linked to the UKCC's PREP implementation recommendations being considered currently by the Secretary of State. The generic route would then build the main educational and practice components of the special registers into subsequent continuing professional curricula. This fits the conceptual paradigm of the UKCC's nurse specialist and advanced practitioner recommendations. It can be hypothesised that child health nursing more easily equates to specialist and advanced practitioner status than it would otherwise, when linked to pre-registration diploma status courses.

The total integration of nurse education into the tertiary educational sector paves the way for the development of innovative curricular activities which could, within a short time span, change irrevocably the face of nursing. The assertion by Biley[2] that nurse education must adopt progressive nurse education strategies is absolutely correct and is linked to eventual improvements in the quality of nursing care.

There remains much speculation related to the long term future of the specialist registers. The impact of Project 2000, re-profiling and economic austerity on the development of nursing as a profession continues to be the subject of longer term evaluation. What is quite clear is that there will continue to be a contraction of student numbers throughout the UK. The crisis in nurse education has been further fuelled by the recent inflammatory remarks of Keele University's Professor Roger Dyson who has called for a suspension of Project 2000 and a complete overhaul of nurse education. Re-profiling exercises and the resultant concluding inferential statistics demonstrating the over-capacity of certain specialist nurses are crude in the extreme. It has, for example, been claimed that there is an over-capacity of RSCNs in some regions of the order of magnitude of 120%. The recently published Audit Commission report relating to child care belies these suggestions and highlights the lack of RSCNs.[3] The debate as to the future of child health nursing should ideally be given a public airing. The proposition that the specialist registers should be built onto a generic nurse undergraduate programme at postgraduate diploma or master's level is contentious. Some professionals believe that to move to an all graduate generic workforce will disenfranchise those able, but less academically gifted individuals who wish to pursue nursing as a career.

However, a utilitarian approach should be adopted and the termination of the monotechnic status of college of nursing through the phased incorporation of such into the higher education sector has important ramifications for the future of the profession. The general acceptance of the credit accumulation and transfer scheme, the assessment of prior learning and experiential learning (CATS, APL and APEL) should allow these individual students not entering higher education through the normal route, improved access to undergraduate courses. The huge investment in NVQ and GNVQ schemes will ultimately lead to a more educated workforce who are better equipped to take advantage of the predicted explosion in higher education. In any event, the large numbers of students with appropriate 'A' level passes applying for the limited undergraduate nursing places thorughout the UK gives some confidence for predicting that Project 2000 at diploma level could be abandoned. Restructuring existing diploma level Project 2000 courses (240 CATS) would not be difficult and should be encouraged. The numbers of existing Project 2000 diplomate students who intend to go on after registration to complete a degree, belies the suggestion that the uptake for post-registration baccalaureate programmes will be minimal. The profession may wish to pursue the Australian model in which the transition from diploma to degree was achieved with little fuss and very quickly. In many instances the Australian diploma curricula were revalidated with minor modifications to degree level. Were this to happen in the UK the thorny issue of three-year degree programmes (currently under review by the ENB), would need to be addressed and resolved. The main point to be made from this debate is that a window of opportunity may exist, first to develop a generic nurse preparation programme and secondly, to launch this at undergraduate level. It is salutary to note that nursing is now one of the only non-graduate health care professions in the UK. Unless the graduate path is followed, it is difficult to see how the profile of nursing as a profession will be raised. Child health nursing can, therefore, follow one of two paths. Path one would link the existing RSCN qualification to a post-generic nursing post-graduate diploma/masters programme and is probably the option of choice. Path two would argue that option one is not feasible in the near future. It would press instead for an all graduate child health workforce. Given the small number of students undertaking the child branch components of Project 2000 diplomate courses and the oversubscription of students applying for undergraduate child branch nursing degrees, this is eminently feasible and is commensurate with the growing body of knowledge that represents the art and science of child health nursing. Greater interface with other child health professionals, health visitors and school nurses, must be pursued and satisfactorily resolved as the current artificial barriers that do exist, will obstruct the development of this important branch of nursing. No doubt this debate will continue.

Research, development and practice

Although the first undergraduate degree in nursing was launched by the University of Edinburgh as long ago as 1960, the route taken by nurses towards higher education has been protracted. It would appear that higher education offers nursing students greater professional status and autonomy. In addition, it facilitates a robust research base and framework for continuing professional education. We should, however, be aware of the recent HEFC (Higher Education Funding Council) research selectivity exercise which placed nursing research very low in a national league of excellence. Professor David Marsland highlights the crudeness of this exercise when he states: 'Nothing could be more helpful to our rivals than to have top nursing researchers admitting that the ratings were valid and accurate'.[4] Health care research is jealously protected and intensively competitive. Nurses are competitive newcomers in the pond and there are other large fish striving to survive in the increasingly depleted pool that is research funding. Other professionals such as psychologists, sociologists, social policists, health economists and the professions allied to medicine are involved with health care research and view with guarded suspicion the entry of a new intruder to the field. Some of these professional groups have a long history of robust research within the area of child health and, if nurses wish to compete on a level playing field, they must equip themselves with the necessary research skills. This can be achieved through an appropriate educational strategy which encourages reflective practice. The raison d'être of the child health nurse practitioner in the 1990s is innovation in practice. This operates on three fronts, namely tertiary, secondary and primary health care.

Changing patterns of research

Research design in the early years of academic nursing closely paralleled methodologies used in the traditional sciences. Having little or no tradition of their own, such nurse researchers had no choice but to rely on those time-tested methods which would gain respectability within a multidisciplinary forum. The obsessive search for a theory of nursing which would underpin the art of nursing, was pursued for many years and was probably responsible for the so called theory–practice gap. Nolan[5] states, 'The manifest failure of the theoretical and research based literature to make substantial inroads into the world of practice has become known as the theory–practice gap.' The divorce between the researchers and the innovators is cause for considerable concern and must be addressed as a matter of some urgency. The new nursing curricula, which are emerging with the advent of Project 2000, coupled with the PREP framework of continuing education, are already endeavouring to reduce the theory–practice gap.

The profound reorganisation of research activity within the National Health Service, spearheaded by Professor Sir Michael Peckham, is committed to linking research to practice. This more pragmatic approach to health care research is inextricably linked to the *Health of the Nation* recommendations, with its emphasis on the burden of disease and health gain. This more utilitarian approach to research is more closely associated with innovation in practice and favours multidisciplinary co-operation. Although 'blue skies' research will continue to be funded, nursing as a practice-based discipline must look to its various client groups for research inspiration. Evaluation research and action research methodologies are effective in involving practitioners and, therefore, should be pursued whenever possible. Action research promotes innovation, with the participating researcher actively involved in the process of change.

Primary health care

The emphasis of recent reorganisations within the health service has been the transition of care from the tertiary to the primary health care sector. Such a philosophy underpins the government White Paper *Working for Patients* and its subsequent working papers, including the Community Care Act, which have dramatically altered the face of UK health care. The move away from mechanistic medical care to a more holistic approach can be seen with the publication of the Patient's Charter, which for the first time reaffirms the position of patients/parents as consumers of health care. In many industrialised western societies there are beginning to emerge reforms which fundamentally alter the traditional doctor, nurse, patient paradigm which has bedevilled health care for so long. Patient's charters or patient's bills of rights are the precursors to advocacy and empowerment. Child health nurses have endeavoured to act as advocates for families by providing appropriate information in the quest for empowerment. Indeed, information is the very key to empowerment. However, some factors have impeded child health nurses in their quest for family advocacy, and chief among these are the remnants of a past history of medical paternalism. Such an approach sought to protect families from the harsh realities of childhood illness, and its roots belong to an era prior to the advent of antibiotics when childhood mortality was high. The move towards reflective practice in nursing is eroding this outmoded concept and allows nurses to be more assertive in practice. The pursuit of strategies which coordinate and facilitate quality measurement helps promote advocacy. This in turn has refocused attention on parents as partners in care. Partnership is now firmly embedded within the ethos of child health nursing, especially among the groups of community nurses involved with child care. Health visitors, paediatric community nurses and school nurses are responsible for the proactive stance which has repudiated the traditional role of parents as passive bystanders in the care of their children. The concept of parents/children as equal partners in care has spread more slowly within the tertiary inpatient sectors of health care. This is beginning to change and the work of Casey[6] at the Hospital for Sick Children, London, is now embodied within the curricular design of a number of diplomate and undergraduate child branch courses throughout the UK.

The growth of surgical day care, coupled with earlier discharge from hospital, has increased the workload of the primary health care team. Although such moves have been argued on a psychological level, that is the best place to care for a child is at home, nurses must be vigilant that economic factors do not prevail as the main reason. The burden and impact of nursing a sick child at home will be the subject of continuing evaluation. The shifting emphasis towards research by nurses in this field will figure prominently throughout the 1990s. Neylon[7] has demonstrated the value of health promotion for school children and ratifies the important role that this group of community nurses has to offer. The projects which lead to greater empowerment for the designated client group under investigation will, undoubtedly, continue to attract the patronage of the funding bodies. Neylon's study demonstrated that health promotion given to children was effective in 75% of cases and argues the case for school child health interviews as a method of health education.

Secondary health care

Once the backwater of child health care, this area is assuming greater importance. The development of the purchasers and provider scenario, under the auspices of NHS trusts and health commissions, has been reinforced by the sanctioning of GP fundholders. GP fundholding is likely to affect the development of secondary care for children to a considerable degree. Day care units and outpatient departments, in addition to accident and emergency departments, are already re-evaluating their role and are responding to the changes sweeping the health service. Some general practitioners are demanding an improvement in the way that referrals to children's outpatients are co-ordinated. After years in the doldrums, the spotlight is now firmly on the OPDs as areas of innovation. The work of Campbell and Lowson,[8] in developing the first paediatric nursing development unit at Southampton, has raised the profile of children's outpatient departments as areas of innovation. Such developments are timely, given the publication of the recent Caring for Children in the Health Services' *Bridging the Gaps*.[9] This exploratory study of the interfaces between primary and specialist care for children within the health services augments the need for a sharing of information with families and intrinsically supports the notion of family information centres. Child health nurses working in secondary care settings will find the embodied standards of care in the document a source of inspiration.

The outpatient department is often the first point of contact for families with the hospital and, like the accident and emergency department, is the shop window of potential innovatory change. Although publications such as *Bridging the Gaps* act as powerful agents of change, they themselves are based on 'best practice' in a variety of units around the UK and elsewhere. It is absolutely clear from even a cursory glance at the literature that child health nurses do not need to work in large well endowed prestigious units to promote change. Excellent action research within the realms of secondary care is being carried out, often in small uninspiring units. A good team approach to local problems can often prevail where single researchers might founder. The sterling work of Hawthorn from Northern Ireland in promoting the care of bereaved relatives is one such example. Hawthorn[10] collected data retrospectively from the parents of bereaved infants and was able to implement pragmatic changes to the infrastructure of the hospital Chapel of Rest and to the way in which parents were counselled at the time of their bereavement and subsequently.

The huge growth of interest in day care has been fuelled by the Caring for Children in the Health Services' publication *Just for the Day*.[11] This document recommends good practice and presents a cogent argument for the future management of children with minor surgical and medical disorders. Clearly any increase in utilisation of day care, for what is becoming a discrete client group in its own right, has important ramifications for the primary health care team. Further evaluation of the impact of day care on the family needs to be undertaken. Such reports do, however, help many nurses working within the field of child health promote recent innovations in care among their colleagues.

The decline in the average length of stay of children in hospital, which has occurred parallel to the growth in day care, has led to an increased utilisation of outpatient departments. The problems of coping with this extra client volume load are proving challenging to nurses working in such areas and will be the subject of continued research and development. Despite this increased utilisation of secondary hospital services, there continue to be major problems with non-attendance by families. This potential serious state of affairs is rarely investigated. The advent of GP fundholding will focus attention on this otherwise ignored, but important problem.

Tertiary health care

Once the high profile area of child health nursing, the title 'registered sick childrens' nurse' symbolises the main thrust of care that was child health nursing not so many years ago. Some members of the profession are seriously questioning the continued use of such a title. Were the generic route to be followed as alluded to earlier, would this make the RSCN title redundant? Will we see postgraduate diplomas/master's degrees which combine the skills of the three groups of nurses who currently come under the umbrella of child health nursing: children's nurse, school nurse and health visitors?

Depsite the swing away from traditional inpatient care, there remain many research and development projects which are designed to enhance the delivery of care. The growth of the clinical nurse specialist is loudly resonated in the UKCC's PREP proposals, and is already a feature of child health nursing in all three clinical domains. The complexity of tertiary care requires specialised nurses. Those children now requiring inpatient care are often very sick and come under the broad umbrella of 'high care'. The sheer diversity of the specialisations within child care dictate a reflection of what is required to ensure an appropriate supply of skilled nurses. There are those who would argue that such a route follows the medical model and indeed, on the surface, this would appear so. However, the specialised nursing needs that the families of very sick children have, make this comparison inevitable. Much innovation has already occurred and the early consensus of nurses relating to the environment of the hospital, the role of parents etc., have been addressed. Yet there is little room for complacency, and research and development bids from nurses working in the tertiary areas continue to be given a high profile.

1 Develop a cogent clearly defined research question.
2 Endeavour to foster a multidisciplinary research team approach (the project is likely to attract funding if several professional groups are involved).
3 Ensure an appropriate research methodology—solicit the support of your local university nursing studies department.
4 Be realistic with costings. Research always costs in terms of time and money. Research on the cheap will be bad research. If the project is worth doing, it is worth supporting, but first you have to convince the funding body! Remember that printing costs money as does secretarial and computer time.
5 Replication of research conducted in other units within the UK or abroad may be strategically valuable, especially if a visit can be arranged beforehand.
6 Educational visits to develop research and development ideas can be sponsored under the auspices of a number of agencies such as the Florence Nightingale Memorial Fund, the ABPN Portex Scholarship or the RCN Cow and Gate Scholarship etc.

Figure 42.1 Attracting research and development sponsorship

The recent Audit Commission's review of children's hospital services[3] has identified a number of problem areas which fall within the remit of children's nursing. Such problems include, among others, a failure to implement the principle of child and family centred care in some children's units, a shortage of RSCNs and the nursing of children on adult wards. Research and development projects designed to promote the recommendations of such reports are likely to attract research and development funding from a variety of funding agencies. Child health nurses must learn to be more competitive in bidding for such funding (*see* Figure 42.1).

The Department of Health publication *A Vision for the Future* (1993)[12] sets out the redefined strategy for nursing and will be a continuous seminal reference paper for those children's nurses wishing to promote research and development activities. The document highlights the importance of clinical practice and urges the professions to work in partnership with academic departments for enhanced patient care practice. The recommendations that all possible units demonstrate areas of care that have improved as a result of research findings will act as a stimulus for change. Children's nurses will be in the forefront of these developments!

Notes

1. Darbyshire, P. (1993) 'Preserving nurse caring in a destitute time' [guest editorial], *Journal of Advanced Nursing*, 1993, **18**, 507–508.

2. Biley, F. (1991) 'The divide between theory and practice', *Nursing*, **4**(29).

3. Audit Commission (1993) *Children First. A Study of Hospital Services*, London, HMSO.

4. Marsland, D. (1993) 'Research and destroy', *Nursing Standard*, **7**(23), 45.

5. Nolan, M. and Grant, G. (1993) 'Action research and quality of care', *Journal of Advanced Nursing*, **18**, 305–311.

6. Casey, A. (1988) 'A partnership with child and family', *Senior Nurse*, **8**, 8–9.

7. Neylon, J. (1993) 'Health promotion for school children', *Nursing Standard*, **7**, 37–40.

8. Campbell, S. *et al.* (1993) 'Families first: the Southampton nursing development unit', *Paediatric Nursing*, **4**, 35–37.

9. Thornes, R. (1993) *Bridging the Gaps*. Caring for Children in the Health Services/ Action for Sick Children, London.

10. Hawthorn, A. (1992) *Give Sorrow Words*, RCN, London.

11. Thornes, R. (1991) *Just for the Day*. Caring for Children in the Health Services. NAWCH, London.

12. DoH/NHSME (1993) *A Vision for the Future*, HMSO, London.

Index